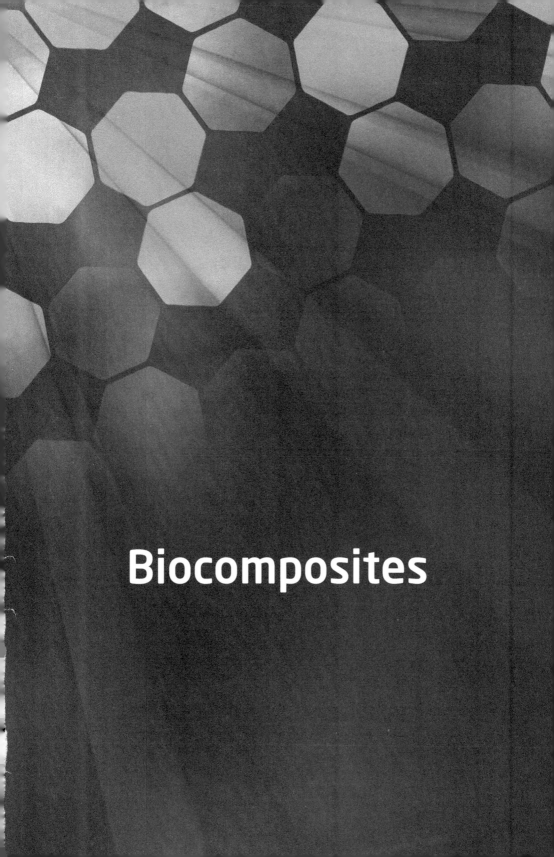

Biocomposites

Biocomposites
Biomedical and Environmental Applications

edited by

**Shakeel Ahmed | Saiqa Ikram
Suvardhan Kanchi | Krishna Bisetty**

PAN STANFORD PUBLISHING

Published by

Pan Stanford Publishing Pte. Ltd.
Penthouse Level, Suntec Tower 3
8 Temasek Boulevard
Singapore 038988

Email: editorial@panstanford.com
Web: www.panstanford.com

British Library Cataloguing-in-Publication Data
A catalogue record for this book is available from the British Library.

Biocomposites: Biomedical and Environmental Applications
Copyright © 2018 by Pan Stanford Publishing Pte. Ltd.
All rights reserved. This book, or parts thereof, may not be reproduced in any form or by any means, electronic or mechanical, including photocopying, recording or any information storage and retrieval system now known or to be invented, without written permission from the publisher.

For photocopying of material in this volume, please pay a copying fee through the Copyright Clearance Center, Inc., 222 Rosewood Drive, Danvers, MA 01923, USA. In this case permission to photocopy is not required from the publisher.

ISBN 978-981-4774-38-3 (Hardcover)
ISBN 978-1-315-11080-6 (Ebook)

Contents

Preface	xix

1. Composites from Natural Fibers and Bio-resins   1
Vimla Paul and Maya Jacob John

1.1	Introduction		2
1.2	Lignocellulosic Fibers		2
	1.2.1	Chemical Treatment of Banana Fiber	6
1.3	Bio-resins		10
	1.3.1	Banana Sap	12
		1.3.1.1 Physical and chemical properties of BS bio-resin	13
1.4	Biocomposites		14
1.5	Biodegradability of Hybrid Biocomposites		17
1.6	Conclusion		18

2. Advancements and Potential Prospects of Polymer/Metal Oxide Nanocomposites: From Laboratory Synthesis to Commercialization   27
Deepali Sharma and Karan Vadehra

2.1	Introduction		28
2.2	Different Approaches for Nanocomposite Synthesis		30
	2.2.1	Template Synthesis	30
	2.2.2	In Situ Synthesis	31
	2.2.3	Melt Mixing	33
	2.2.4	Solution Intercalation	33
	2.2.5	Electrospinning	34
	2.2.6	Click Chemistry	35
2.3	Polymer-Based Metal Oxide Nanocomposites		35
	2.3.1	Polymer–Iron Oxide-Based Nanocomposites	36
	2.3.2	Polymer–Zinc Oxide-Based Nanocomposites	38
	2.3.3	Polymer–Silica-Based Nanocomposites	40

		2.3.4	Polymer–Titanium Oxide-Based Nanocomposites	42
	2.4		Role of Metal Oxide Nanoparticles in Enhancing the Properties of Nanocomposites	43
	2.5		Applications of Nanocomposites	45
		2.5.1	Sensors	45
		2.5.2	Energy Storage	48
		2.5.3	Optoelectronics	49
		2.5.4	Biomedical	51
		2.5.5	Photocatalysis	52
	2.6		Commercial Opportunities for Metal Oxide/ Polymer Nanocomposites	54
	2.7		Conclusion and Future Prospects	55

3. Biomedical Insights of Lipid- and Protein-Based Biocomposites — 65

Aasim Majeed, Raoof Ahmad Najar, Shruti Chaudhary, Sapna Thakur, Amandeep Singh, and Pankaj Bhardwaj

3.1		Introduction		66
3.2		Protein-Based Biocomposites		67
	3.2.1	Medical Applications of Protein-Based Composites		71
		3.2.1.1	Tissue engineering	72
		3.2.1.2	Cancer therapy	75
		3.2.1.3	Wound healing	76
3.3		Lipid-Based Biocomposites		78
	3.3.1	Medical Applications of Lipid-Based Composites		79
		3.3.1.1	Drug delivery	79
		3.3.1.2	Cancer therapy	81
		3.3.1.3	Antimicrobial application	82
		3.3.1.4	Skin protection	83
		3.3.1.5	Dental application	84
		3.3.1.6	Miscellaneous	84
3.4		Conclusion		85

4. Biocomposites for Hyperthermia Applications — 97

Tomy J. Gutiérrez

4.1		Introduction	98
4.2		Synthesis of Iron Nanoparticles	101
	4.2.1	Coprecipitation	102

		4.2.2 Hydrothermal Method	104
	4.3	Magnetite: Tumor Treatment Using External Magnetic Field	105
	4.4	In Vivo Studies Demonstrating the Anticancer Effect of Magnetic Nanocarriers	105
	4.5	In Vitro Studies Demonstrating the Improvement in Intake Rate of Anticancer Agents Loaded into Nanoparticles in Different Tumor Cells	107
	4.6	Saturated Fatty Acids as Coatings for MNPs with Improved Properties as Anticancer Drugs Carriers	108
	4.7	Fabrication, Characterization, and In Vitro Assay of Antitumor Activity of Magnetite Coated with Non-polar Shell Without Using External Magnetic Field	110
	4.8	Biocomposites from Iron Nanoparticles: Biopolymers	111
	4.9	Biocomposites from Iron Nanoparticles: Hydroxyapatite	116
	4.10	Conclusion	119

5. **Biocomposites Based on Natural Fibers: Concept and Biomedical Applications** — 135

   Raoof Ahmad Najar, Aasim Majeed, Gagan Sharma, Villayat Ali, and Pankaj Bhardwaj

5.1	Introduction	136
5.2	Types of Natural Fibers	136
5.3	Natural Fiber–Based Biocomposites	139
5.4	Biomedical Applications of Natural Fibers	142
	5.4.1 Tissue Engineering	143
	5.4.2 Dental Application	146
	5.4.3 Wound Healing	147
	5.4.4 Drug Delivery	148
5.5	Conclusion	151

6. **Algae-Based Composites and Their Applications** — 163

   Richa Mehra, Satej Bhushan, Balraj Singh Gill, Wahid Ul Rehman, and Felix Bast

6.1	Introduction	164

6.2	Bio-based Natural Fibers			165
	6.2.1	Algal versus Other Natural and Synthetic Fibers		166
	6.2.2	Algal Constituents as Biocomposite Candidate		167
		6.2.2.1	Alginate	167
		6.2.2.2	Cellulose	168
		6.2.2.3	Agar	168
		6.2.2.4	Carrageenan	169
6.3	Synthesis of Biocomposites			169
	6.3.1	Algae Culture		169
	6.3.2	Extraction of Algal Fiber		169
	6.3.3	Natural Fiber Processing		170
6.4	Applications of Algae-Based Composites			171
	6.4.1	Biosorption of Heavy Metals		172
	6.4.2	Automotive Industry		172
	6.4.3	Construction Materials		173
	6.4.4	Medical Applications		173
	6.4.5	Packaging Industry		174
	6.4.6	Cosmetics		174
	6.4.7	Textiles		175
	6.4.8	Paper Industry		175
6.5	Challenges and Future Prospects			176

7. Going Green Using Colocasia esculenta Starch and Starch Nanocrystals in Food Packaging — 181

Bruce Saunders Chakara and Shalini Singh

7.1	Introduction			182
7.2	Food Packaging			182
	7.2.1	Conventional Synthetic Packaging		183
	7.2.2	Biofilms, Edible Films, and Coatings		185
7.3	Starch			187
	7.3.1	Potato		189
	7.3.2	Cassava		189
	7.3.3	Maize		190
	7.3.4	Amadumbe		190
7.4	Methods			191
	7.4.1	Starch Extraction		192
		7.4.1.1	Water extraction method	192
		7.4.1.2	Alkaline extraction method	192

7.4.2	Preparation of Starch Nanocrystals	192
7.4.3	Film Preparation	193
7.4.3.1	Scanning electron microscopy	193
7.4.3.2	Transmission electron microscopy	194
7.5	Conclusion	194

8. Bionanocomposite Materials: Concept, Applications, and Recent Advancements — 199

Nafees Ahmad, Saima Sultana, Suhail Sabir, Ameer Azam, and Mohammad Zain Khan

8.1	Introduction	200
8.2	Types of Bionanocomposites	201
8.2.1	Polysaccharide-Based Bionanocomposites	201
8.2.1.1	Chitosan-based bionanocomposites	201
8.2.1.2	Cellulose-based bionanocomposites	202
8.2.1.3	Starch-based bionanocomposites	202
8.2.1.4	Chitin-based bionanocomposites	202
8.2.2	Nanoclay-Based Nanocomposites	203
8.2.3	Hallyosite-Based Nanocomposites	203
8.3	Preparation and Modifications	204
8.4	Special Properties of Bionanocomposites	205
8.4.1	Mechanical and Barrier Properties	205
8.4.1.1	Young's modulus and tensile strength	206
8.4.1.2	Toughness and strain	206
8.4.2	Biological Properties	206
8.4.3	Thermal Properties	206
8.4.4	Antimicrobial Properties	207
8.5	Recent Advances in the Field of Bionanocomposites	207
8.6	Applications of Bionanocomposites	208
8.6.1	Electronic, Sensor, and Energy Generation	208
8.6.2	Biomedical Applications	209

		8.6.3	Packaging Applications	209
8.7	Challenges			210
8.8	Conclusion and Future Trends			210

9. Plant Fiber–Reinforced Thermoset and Thermoplastic-Based Biocomposites   217

T. P. Mohan and Krishnan Kanny

9.1	Introduction			218
9.2	Natural Fibers as Reinforcement			218
9.3	Woven and Non-woven Fabric			223
	9.3.1	Woven Fabric		223
	9.3.2	Non-woven Fabric		224
9.4	Comparison of Non-woven and Woven Fabrics			225
9.5	Mechanical Properties: Woven versus Non-woven Kenaf Fibers			226
9.6	Types of Plant Fibers and Chemical Treatments			228
	9.6.1	Types of Plant Fibers		228
	9.6.2	Chemical and Thermal Treatment of Fibers		229
		9.6.2.1	Alkali treatments	230
		9.6.2.2	Acid treatments	231
		9.6.2.3	Pyrolysis treatments	232
		9.6.2.4	Coating with silane treatment	233
		9.6.2.5	Benzoylation treatment	234
9.7	Plant Fiber–Reinforced Thermoplastic Composites			234
	9.7.1	Processing and Characterization for the Processing of Natural Fiber–Reinforced Thermoplastics		235
		9.7.1.1	Polymer solution casting	236
		9.7.1.2	Compression molding	238
		9.7.1.3	Injection molding	239
	9.7.2	Mechanical, Thermal, and Physical Properties		241
	9.7.3	Flame-Retardant Properties of NFPCs		243
	9.7.4	Biodegradability of NFPCs		244
	9.7.5	Energy Absorption of NFPCs		244
	9.7.6	Water Absorption Characteristics of NFPCs		245

9.8	Products and Applications of Plant Fiber-Reinforced Thermoplastics		247
9.9	Plant Fiber–Reinforced Thermoset Composites		249
	9.9.1	General Characteristics of NFPCs	250
	9.9.2	Vacuum-Assisted Resin Transfer Molding	252
	9.9.3	Resin Transfer Molding	255
	9.9.4	Benefits of RTM	256
	9.9.5	Mechanical Properties of NFPCs	257
	9.9.6	Viscoelastic Behavior of NFPCs	257
9.10	Applications of Natural Fiber Polymer Composites		259
	9.10.1	Natural Fiber Applications in the Industry	260
9.11	Rubber Composite Materials (Natural Fibers)		262
	9.11.1	Properties of Rubber Composites	263
	9.11.2	Manufacturing Process of Rubber Composites	265
	9.11.3	Applications of Rubber Composites	265
9.12	Conclusion and Future Scope		266

10. Multifaceted Applications of Nanoparticles and Nanocomposites Decorated with Biopolymers — **275**

Natarajan Kumari Ahila, Arivalagan Pugazhendhi, Sutha Shobana, Indira Karuppusamy, Vijayan Sri Ramkumar, Ethiraj Kannapiran, Periyasamy Sivagurunathan, and Gopalakrishnan Kumar

10.1	Introduction		276
10.2	Biosynthesis of Metal Nanocomposites		279
	10.2.1	Gold Nanoparticles	279
	10.2.2	Silver Nanoparticles	282
	10.2.3	Platinum Nanoparticles	283
	10.2.4	Copper Nanoparticles	283
	10.2.5	Titanium Oxide Nanoparticles	284
10.3	Biopolymers		285
	10.3.1	Nanocomposites from Bacteria	287
	10.3.2	Polyhydroxyalkanoates	288
	10.3.3	Application of Biopolymer–Metal Nanocomposites	289

10.4	Biomedical Applications		289
	10.4.1	Tissue Engineering	289
	10.4.2	Drug-Delivery Systems	291
10.5	Conclusion		292

11. Bionanocomposites, Their Processing, and Environmental Applications — 297

Sagar Roy and Chaudhery Mustansar Hussain

11.1	Introduction: Biodegradable Polymers		298
11.2	Conventional Polymers versus Biodegradable Polymers		300
11.3	Classification and Properties of Biodegradable Polymers		301
	11.3.1	Natural Biodegradable Polymers	302
		11.3.1.1 Polysaccharides	302
		11.3.1.2 Lignocellulosic complex (fibers)	303
		11.3.1.3 Starch	304
		11.3.1.4 Chitin and chitosan	305
		11.3.1.5 Alginic acid	306
	11.3.2	Polypeptides of Natural Origin	307
		11.3.2.1 Collagen and gelatin	307
		11.3.2.2 Corn zein	308
		11.3.2.3 Wheat gluten	308
		11.3.2.4 Soy protein	309
		11.3.2.5 Casein and caseinate	309
		11.3.2.6 Whey proteins	309
	11.3.3	Biopolymers Synthesized from Bio-derived and Synthetic Monomers	310
		11.3.3.1 Poly(lactic acid) or polylactide	310
		11.3.3.2 Poly(glycolic acid)	310
		11.3.3.3 Poly(ε-caprolactone)	311
		11.3.3.4 Poly(butylene succinate) and its copolymer	311
		11.3.3.5 Poly(p-dioxanone)	312
		11.3.3.6 Poly(hydroxyalcanoate)	312
	11.3.4	Other Important Biodegradable Polymers	313

		11.3.4.1	Bacterial cellulose	313
		11.3.4.2	Poly(vinyl alcohol) and Poly(vinyl acetate)	313
		11.3.4.3	Poly(carbonate)	314
		11.3.4.4	Polyurethanes	314
		11.3.4.5	Polyamide and poly(ester-amide)	315
		11.3.4.6	Polyanhydrides	315
	11.4	Nanofillers for Bionanocomposites		316
		11.4.1	Cellulose-Based Nanofillers	317
		11.4.2	Carbon Nanotubes	318
		11.4.3	Nanoclays	318
	11.5	Processing Aspects of Bionanocomposites		319
		11.5.1	Conventional Manufacturing Techniques	319
		11.5.2	In Situ Intercalative Polymerization	321
		11.5.3	Exfoliation–Adsorption	321
		11.5.4	Melt Intercalation	322
		11.5.5	Foam Processing Using Supercritical CO_2	322
		11.5.6	Template Synthesis	323
	11.6	Environmental Applications of Bionanocomposites		323
	11.7	Conclusion		325
12.	**Bionanocomposites in Water and Wastewater Treatment**			**329**

Gulshan Singh, Deepali Sharma, and Thor Axel Stenström

	12.1	Introduction		330
	12.2	Polymer Bionanocomposites		333
		12.2.1	Polysaccharide-Based Bionanocomposites	336
			12.2.1.1 Chitosan-based polymer bionanocomposites	337
			12.2.1.2 Gum polysaccharide–based bionanocomposites	341
			12.2.1.3 Cellulose nanocomposites	347
		12.2.2	Protein-Based Bionanocomposites	353
	12.3	Conclusion and Future Perspectives		353

13. **Gamma Radiation Studies on Thermoplastic Polyurethane/Nanosilica Composites** 363
    Abitha V. K., Rane Ajay Vasudeo, Krishnan Kanny, Sabu Thomas, Niji M. R., and K. Rajkumar
    13.1 Introduction 364
    13.2 Preparation of Thermoplastic Polyurethane/ Nanosilica Composite 367
        13.2.1 Preparation of Nanocomposites 367
    13.3 Results and Discussions 368
        13.3.1 Mechanical Properties 368
        13.3.2 Electrical Properties 369
            13.3.2.1 Comparison of mechanical properties with normal silica versus nanosilica 371
        13.3.3 Thermal Analysis of Nanosilica Composites 371
            13.3.3.1 Comparison of thermal properties with nanosilica versus normal silica 372
    13.4 Conclusion 373

14. **Removal of Heavy Metals and Textile Dyes in Industrial Wastewater Using Biopolymers and Biocomposites** 375
    May Myat Khine, Nang Seng Moe, Kyaw Nyein Aye, and Nitar Nwe
    14.1 Introduction 376
    14.2 Removal of Heavy Metals in Industrial Wastewater Using Biopolymers and Biocomposites 377
        14.2.1 Types of Heavy Metals in Industrial Wastewater 377
        14.2.2 Removal of Heavy Metals Using Biopolymers 377
        14.2.3 Removal of Heavy Metals Using Biocomposites 378
        14.2.4 Method for Treatment of Heavy Metals in Wastewater 381
        14.2.5 Adsorption Process 381
        14.2.6 Advantages and Disadvantages of Heavy Metal–Removal Techniques 386

		14.2.7	Types of Heavy Metals and Their Effect on Human Health	388
	14.3		Removal of Textile Dyes in Industrial Wastewater Using Biopolymers and Biocomposites	391
		14.3.1	Classification of Dyes Based on Their Applications	391
		14.3.2	Types of Textile Dyes in Industrial Wastewater	392
		14.3.3	Removal of Textile Dyes in Industrial Wastewater Using Biopolymers	393
		14.3.4	Removal of Textile Dyes in Industrial Wastewater Using Biocomposites	394
		14.3.5	Method for Treatment of Textile Dye in Wastewater	395
		14.3.6	Advantages and Disadvantages of Various Dye-Removal Techniques	396
	14.4	Conclusion		397
15.	**Bio-based Material Protein and Its Novel Applications**			**405**

Tanvir Arfin and Pooja R. Mogarkar

	15.1	Introduction			406
	15.2	Amino Acids			407
		15.2.1	Classification of Amino Acids		407
	15.3	Classification of Proteins			408
		15.3.1	Simple Proteins		409
			15.3.1.1	Fibrous proteins	410
			15.3.1.2	Globular proteins	410
		15.3.2	Conjugated Proteins		410
			15.3.2.1	Glycoproteins or mucoproteins	411
			15.3.2.2	Lipoproteins	411
			15.3.2.3	Nucleoproteins	411
			15.3.2.4	Phosphoproteins	412
			15.3.2.5	Chromoproteins or metalloproteins	412
		15.3.3	Derived Proteins		412
	15.4	Structure of Protein			413
		15.4.1	Primary Structure		413
		15.4.2	Secondary Structure		413

		15.4.3	Tertiary Structure	415
		15.4.4	Quaternary Structure	416
	15.5	Properties of Proteins		417
		15.5.1	Electrolytic Properties of Protein	417
		15.5.2	Ionic Characteristics	417
		15.5.3	Solubility	417
		15.5.4	Hydrolytic Characteristic	417
		15.5.5	Putrefaction	418
	15.6	Native Proteins and Their Denaturation		418
		15.6.1	Denaturation	418
	15.7	Protein Gels		420
		15.7.1	Adsorption	420
		15.7.2	Three-Dimensional Network Theories	421
		15.7.3	Particle Orientation Theory	421
	15.8	Food Proteins		421
		15.8.1	Animal Proteins	422
		15.8.2	Vegetable Proteins	422
	15.9	Non-traditional Proteins		423
	15.10	Nutritional Importance of Proteins		424
	15.11	Applications of Protein-Based Biocomposites		426
		15.11.1	Protein-Based Biocomposites as Biodegradable Packaging Materials	426
		15.11.2	Protein-Based Thermoplastics in Biomedical Applications	427
		15.11.3	Agriculture	428
		15.11.4	Tissue Engineering	428
		15.11.5	Textile Industry	429
		15.11.6	Other Applications	429
	15.12	Conclusion and Future Perspectives		430
16.	**Biopolyesters: Novel Candidates to Develop Multifunctional Biocomposites**			**433**
	Hafiz M. N. Iqbal and Tajalli Keshavarz			
	16.1	Introduction		434
	16.2	Biopolyesters		434
	16.3	Physiochemical Characteristics of Biopolyesters		437
	16.4	Poly(3-hydroxybutyrate)		437
	16.5	Biocomposites		439
	16.6	Properties of Biocomposites for Biomedical Applications		440

		16.6.1 Biocompatibility and Biodegradability	440
	16.7	Biomedical and Biotechnological Applications	442
		16.7.1 Biomedical Applications	443
		16.7.2 Biotechnological Applications	445
	16.8	Concluding Remarks and Future Considerations	446

17. Treatment of Industrial Wastewater Using Biopolymers and Biocomposites — 457

Nang Seng Moe, May Myat Khine, Kyaw Nyein Aye, Hiroshi Tamura, Hideki Yamamoto, and Nitar Nwe

	17.1	Introduction	458
	17.2	Wastewater from Various Industries	459
		17.2.1 Wastewater from Food Industries	459
		17.2.2 Wastewater from Distillery Plants	459
		17.2.3 Wastewater from Coffee Processing	460
		17.2.4 Wastewater from Milk Industries	461
		17.2.5 Wastewater from Slaughterhouses	462
		17.2.6 Wastewater from Other Industries	463
	17.3	Methods of Wastewater Treatment	465
		17.3.1 Physical Treatment	465
		17.3.2 Biological Treatment	466
		17.3.3 Chemical Treatment	467
	17.4	Types of Reactors Used in Wastewater Treatment	468
		17.4.1 Membrane Filtration	468
		17.4.2 Fluidization	469
		17.4.3 Complete Mixed Reactor	470
		17.4.4 Anaerobic Filters	471
	17.5	Application of Biopolymer and Biocomposite in Wastewater Treatment	472
		17.5.1 Application of Chitosan in Wastewater Treatment	472
		17.5.2 Application of Alginate in Wastewater Treatment	474
	17.6	Agriculture Byproducts as Low-Cost Biosorbent for Wastewater Treatment	475
	17.7	Conclusion	477

Index — 483

Preface

A biocomposite is a composite material formed by a matrix and a reinforcement of natural fibers. It often mimics the structure of a living material involved in a certain biological process. The matrix provides strength to the biocomposite along with being biocompatible. The matrix is formed by polymers derived from renewable and non-renewable resources. It protects the natural fibers from environmental degradation and mechanical damage, holds the fibers together, and transfers their load on itself. The interest in biocomposites is rapidly growing in terms of industrial and fundamental applications due to the great benefits they offer such as being renewable, cheap, recyclable, and biodegradable.

This book examines the current state of the art, new challenges, opportunities and applications in the field of biocomposites. It highlights recent advances in technology in many areas from chemical synthesis and biosynthesis to end-user applications. These areas have not been covered in any book before and include information on biopolymers' synthesis, modifications, material structures, processing, characterization, properties, and applications. The chapters in this book cover nearly every conceivable topic related to polysaccharides such as biofibers, biothermoplastics, biocomposites, natural rubbers, proteins, gums, and algae polymers.

The book focuses on fiber-based composites applied to biomedical and environmental applications. It addresses three main areas. First, it presents a comprehensive survey of biocomposites from the existing literature paying particular attention to various biomedical and environmental applications. Second, it describes mechanical designs and manufacturing aspects of various fibrous polymer matrix composites. Third, it presents examples of the synthesis and development of bionanocomposites and their applications.

There are already a number of fine texts that comprehensively cover the subject of biopolymers and their various applications in great details, but the content of this book is unique. It covers an up-to-date record on the major findings and observations in the field of biocomposites and will be a useful reference for all who are related to this field.

Shakeel Ahmed
Saiqa Ikram
Suvardhan Kanchi
Krishna Bisetty
Autumn 2017

Chapter 1

Composites from Natural Fibers and Bio-resins

Vimla Paul[a] and Maya Jacob John[b,c]
[a]*Department of Chemistry, Faculty of Science, Durban University of Technology, PO Box 1334, Durban 4000, South Africa*
[b]*CSIR Materials Science and Manufacturing, Polymers and Composites Competence Area, PO Box 1124, Port Elizabeth 6000, South Africa*
[c]*Department of Chemistry, Faculty of Science, Nelson Mandela Metropolitan University, PO Box 1600, Port Elizabeth 6000, South Africa*
vimlap@dut.ac.za, mjohn@csir.co.za

There is an increasing urgency worldwide to develop bio-based products that can ease the widespread dependence on fossil fuels. The use of natural fibers and natural bio-based resin systems for the production of biocomposites has been pursued by researchers as they address environmental concerns.

This chapter focuses on biocomposites produced from natural fibers and bio-resins, specifically using banana fibers and banana sap (BS)-based bio-resin. More importantly, natural fibers and bio-resins from agricultural waste were utilized to produce the biocomposites. The biodegradability tests of the biocomposite via

---

Biocomposites: Biomedical and Environmental Applications
Edited by Shakeel Ahmed, Saiqa Ikram, Suvardhan Kanchi, and Krishna Bisetty
Copyright © 2018 Pan Stanford Publishing Pte. Ltd.
ISBN 978-981-4774-38-3 (Hardcover), 978-1-315-11080-6 (eBook)
www.panstanford.com

respirometric methods confirmed that banana fiber with the BS bio-resin degraded over a period of time.

1.1 Introduction

Over decades, composites have become an indispensable part of our lives with their various applications such as packaging, sporting equipment, agriculture, consumer products, medical applications, building materials, auto-industry, and aerospace materials among others. Although petroleum-derived thermosetting polymers (namely, vinyl ester, polyester, and epoxy) have the desired properties for these applications, they are invariably costly. These traditional synthetic resins are also unsustainable as petroleum resources are being depleted [1, 2]. Furthermore, they cannot be easily disposed of at the end of their useful lives and simply accumulate causing significant damage to the environment. The occurrence of plastics in the environment, the lack of landfill space, CO_2 emission during incineration of the plastics, and the ingestion and entrapment hazards have created an enormous negative environmental impact [1]. There is, therefore, an increasing urgency to develop bio-based products that can ease the widespread dependence on fossil fuels. The use of natural fibers and natural bio-based resin systems for the production of biocomposites has been pursued by researchers worldwide as they address environmental concerns [1, 2]. However, it is a challenge to replace conventional glass-reinforced composites with biocomposites as they present the disadvantage of low impact strength, water absorption properties, fiber degradation during processing, and fiber orientation and distribution.

Our contribution in this chapter focuses on biocomposites from natural fibers and bio-resins specifically using banana fibers and BS-based bio-resin. Particular attention is paid to the studies in which banana fibers and bio-based resins were characterized.

1.2 Lignocellulosic Fibers

The use of natural fibers dates back to at least 5500 years ago when ancient Egyptians pressed thin stems of papyrus on which to write [3]. There are about 2000 species of fibers in various parts of the world used for various applications, classified into three major types as animal fibers, vegetable fibers, and mineral fibers.

The following advantages of natural fibers make them a potential replacement for synthetic fibers in composites [4–7]:

- Readily available, abundant, low density, low cost, and biodegradable.
- Plant fibers are obtained from renewable resources. Low energy is required during production and show carbon dioxide neutrality.
- Natural organic products. There is no dermal issue for their handling compared to glass fibers and do not pose a biohazard upon disposal.
- Natural fibers are non-abrasive and exhibit great formability.
- Light in weight (less than half the density of glass fibers).
- Cheap compared to glass fibers.
- Exhibit good thermal insulating and acoustic properties due to their hollow tubular structures.

All plant fibers are composed of cellulose and are stronger and stiffer than animal fibers. Since they are more suitable for use in composite material, this study will focus on plant fibers. Biofibers are hollow cellulose fibrils held together by lignin and hemicellulose [8]. The main components of natural fibers are cellulose, hemicellulose, lignin, pectin, and waxes [6, 9–11].

Cellulose is regarded as the most abundant polymer in nature, which is found in plants, green algae, and some bacteria [12]. Cellulose is a linear, high-molecular-weight polymer that can be described as natural, renewable, and biodegradable [13]. Cellulose is a natural polymer consisting of 1,4-β-D-anhydroglucose ($C_6H_{11}O_5$) repeating units joined by 1,4-β-D-glycosidic linkages at C_1 and C_4 positions, in which each single unit contains three hydroxyl groups, as shown in Fig. 1.1 [14, 15]. The hemicellulose is responsible for the biodegradation, moisture absorption, and thermal degradation of the fiber. It is made up of polysaccharides composed of a combination of five and six carbon ring sugars.

Lignin is a complex hydrocarbon polymer with both aliphatic and aromatic constituents. Lignin, an amorphous polymer, is thermally stable but is responsible for UV degradation. It is a complex three-dimensional copolymer of aliphatic and aromatic constituents of very high molecular weight [9, 14]. Pectin, whose function is to hold the fiber together, is a polysaccharide like cellulose and hemicellulose. The mechanical strength of the plant fiber is related to the distribution of lignin between hemicellulose and cellulose, causing binding and stiffening of the plant fibers to occur.

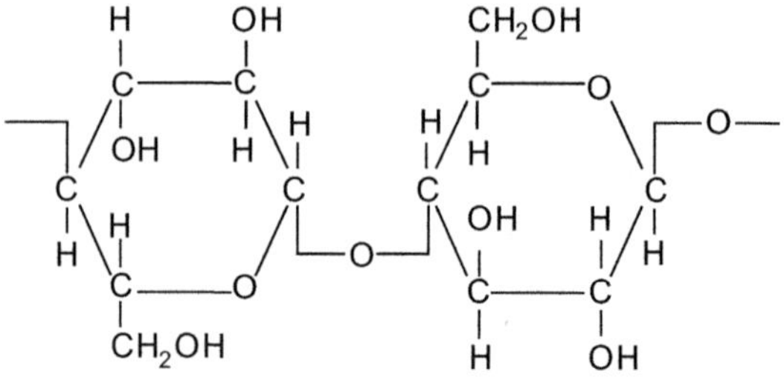

Figure 1.1 Schematic drawing of cellulose.

Bananas are a major food crop globally and are grown and consumed in more than 100 countries throughout the tropics and subtropics [17]. It is the fourth most widespread fruit crop in the world [18]. Bananas are said to be native to tropical South and Southeast Asia. They are among the most important commercial subtropical fruits grown in South Africa and are planted for sale in local markets or self-consumption [19]. Since only a fraction of all bananas are sold in the world markets, according to the Agri-food Business Development Centre, South Africa ranks 29th in the world, producing 250,000 metric tons of bananas [19, 20].

Bananas are mainly produced in Mpumalanga, Limpopo, and both the North and South Coasts of KwaZulu-Natal. In KwaZulu-Natal, the major banana-growing area is the North Coast with 15% (1700 ha) of the total area cultivated with bananas in 2010 [19]. South African records refer only to banana used for consumption, and there are no records of the use of the wasted banana plant once the fruit is harvested.

The banana plant is a large herbaceous flowering plant of the genus *Musa*. Each pseudostem can produce only a single bunch of bananas. After harvesting of the single bunch of bananas, the pseudostem dies and great amounts of agricultural residues are produced, causing environmental pollution [21, 22]. Exploitation of waste banana plants will be favorable to the environment and will have profitable economic benefits [23]. Since there is no further use for the plant, it was decided to use this waste material to produce a biocomposite material. Figure 1.2 shows typical mature local banana plants and banana fibers extracted from pseudostem. The fibers have many uses such as making cloth, string, rope, cordage, and paper making [24]. Applications for the banana plant residues represent an important contribution to increase the economic importance of banana plantations [21].

Table 1.1 shows that banana fibers consist of 58.92% cellulose, 16.11% hemicellulose, and 7.31% lignin. These results are consistent with the results obtained by others [25], where 63% cellulose, 19% hemicellulose, and 5% lignin in banana fibers were reported.

Table 1.1 Chemical assay of banana fibers

Av dry matter (%)	93.89
Ash (%)	3.28
Crude protein (%)	1.62
Cellulose (%)	58.92
Hemicellulose (%)	16.11
Lignin (%)	7.31
Starch (%)	11.72
Crude fat (%)	1.06
Gross energy (%)	40.36
Arabinose (%)	2.93
Galactose (%)	1.26
Glucose (%)	53.65
Xylose (%)	8.82
Mannose (%)	1.01

Note: Results obtained in accordance to ASTM conducted at the Animal Sciences Department at the North Dakota State University

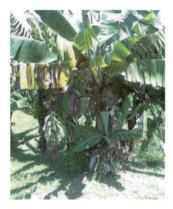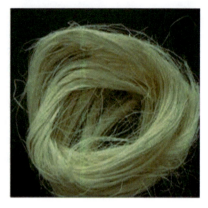

Figure 1.2 Mature local banana plants (left). Extracted banana fibers (right).

1.2.1 Chemical Treatment of Banana Fiber

Lignocellulosic fibers pose a major drawback of poor compatibility with commonly used non-polar matrices because of its hydrophilic character resulting in inferior mechanical properties as a result of moisture absorption. To circumvent this drawback, the surface of the fiber should be modified in order to obtain an efficient hydrophobic barrier and to reduce the interfacial energy with the non-polar matrix resulting in optimum adhesion [26].

Bogoeva-Gaceva investigated various chemical treatments of fibers such as dewaxing, mercerization, bleaching, cyanoethylation, silane treatment, benzoylation, peroxide treatment, isocyanate treatment, acrylation, latex coating, and steam-explosion [4]. Furthermore, Nassif used 10% NaOH to chemically treat banana fibers and reported that the dielectric strength and thermal conductivity increased by 29% and 139%, respectively [27]. Li et al. suggested that alkaline treatment was one of the most-used classical treatments that partially remove lignin, wax, and oils from the fiber cell wall [7]. Moreover, Herrera and George et al. explain that the purpose of the alkaline treatment was to increase the surface roughness and the amount of cellulose exposed on the fiber surface, resulting in better mechanical interlocking and increased number of reaction sites [15, 28]. Hydrogen bonding broken in the network structure increases the surface roughness. Fiber treatment, therefore, improves the bonding strength between the fiber and the matrix, which is of utmost importance in the formation of composites [29]. This bonding strength is determined by measuring the force required to pull out a fiber embedded in the matrix.

Paul and co-workers used an alkali chemical modification to enhance the compatibility of the resin with the banana fiber [30]. Figure 1.3A shows the SEM image of untreated fiber. A smooth surface containing lignin, pectin, cellulose, and hemicellulose was observed. The treatment of banana fiber with 2% NaOH resulted in a rough surface where hemicellulose and pectin were removed and hydrogen bonds were broken (Fig. 1.3B).

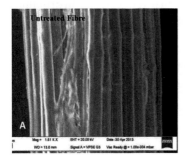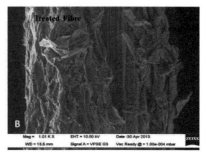

Figure 1.3 SEM images of banana fibers: (A) untreated and (B) treated with 2% NaOH.

FTIR scans in Fig. 1.4 show the functional groups of the untreated and treated fibers. For the untreated fiber, the broad band observed at 3439 cm^{-1} is related to the stretching vibration of the OH groups from the cellulose (carbon 2, 3, and 6 of the glucose) [31, 32]. After the alkali treatment, the intensity of this band was reduced due to the hydrogen bonding caused by the OH group. The peak at 2908 cm^{-1} assigned to the C–H aliphatic stretching band of the fiber was reduced after the alkali treatment due to the removal of the hemicellulose [33]. In the untreated BF, the peak at 1627 cm^{-1} corresponded to the C=O stretching of hemicellulose. After alkali (NaOH) treatment, a major reduction in peak intensity was observed, possibly indicative of the removal of hemicellulose and lignin from the fiber surface, a result analogous to the alkali treatment of kenaf fibers reported by El-Shekeil et al. [34]. The reduction in intensity of the absorption band at 1627 cm^{-1} may be attributed to a decrease in lignin and consequently a reduction in the C=O functionality. A similar observation was made by Barreto et al. with alkali treatment of sisal fibers [35]. The sharp peak observed at 1313 cm^{-1} was assigned to the C–H asymmetric deformation and disappeared after alkylation, thus indicating crosslinking. The prominent peak at 1014 cm^{-1} was due to the vibration of the –C–O–C–. The intensity of this peak increased after alkali treatment possibly due to the relaxation of crosslinking that increased the intensity and resolution [11]. From the FTIR analysis, it was evident that the alkali treatment removed the lignin and hemicellulose from the surface of the fiber. The NaOH breaks the intermolecular H-bonding of the fiber and formed –ONa bonds on the fiber surface, which in turn reduced the hydrophilic behavior of the fiber as shown in the following reaction [36]:

$$\text{Fiber–OH} + \text{NaOH} \longrightarrow \text{Fiber–O}^-\text{Na}^+ + \text{H}_2\text{O} \qquad (1.1)$$

This resulted in the surface becoming less crystalline, which was further suggested by the less resolute FTIR peaks, thereby allowing improved fiber/matrix adhesion. In comparison, the untreated fiber was more crystalline or more orderly structured as seen by the high resolute peaks.

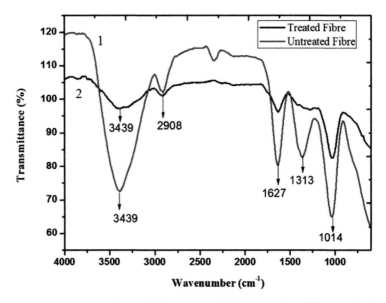

Figure 1.4 A comparison of FTIR spectra of (1) untreated and (2) treated with 2% NaOH.

Fiber length and fiber diameter are important parameters to consider when processing fibers for composites. The aspect ratio (length/diameter) is another important parameter that has an influence on mechanical properties [37]. The higher the aspect ratio, the higher the strength properties of natural fiber-based composites. The fiber strength is an important factor in selecting a specific natural fiber for a specific application. Paul et al. have shown that fibers become stronger and harder with retting, while elasticity and elongation simultaneously decrease [38].

The comparable strength of natural fibers to high-tensile steel [39] makes it a suitable reinforcement with bio-based resins in composite material. Extensive work done by Jacob et al. describes the reinforcement of various lignocellulosic fibers such as coir, bamboo, sisal, oil palm, grass fiber, pineapple, and jute with natural rubber [40]. It was concluded that the reinforcement of natural fibers with rubber generally decreased the tensile strength. The compatibility of the hydrophobic rubber and hydrophilic fiber was improved through chemical treatment of the fiber or modification of the polymer. Chemical treatment of natural fibers such as banana and oil palm fibers can result in superior mechanical properties as shown by Thomas and co-workers [41]. Isora, a novel fiber, was seen as a potential reinforcement with natural rubber with improved mechanical properties [42]. Paul and co-workers have extensively shown the use of reinforcement of banana fibers with a novel hybrid bio-based resin using BS extracted from the pseudostem of the plant, in the resin formulation [30]. Mechanical properties of the biocomposite improved with the BS bio-resin as compared to a control resin. The authors observed that alkali treatment of the banana fibers improved adhesion to the matrix.

Although hybrid-fiber-reinforced composites are gaining awareness, the mechanical and physical properties only tentatively reach the characteristic values of glass-fiber-reinforced systems. By using hybrid composites made of natural fibers and carbon fibers or natural fibers and glass fibers, the properties of natural-fiber-reinforced composites can be improved further. Using a hybrid composite that contains two or more types of different fibers, the advantages of one type of fiber could complement what are lacking in the other. Many researchers have investigated improved properties of hybrid-fiber-reinforced composites. Mohan et al. reported that jute fibers enhanced the mechanical properties of the jute/glass fiber hybrid composite [43]. Thwe and Laio reported that bamboo fibers hybridized with stronger and more corrosion-resistant synthetic fiber, for example, glass or carbon fiber, can also improve the stiffness, strength, as well as moisture resistance of the composite [44]. The addition of small volume fraction (0.05) of glass to coir biocomposites enhanced the tensile strength by about 100%, flexural strength by more than 50%, and impact strength by more than 100% [45].

1.3 Bio-resins

The American Society for Testing and Materials (ASTM) defines a bio-based material as "an organic material in which carbon is derived from a renewable resource via biological processes. Bio-based materials include all plant and animal mass derived from CO_2 recently fixed via photosynthesis" [46].

The schematic classification of bio-based polymers is represented in Fig. 1.5.

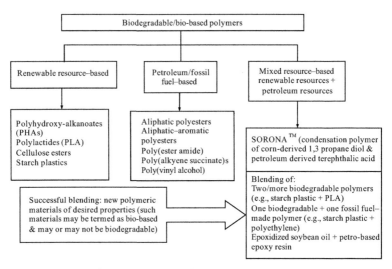

Figure 1.5 Classification of bio-based polymers. Reprinted from Ref. [47], with permission from Taylor and Francis Group LLC Books.

The term "bio-resin" refers to a resin that is made of raw materials derived from renewable resources such as plant oils (soybean oil, pine oil, castor oil), polysaccharides (starch, cellulose), and proteins [4, 48]. Rubber, tannins, lignin, soybean oil, epoxidized pine oil waste, castor oil, furfural alcohol-based resins, lactic acid, cashew nut shell liquid (CNSL), carbohydrates, proteins, and bio-alkyds are some of the raw materials used in the manufacturing of commercial thermosetting resins [48]. Table 1.2 shows selected bio-resins, which have been used to replace synthetic resins.

Table 1.2 Selected bio-resins showing their origin and uses

Bio-resin	Origin, properties, uses	Reference
Natural rubber	Milky white fluid known as latex from a tropical rubber tree.	[49]
Tannin-based adhesives	From timber species such as wattle or mimosa bark extract and pine. Used for exterior wood bonding.	[46, 50–52]
Lignin	From woody plant glue. Lignin with hemp and flax used for car dashboard panels, computer, and television frames.	[53]
Cashew nut shell liquid (CNSL)	Phenolic-based for uses such as resins, friction lining material, surface coating. CNSL with hemp fibers gave low cost, mechanically robust materials.	[54–56]
Polysaccharides	Blends from starch with aliphatic polyesters, PLA, polycaprolactone, PVA, or cellulose acetate. Uses: single-use microwavable dishes, catering utensils, horticultural applications, mulch bags, shopping bags.	[53]
Cellulose-derived biopolymers	From wood and sugarcane bagasse. Used for cellophane films, membranes for reverse osmosis, packaging.	[46]
Furfural	By-product of sugarcane bagasse, oats, wheat bran, and corncobs. Used for binding glass, rockwool, and carbon fibers.	[57]

(*Continued*)

Table 1.2 (Continued)

Bio-resin	Origin, properties, uses	Reference
Soybean and palm oil	From soybean and oil palm trees. Used for particle boards, thermoset resins, foams, household and furniture applications	[58, 59]
Polylactic acid (PLA)	From lactic acid. Used in medical applications, packaging among others.	[60–62]
Aliphatic polymers	From polycondensation of aliphatic glycol and aliphatic dicarboxylic acid. Used in medical application, films, compost bags, bottles among others.	[63]

1.3.1 Banana Sap

Banana sap is a clear liquid extracted from the pseudostem of the banana plant and has been successfully used to synthesize a hybrid bio-resin [30]. Studies on the chemical composition of BS from the pseudostem, such as carbohydrates, fiber composition, and mineral content, have been reported [18, 21, 64, 65]. It is also reported that the moisture content of fresh banana pseudostem is about 96% [22]. Furthermore, Aziz and co-workers reported the presence of polyphenols and flavonoids in the sap [18]. Oxidative browning takes place when the sap is exposed to air, implying the presence of phenolic compounds. Paul and co-workers [30] identified monosaccharides (glucose and fructose) and disaccharide (sucrose) in BS, the structures of which are shown in Fig. 1.6. With reference to other research [66] on the use of saccharides in the formation of ester-carboxylic derivatives, it was predicted that these sugars actually attach themselves to the backbone of the maleate polymer. Hirose and co-workers dissolved glucose in ethylene glycol and added it to succinic anhydride and dimethylbenzylamine to form a saccharide polyacid and consequently the thermal stability increased [66].

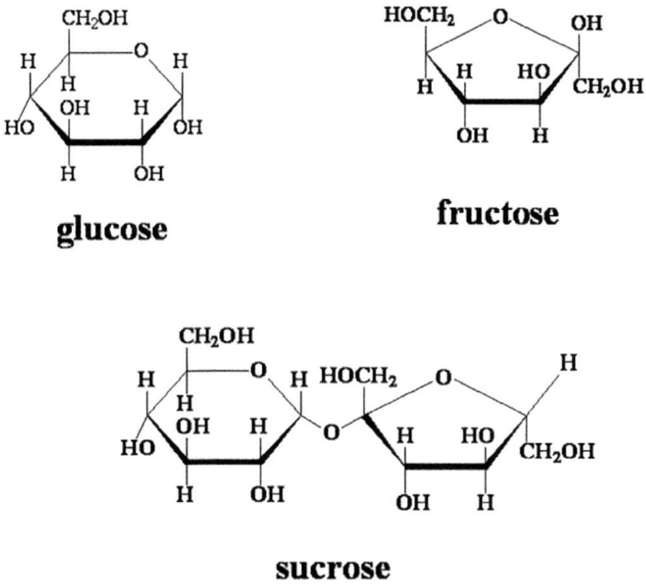

glucose

fructose

sucrose

Figure 1.6 Structures of glucose, fructose, and sucrose found in banana sap [67].

1.3.1.1 Physical and chemical properties of BS bio-resin

During the condensation polymerization process, propylene glycol and maleic anhydride reacted with the BS to form a hybrid unsaturated polyester resin and water as by-product. The BS bio-resin formulated by Paul et al. [30] was referred to as BSM, and a control sample without the BS was referred to as the control. It was proven by the authors that the crosslinking of the sugars from the BS with the polyester resin contributed higher physical (Table 1.3), chemical, and mechanical properties.

Table 1.3 Specifications of the control and BSM resins

Test	Control resin	BSM resin
Acid value (mg KOH/g resin)	44	43
Volatile content	39	40
Viscosity at 25°C (Brookfield sp3 500 rpm)	300	200

(Continued)

Table 1.3 (Continued)

Test	Control resin	BSM resin
Stability at 120°C (hours)	4	2.5
at ambient (months)	—	—
Rel. density at 25°C (g/cm^3)	1.098	1.093
Time to gel (min)	28	20
Time to peak (min)	36	31
Peak exotherm (°C)	203	207

1.4 Biocomposites

Broadly defined, biocomposites are composite materials made from natural or biofiber and non-biodegradable polymers such as polypropylene (PP), polyethylene (PE), and epoxies, or with biopolymers such as polylactic acid (PLA) and polyhydroxyalkanoates (PHAs) [47, 68].

Several researchers have contributed to the knowledge of biocomposites. For instance, Thomas and Pothan present a book on natural fiber–reinforced polymer composites. In particular, natural fiber surface modification, nanocomposites based on natural fibers, and fiber-reinforced rubber composites, to name a few, are discussed in detail [69]. A number of high-quality chapters have been included in the book. Meier et al. reviewed plant oil renewable resources as green alternatives with emphasis on using plant oils as raw materials for monomers and polymers [70]. Puglia et al. reviewed natural fiber-based composites with emphasis on natural fibers with matrices ranging from thermosets, thermoplastic, and biodegradable biocomposites [71]. John and Thomas reviewed various aspects of biofibers and biocomposites in their review article [9] where they classified biocomposites into green, hybrid, and textile and highlighted the applications of these biocomposites. Finally, they discuss that the material revolution of this century may be provided by green composites.

Mwaikamboa and Ansell have used CNSL as a useful bio-resin isolated from cashew nut shells as a by-product of the cashew nut processing industry, which has environmental advantages [56]. They found that hemp fibers with natural monomers containing similar phenolic compounds such as CNSL provided a compatible interaction on polymerization, hence improved mechanical properties. Furthermore, other researchers showed that the phenol derivative of CNSL as a bio-resin showed comparable properties to the commercially available CNSL-formaldehyde resin [54, 55]. In another study by Aziz and Ansell, a general trend was observed for the overall mechanical test results of the composites of a mixture of hemp and kenaf with CNSL, whereby high flexural modulus and high flexural strength were associated with a low work of fracture [72].

In addition, Savistano reported on the mechanical properties of Kraft pulp made from waste sisal and banana fibers reinforced cement composites [73]. They reported that the composites had flexural strength of 20 MPa and fracture toughness values in the range 1.0–1.5 kJ/m². The aforementioned researchers have used banana fiber in a synthetic resin system compared to a natural/hybrid resin system used in the current study. Majhi et al. made a biocomposite of polylactic acid and banana fiber at 30% fiber loading, and they reported that a tensile strength of 35 MPa was possible for a natural fiber/natural resin system [74].

Researchers Niedermann et al. [75] developed sandwich structures for aircraft interior applications from jute-fabric-reinforced bio-based epoxy resin (glucofuranoside) skins and polymethacrylimide foam core. Bending results indicated that the use of thinner core (6.5 mm) resulted in an increase in the bending strength by 25% when compared to conventional epoxy resin panels. The use of a thicker core (20 mm) resulted in higher flexural strength for the conventional epoxy resin, while the modulus values remained the same. During flexural testing, the upper skins underwent cracks resulting in catastrophic failure for the thicker core samples, while a catastrophic failure was recorded for the thinner core. The authors concluded that the sandwich panels developed from the bio-based resin could be used for flooring applications inside aircraft.

In an interesting study by Rosa et al. [76], an eco-sandwich material containing cork, flax fibers, and bio-based epoxy resin was fabricated and life cycle assessment (LCA) was applied to evaluate the environmental impact of the system. The panels were manufactured by the process of resin infusion technique. The authors observed that eco-sandwich panels exhibited lower thermal conductivity values (0.074–0.081 W/mK) compared to cement (0.9 W/mK) and weight when compared to other PVC foam board and cement-coated cork panel. The LCA results showed that the environmental performance was lower when compared to conventional materials.

Poly(furfuryl alcohol) (PFA) has emerged as an interesting bio-based renewable resource polymer that possess excellent properties such as high heat distortion temperature, high chemical resistance, and hydrophobicity. PFA is derived from a furfuryl alcohol (FA) precursor, which is a main chemical product produced from furfural. Furfural is an aldehyde obtained from hydrolysis of agricultural residue of sugarcane, rice hulls, hazelnut shells, wheat, corn, and birch wood. In addition, nearly 85–90% of the furfural produced globally is being transformed into furfuryl alcohol by an inexpensive derivation route, and a cationic condensation reaction is used to polymerize the furanic monomer.

In a study dealing with kenaf fiber/PFA composites [77], moisture absorption behavior was found to increase with increasing kenaf fiber content with a maximum water uptake of 7.8% at saturation point. This was attributed to the high hydrophilic nature of natural fibers. The researchers found that the best properties of the green composites were achieved at 20 wt.% fiber loading and showed significant increases in the flexural (48%) and tensile (310%) strength as well as the storage modulus (123%). Interestingly, retention after moisture absorption of up to 89% for flexural, 82% for impact, and 83% for tensile strength was observed after the composites were subjected to hot water immersion studies.

Although very little reviews have been found on banana fiber with natural-based bio-resins, research is growing with regards to banana fiber as reinforcement with synthetic resin especially unsaturated polyester resin, which is the type of resin used in the study by Paul and co-workers [30]. The mechanical properties of the biocomposite and the control samples are shown in Table 1.4.

Table 1.4   Mechanical properties of BSM and control biocomposites

Mechanical property	BSM biocomposite	Control biocomposite
Tensile strength (MPa)	26.1 ± 1.14	22.0 ± 0.82
Flexural strength (MPa)	32.3 ± 2.32	30.4 ± 3.5
Tensile modulus (MPa)	2968 ± 148.3	2609 ± 218.2
Flexural modulus (MPa)	1994 ± 122	5.2

1.5 Biodegradability of Hybrid Biocomposites

The primary aim of replacing traditional fibers with lignocellulosic fibers is to address landfill problems, environmental issues, and minimize dependence on petroleum-based products. Scientists worldwide have made tremendous effort to develop non-petroleum-based composites that are environmentally friendly and sustainable, using agri-fibers and resins. The advantage of biocomposites is that they can be easily disposed of or composted at the end of their life [78].

Biodegradability is defined as the degradation results from the action of naturally occurring microorganisms such as bacteria, fungi, and algae (according to ASTM D6400-99) [79, 80]. A compostable plastic is one that undergoes degradation by biological processes during composting to yield CO_2, water, inorganic compounds, and biomass and leaves no visible, distinguishable, or toxic residue. The consumption of oxygen or the formation of CO_2 is also a good indicator of polymer degradation [81, 82].

Smith classified biodegradable polymers according to their chemical composition, synthesis method, processing method, economic importance, applications, etc. [83]. Furthermore, these polymers can be obtained from natural resources, or they can be synthesized from crude oil [79, 83]. Biodegradation of polymers can be monitored by visual observations (roughening of the surface, formation of holes or cracks, defragmentation, changes in color, or formation of biofilms on the surface. Degradation mechanism can be obtained by scanning electron microscopy (SEM) or atomic force microscopy (AFM). Paul and co-workers did extensive work on various biodegradability tests such as soil burial test, microbial growth test, and respirometric tests on the banana fiber/BS bio-resin biocomposites [30]. The authors determined that the biocomposites with banana fiber and BS bio-resin degraded by 17.6% and the BS bio-resin by 7.1% over a period of 55 days. The SEM image in Fig. 1.7 shows the visual observation of roughening of the surface and the formation of cracks.

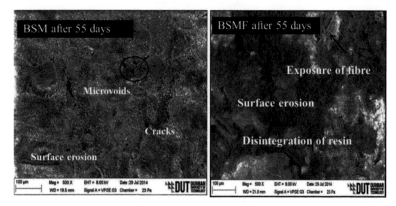

Figure 1.7 SEM images of composted bio-resin (left) and biocomposites (right).

1.6 Conclusion

The production of natural-fiber-reinforced bio-resin composites has drawn tremendous interest due to their versatility, biodegradability, low cost, low density, and significant processing advantages. Furthermore, these biocomposites are produced mostly from agricultural wastes, eliminating cost issues. They provide a solution to environmental issues by reducing synthetic and agricultural wastes.

Natural fiber biocomposites have been used in various industrial and automotive industries. There is still a great potential for biocomposite materials with improved mechanical strength.

Acknowledgments

The authors thank the National Research Fund for financial assistance.

References

1. Pothan, L. A., Z. Oommen, and S. Thomas, Dynamic mechanical analysis of banana fiber reinforced polyester composites. *Composites Science and Technology*, 2003, **63**(2): pp. 283–293.

2. Yu, L., K. Dean, and L. Li, Polymer blends and composites from renewable resources. *Progress in Polymer Science*, 2006, **31**(6): pp. 576–602.
3. Jourdan, F. The papyrus and its origins. [1 August 2012]; Available from: http://www.ptahhotep.com/articles/Papyrus.html.
4. Bogoeva-Gaceva, G., et al., Natural fiber eco-composites. *Polymer Composites*, 2007, **28**(1): pp. 98–107.
5. Peijs, T. Composites turn green. Department of Materials, Queen Mary, University of London 2002; Available from: http://www.e-polymers.org/.
6. Saheb, D. N. and J. Jog, Natural fiber polymer composites: A review. *Advances in Polymer Technology*, 1999, **18**(4): pp. 351–363.
7. Li, X., L. G. Tabil, and S. Panigrahi, Chemical treatments of natural fiber for use in natural fiber-reinforced composites: A review. *Journal of Polymers and the Environment*, 2007, **15**(1): pp. 25–33.
8. Jayaraman, K., Manufacturing sisal–polypropylene composites with minimum fibre degradation. *Composites Science and Technology*, 2003, **63**(3): pp. 367–374.
9. John, M. J. and S. Thomas, Biofibres and biocomposites. *Carbohydrate Polymers*, 2008, **71**(3): pp. 343–364.
10. Westman, M. P., et al., *Natural Fiber Composites: A Review*. 2010: Pacific Northwest National Laboratory.
11. Elanthikkal, S., et al., Cellulose microfibres produced from banana plant wastes: Isolation and characterization. *Carbohydrate Polymers*, 2010, **80**(3): pp. 852–859.
12. Jonas, R. and L. F. Farah, Production and application of microbial cellulose. *Polymer Degradation and Stability*, 1998, **59**(1): pp. 101–106.
13. Heydarzadeh, H., G. Najafpour, and A. Nazari-Moghaddam, Catalyst-free conversion of alkali cellulose to fine carboxymethyl cellulose at mild conditions. *World Applied Sciences Journal*, 2009, **6**(4): pp. 564–569.
14. Nevell, T. P. and S. H. Zeronian, Cellulose chemistry fundamentals, in *Cellulose Chemistry and Its Applications*, T. P. Nevell and S. H. Zeronian (Eds.), 1985, Ellis Horwood Ltd: England. pp. 15–30.
15. Herrera, F. P. J. and A. Valadez-Gonzalez, Fibre-matrix adhesion in natural fiber composites, in *Natural Fibers, Biopolymers, and Biocomposites*, A. K. Mohanty, M. Mishra, and L. T. Drzal (Eds.), 2005, CRC Press, Taylor Francis Group: USA, pp. 177–230.

16. Chloe Van. Cellulose. [online] 2010 [cited 2014.]; Available from: https://myorganicchemistry.wikispaces.com/Cellulose.
17. INIBAP (International Network for the Improvement of Banana and Plantain), International Plant Genetic Resources Institute. 2000; Available from: http://www.bioversityinternational.org/fileadmin/bioversity/publications/pdfs/664_Networking_Banana_and_Plantain.pdf.
18. Aziz, N., et al., Chemical and functional properties of the native banana pseudo-stem and pseudo-stem tender core flours. *Food Chemistry*, 2011, **128**(3): pp. 748–753.
19. Department of Agriculture. A profile on the South African banana market value chain. 2011 [cited 2012]; Available from: http://www.nda.agric.za/docs/AMCP/Bananamvcp2011-12.pdf.
20. NationMaster. Agriculture statistics: Banana production (most recent) by country. 2000 [cited 2012]; Available from: http://www.nationmaster.com/red/graph/agr_ban_pro-agriculture-banana-production&b_map=1.
21. Oliveira, L., et al., Chemical composition of different morphological parts from 'Dwarf Cavendish' banana plant and their potential as a non-wood renewable source of natural products. *Industrial Crops and Products*, 2007, **26**(2): pp. 163–172.
22. Li, K., et al., Analysis of the chemical composition and morphological structure of a banana psuedo-stem. *BioResources*, 2010, **5**(2).
23. De Beer, Z. and A. Sigawa. Banana (Musa spp.) juice production in South Africa. 2008.
24. Wigglesworth. Uses of Abaca. 2007; Available from: http://www.wigglesworthfibres.com/products/abaca/usesofabaca.html.
25. Joseph, S., et al., A comparison of the mechanical properties of phenol formaldehyde composites reinforced with banana fibres and glass fibres. *Composites Science and Technology*, 2002, **62**(14): pp. 1857–1868.
26. Belgacem, M. N. G., A., Natural fibre-surface modification and characterisation, in *Natural Fibre Reinforced Polymer Composites*, S. P. Thomas and L. A. Pothan (Eds.), 2009, Old City Publishing, Inc.: USA. pp. 14–46.
27. Nassif, R. A., Effect of chemical treatment on some electrical and thermal properties for unsaturated polyester composites using banana fibers. *Matrix*, 2010, **1**: pp. 7.

28. George, J., S. Bhagawan, and S. Thomas, Effects of environment on the properties of low-density polyethylene composites reinforced with pineapple-leaf fibre. *Composites Science and Technology*, 1998, **58**(9): pp. 1471–1485.

29. Wang, C., Fracture mechanics of single-fibre pull-out test. *Journal of Materials Science*, 1997, **32**(2): pp. 483–490.

30. Paul, V., K. Kanny, and G. Redhi, Formulation of a novel bio-resin from banana sap. *Industrial Crops and Products*, 2013, **43**: pp. 496–505.

31. Calado, V., D. Barreto, and J. d'Almeida, The effect of a chemical treatment on the structure and morphology of coir fibers. *Journal of Materials Science Letters*, 2000, **19**(23): pp. 2151–2153.

32. Fan, M., D. Dai, and B. Huang, Fourier transform infrared Spectroscopy for natural Fibres. *Fourier Transform–Materials Analysis*. Intech, 2012.

33. Bessadok, A., et al., Effect of chemical treatments of Alfa (*Stipa tenacissima*) fibres on water-sorption properties. *Composites Science and Technology*, 2007, **67**(3): pp. 685–697.

34. El-Shekeil, Y., et al., Influence of fiber content on the mechanical and thermal properties of Kenaf fiber reinforced thermoplastic polyurethane composites. *Materials & Design*, 2012, **40**: pp. 299–303.

35. Barreto, A. C. H., et al., Properties of sisal fibers treated by alkali solution and their application into cardanol-based biocomposites. *Composites Part A: Applied Science and Manufacturing*, 2011, **42**(5): pp. 492–500.

36. Indira, K. N., et al., Adhesion and wettability characteristics of chemically modified banana fibre for composite manufacturing. *Journal of Adhesion Science and Technology*, 2011, **25**(13): pp. 1515–1538.

37. Joseph, S., M. Jacob, and S. Thomas, Natural fiber-rubber composites and their applications, in *Natural Fibers, Biopolymers, and Biocomposites*, A. K. Mohanty, M. Mishra, and L. T. Drzal (Eds.), 2005, CRC Press: New York. pp. 177–230.

38. Paul, S. A., L. A. Pothan, and S. Thomas, Advances in the characterization of interfaces of lignocellulosic fiber reinforced composites, in *Characterization of Lignocellulosic Materials*, T. Q. Hu (Ed.), 2008, Blackwell Publishing: UK.

39. Munder, F., C. Fürll, and H. Hempel, Processing of bast fiber plants for industrial application, in *Natural Fibers, Biopolymers, and Biocomposites*, A. K. Mohanty, M. Mishra, and L. T. Drzal (Eds.), 2005, CRC Press: New York. pp. 177–230.

40. Jacob, M., R. D. Anandjiwala, and S. Thomas, Lignocellulosic fiber reinforced rubber composites, in *Natural Fibre Reinforced Polymer Composites: From Macro to Nanoscale*, S. Thomas and L. A. Pothan (Ed.), 2009, Old City Publishing, Inc.: USA.

41. Joseph, S., K. Joseph, and S. Thomas, Green composites from natural rubber and oil palm fiber: Physical and mechanical properties. *International Journal of Polymeric Materials*, 2006, **55**(11): pp. 925-945.

42. Mathew, L., K. U. Joseph, and R. Joseph, Isora fibres and their composites with natural rubber. *Progress in Rubber, Plastics and Recycling Technology*, 2004, **20**(4): pp. 337-349.

43. Mohan, K., Microbial deterioration and degradation of polymeric materials. *Journal of Biochemical Technology*, 2011, **2**(4): pp. 210-215.

44. Thwe, M. M. and K. Liao, Durability of bamboo-glass fiber reinforced polymer matrix hybrid composites. *Composites Science and Technology*, 2003, **63**(3): pp. 375-387.

45. Pavithran, C., P. Mukherjee, and M. Brahmakumar, Coir-glass intermingled fibre hybrid composites. *Journal of Reinforced Plastics and Composites*, 1991, **10**(1): pp. 91-101.

46. Celluwood, *Bio-resin systems*. 2008 (ID: ECO/10/277331): pp. 40-48.

47. Mohanty, A., et al., Natural fibres, biopolymers and biocomposites: An introduction, in *Natural Fibers, Biopolymers, and Biocomposites*, A. K. Mohanty, M. Mishra, and L. T. Drzal (Eds.), 2005, CRC Press: New York. pp. 1-36.

48. Laine, L. and L. Rozite. Eco-efficient composite materials. 2010 [2 February 2013]; Available from: http://www.ketek.fi/anacompo/STATE%20OF%20THE%20ART.pdf.

49. Strong, B., Microstructures in polymers, in *Plastics Materials and Processing*, D. Yarnell (Ed.), 2006, Pearson Prentice Hall: New Jersey. pp. 73-117.

50. Kim, S. and H.-J. Kim, Curing behavior and viscoelastic properties of pine and wattle tannin-based adhesives studied by dynamic mechanical thermal analysis and FT-IR-ATR spectroscopy. *Journal of Adhesion Science and Technology*, 2003, **17**(10): pp. 1369-1383.

51. Kim, S. and H.-J. Kim, Evaluation of formaldehyde emission of pine and wattle tannin-based adhesives by gas chromatography. *Holz als Roh- und Werkstoff*, 2004, **62**(2): pp. 101-106.

52. Kim, S., et al., Physico-mechanical properties of particleboards bonded with pine and wattle tannin-based adhesives. *Journal of Adhesion Science and Technology*, 2003, **17**(14): pp. 1863–1875.
53. Clarinval, A. and C. Halleux, Classification of biodegradable polymers, in *Biodegradable Polymers for Industrial Applications*, R. Smith (Ed.), 2005, Woodhead Publishing: Cambridge, GBR. pp. 3–29.
54. Lubi, M. C. and E. T. Thachil, Cashew nut shell liquid (CNSL): A versatile monomer for polymer synthesis. *Designed Monomers and Polymers*, 2000, **3**(2): pp. 123–153.
55. Ikeda, R., et al., Synthesis and curing behaviors of a crosslinkable polymer from cashew nut shell liquid. *Polymer*, 2002, **43**(12): pp. 3475–3481.
56. Mwaikambo, L. and M. Ansell, Hemp fibre reinforced cashew nut shell liquid composites. *Composites Science and Technology*, 2003, **63**(9): pp. 1297–1305.
57. Harlin, A., et al., Industrial biomaterial visions. *VIT Research Notes*, 2009, **2522**: pp. 1–94.
58. Nava, H., S. Brooks, and T. Skrobacki, Soybean based hybrid unsaturated polyester resin system. *Technical Paper at Composites*, 2010.
59. Oprea, S. and F. Doroftei, Biodegradation of polyurethane acrylate with acrylated epoxidized soybean oil blend elastomers by *Chaetomium globosum*. *International Biodeterioration & Biodegradation*, 2011, **65**(3): pp. 533–538.
60. Iovino, R., et al., Biodegradation of poly(lactic acid)/starch/coir biocomposites under controlled composting conditions. *Polymer Degradation and Stability*, 2008, **93**(1): pp. 147–157.
61. Kumar, R., M. Yakubu, and R. Anandjiwala, Biodegradation of flax fiber reinforced poly lactic acid. *Express Polymer Letters*, 2010, **4**(7): pp. 423–430.
62. Narayanan, N., P. K. Roychoudhury, and A. Srivastava, L (+) lactic acid fermentation and its product polymerization. *Electronic Journal of Biotechnology*, 2004, **7**(2): pp. 167–178.
63. Vert, M., Aliphatic polyesters: Great degradable polymers that cannot do everything. *Biomacromolecules*, 2005, **6**(2): pp. 538–546.
64. Cordeiro, N., et al., Chemical composition and pulping of banana pseudo-stems. *Industrial Crops and Products*, 2004, **19**(2): pp. 147–154.
65. Mukhopadhyay, S., et al., Banana fibers: Variability and fracture behaviour. *Cellulose*, 2008, **31**: pp. 3.61.

66. Hirose, S., T. Hatakeyama, and H. Hatakeyama. Synthesis and thermal properties of epoxy resins from ester-carboxylic acid derivative of alcoholysis lignin, in *Macromolecular Symposia*. 2003, Wiley Online Library.

67. Labcat. Simple sugars: Fructose, glucose and sucrose [online], 2009 [cited 20 September 2014.]; Available from: https://cdavies. wordpress.com/2009/01/27/simple-sugars-fructose-glucose-and-sucrose/.

68. Glenn, G., et al., Green composites derived from natural fibres, in *Natural Fibre Reinforced Polymer Composites: From Macro to Nanscale*, S. Thomas and L. A. Pothan (Eds.), 2009, Old City Publishing, Inc.: Philadelphia, USA. pp. 113–139.

69. Thomas, S. and L. A. Pothan, *Natural Fibre Reinforced Polymer Composites: From Macro to Nanoscale*. 2009, Old City Publishing, Inc.: Philadelphia, USA.

70. Meier, M. A., J. O. Metzger, and U. S. Schubert, Plant oil renewable resources as green alternatives in polymer science. *Chemical Society Reviews*, 2007, **36**(11): pp. 1788–1802.

71. Puglia, D., J. Biagiotti, and J. Kenny, A review on natural fibre-based composites—Part II. *Journal of Natural Fibers*, 2005, **1**(3): pp. 23–65.

72. Aziz, S. H. and M. P. Ansell, The effect of alkalization and fibre alignment on the mechanical and thermal properties of kenaf and hemp bast fibre composites: Part 2–cashew nut shell liquid matrix. *Composites Science and Technology*, 2004, **64**(9): pp. 1231-1238.

73. Savastano Jr, H., P. Warden, and R. Coutts, Brazilian waste fibres as reinforcement for cement-based composites. *Cement and Concrete Composites*, 2000, **22**(5): pp. 379–384.

74. Majhi, S. K., et al., Mechanical and fracture behavior of banana fiber reinforced polylactic acid biocomposites. *International Journal of Plastics Technology*, 2010, **14**: pp. 57–75.

75. Niedermann, P., G. Szebényi, and A. Toldy, Characterization of high glass transition temperature sugar-based epoxy resin composites with jute and carbon fibre reinforcement. *Composites Science and Technology*, 2015, **117**: pp. 62–68.

76. La Rosa, A., et al., Environmental impacts and thermal insulation performance of innovative composite solutions for building applications. *Construction and Building Materials*, 2014, **55**: pp. 406–414.

77. Deka, H., M. Misra, and A. Mohanty, Renewable resource based "all green composites" from kenaf biofiber and poly (furfuryl alcohol) bioresin. *Industrial Crops and Products*, 2013, **41**: pp. 94–101.
78. Goda, K., H. Takagi, and A. N. Netravali, Fully biodegradable green composites reinforced with natural fibers, in *Natural Fibre Reinforced Polymer Composites: From Macro to Nanoscale*, S. P. Thomas and L. A. Pothan (Eds.), 2009, Old City Publishing, Inc.: Philadelphia, USA. pp. 329–355.
79. Environment and Plastics Industry Council, *Biodegradable Polymers: A Review*. 2000, EPIC.
80. Müller, R. J., Biodegradability of polymers: Regulations and methods for testing. *Biopolymers Online*, 2005.
81. Puechner, P., W.-R. Mueller, and D. Bardtke, Assessing the biodegradation potential of polymers in screening- and long-term test systems. *Journal of Environmental Polymer Degradation*, 1995, **3**(3): pp. 133–143.
82. Hoffmann, J., et al., Manometric determination of biological degradability of substances poorly soluble in aqueous environments. *International Biodeterioration & Biodegradation*, 1997, **39**(4): pp. 327–332.
83. Smith, R., *Biodegradable Polymers for Industrial Applications*. 2005, CRC Press.

Chapter 2

Advancements and Potential Prospects of Polymer/Metal Oxide Nanocomposites: From Laboratory Synthesis to Commercialization

Deepali Sharma[a] and Karan Vadehra[b]
[a]*Department of Pharmaceutical Sciences, College of Health Sciences, University of KwaZulu-Natal, Durban 4000, South Africa*
[b]*Department of Mechanical Engineering, DAV Institute of Engineering and Technology, Jalandhar 144001, India*
dpschem@gmail.com

For a nanometer scale there is no richer storehouse of interesting ideas and strategies than biology.
—George Whitesides

Nanocomposites generated by the combination of polymer and metal oxide nanoparticles have gained attraction of researchers owing to the remarkable properties exhibited by them. The multifunctionality of nanocomposites has been exploited in many commercial applications with prominent results. The synergistic effects of the combination of the constituent polymers and varied metal oxide nanoparticles have attracted wide interest as sensors, energy storage devices, optoelectronics, and photocatalytic materials. This chapter focuses on the different approaches of synthesis of nanocomposites, types of nanocomposites with their important applications. The properties of nanocomposites depend on the polymer–nanoparticles as well as nanoparticle–nanoparticle interactions, which determine the load transfer between the polymer and the nanoparticles. The last section of the chapter highlights the growth of a commercial market for polymer nanocomposites with future prospects thereby finding an effort put at academic and industrial levels.

2.1 Introduction

Nanocomposites are solid materials with multiphase domains, which are in the nanoscale dimension of 1–100 nm. They are fabricated by combining the properties of organic and inorganic constituents, thereby generating new properties to meet the current and future demands of these functional materials. They can have novel chemical and physical properties depending on the morphology and interfacial properties of their constituent materials. The constituent materials can be nanoparticles (three nanoscale dimension), nanofibers (two nanoscale dimension), and nanoclays (one nanoscale dimension). Nanocomposites have emerged as suitable alternatives to the challenges possessed by the composites with regards to anisotropy, strength, optical, electrical, and chemical properties. In terms of uniqueness of design and properties, they have been reported as 21st century materials.

The history of nanocomposites dates back before 1980s with the first development of nanocomposite in 1950 reported by Carter et al. They developed organoclays with several organic onium bases to reinforce latex-based elastomers [1]. In 1991, Toyota introduced the first polymer/clay auto parts where nylon was filled with montmorillonite (MMT) for automobile timing belts [2]. In the 1990s, nylon nanocomposites containing carbon nanotube fillers were widespread for their applications such as static dissipative components in auto fuel systems as well as computer read–write heads. The other achievements in the history of nanocomposites include the development of the first nanomagnetic compound,

Finemet, by Hitachi Metals (1988) for the fabrication of low-loss transformers; the first commercial ceramic nanocomposites, Nanox 2613 thermal spray patented by Inframat LLC (1998); and nanobiocomposite solar cells (2005). The timeline of development of nanocomposites is depicted in Fig. 2.1.

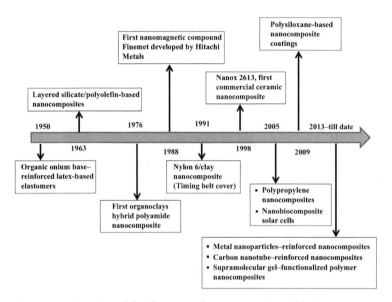

Figure 2.1 Overview of development of nanocomposites with time.

Nanocomposites are the fourth-generation composites. It has been reported that as the particle size changes, the properties of nanocomposites also change due to the improvement in the interactions at phase interfaces [3]. Two main parameters are important for reinforcement: (i) particle–particle interactions and (ii) polymer–particle interactions. It has been reported that higher anisotropy and smaller size lead to higher polymer–particle (high surface area) and particle–particle (more particle number) interactions thereby observing the highest changes in property [4].

Nanoparticles in the size range of 1–100 nm have been used for a decade owing to their unique structural and optical properties. With the increasing development in the area of nanoparticle synthesis, the challenge to have control over size and shape is overcome. The control over nanoparticle assemblies has opened up opportunities for the incorporation of other functional building blocks into nanocomposites to introduce properties complimentary to nanoparticles [5]. The ability to control the location of the nanoparticle's position within a polymeric matrix will allow to enhancing and tailoring the properties of resulting hybrid nanocomposites [6]. They act as fillers in the polymer matrices and alter the mechanical and thermal properties of the polymers, thus changing the properties of the nanocomposites. Current research is targeted on the use of fillers in the nanometer range as they are found to improve the properties of polymers [7]. Metallic nanoparticles have been used as fillers in the fabrication of nanocomposites, and a lot of research has been carried out, but still some of the aspects of the metallic nanoparticle filler modified polymer matrix nanocomposites still remain uncovered. Consequently, in this chapter, the use of metal oxide nanoparticles as fillers in the polymer matrices will be discussed along with highlighting the commercial availability of these nanocomposites.

2.2 Different Approaches for Nanocomposite Synthesis

Nanocomposites can be synthesized by different approaches, which can be categorized as follows:
- Template synthesis
- In situ synthesis
- Melt mixing
- Solution intercalation
- Electrospinning
- Click chemistry

2.2.1 Template Synthesis

Also known as sol–gel technology, this method involves the synthesis of inorganic materials in the presence of polymer matrix. It is mainly used for the synthesis of double-layered hydroxide-based nanocomposites. The precursors used in this process can be either metal alkoxides, inorganic or organic salts. In particular, metal alkoxides are preferred more as they induce electronic, magnetic, or catalytic properties and have highly electronegative –OR groups, which can stabilize the metal atom in its highest oxidation state, thereby making it susceptible to nucleophilic attack [8]. The metal alkoxides undergo hydrolysis and condensation reactions, forming three-dimensional network of inorganic or organic–inorganic hybrid materials. The hydrolysis and condensation reactions are as follows:

Hydrolysis

$$M(OR)_4 + H_2O \longrightarrow M(OR)_x (OH)_{4-x} + R\text{-}OH \quad (2.1)$$

Condensation

$$M\text{-}OR + M\text{-}OH \longrightarrow M\text{-}O\text{-}M + R\text{-}OH \quad (2.2)$$

$$M\text{-}OH + M\text{-}OH \longrightarrow M\text{-}O\text{-}M + H\text{-}OH \quad (2.3)$$

The template-assisted synthesis has been divided into two classes on the basis of the interactions between the polymer and inorganic materials: Class I comprises the systems where only the physical interactions take place between the organic and inorganic components, whereas in Class II, chemical interactions exist between the different phases [9].

This approach is used to obtain layered nanocomposites directly via one-pot reaction with solution phase precursors at ambient temperature. $NiPS_3$ nanocomposites with polyethylenimine (PEI), polyvinyl alcohol (PVA), and polyvinylpyrrolidone (PVP) have been reported to be synthesized via the template approach [10]. The nanocomposites exhibit zigzag monolayers and could generate denser interlayers as compared to other methods (topotactic). The polymer assists in the nucleation and growth of the inorganic particles that get trapped within the layers as they grow [11].

2.2.2　In Situ Synthesis

In the last few years, there has been an elevated interest in embedding inorganic nanoparticles into the polymer matrix. The introduction of inorganic nanoparticles into the polymer gives rise to magnetic, optical, and thermal properties in the nanocomposites. During in situ polymerization, there is in situ synthesis of nanoparticles followed by the polymerization of monomer, which acts as a solvent. Thus, there is a formation of intercalated nanocomposites [12]. In this process, the nanoparticle aggregation can be avoided since the nucleation process takes place inside the polymer matrix and particles grow within the matrix. Additionally, polymer chains have functional groups, which have a stabilizing effect on the formation of nanoparticles. Thus, this effect provides a uniform spatial distribution of nanoparticles in the polymer matrices, thereby preventing their aggregation. Stable nanocomposites are formed with potential properties. The strong interaction between the inorganic precursors and polymer matrix is the predominant factor for controlling the particle size and polydispersity. Polyurethane-TiO_2 nanocomposites have been reported to be synthesized by the in situ synthesis approach with improved nanoparticle dispersion where the nanoparticles were prepared in a solution of pre-polymer hydroxyl-terminated polybutadiene (HTPB). The resulting nanocomposite showed a higher performance as solid propellant binder than the nanocomposite fabricated by conventional powder or solution methods [13].

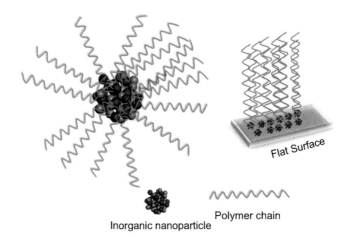

Figure 2.2 Diagram of a polymer brush.

An extensive research is being carried out to embed nanoparticles in polymer brushes to fabricate nanocomposites in order to develop functional surfaces. Polymer brushes are layers of ultrathin polymers tethered to a surface. Inorganic particles are generated in situ in the polymer brushes (Fig. 2.2). Since nanoparticles are generated inside the polymer brush, the particles are confined in the colloidal carrier, and hence, they are stabilized against repulsion without the need of using stabilizing agents, which limit the activity of nanoparticles [14]. Kim et al. used the in situ approach for the synthesis of ruthenium oxide/reduced graphene oxide (RGO) nanocomposites. This was based on coupled reactions involving simultaneous reduction of graphene oxide to RGO and oxidation of Ru^{3+} ions to RuO_2. It was found that as the C/O ratio increased, the number density of RuO_2 nanoparticles decreased due to the decrease in the number of surface functional groups that might act as nucleating and anchoring sites for oxide formation [15].

2.2.3 Melt Mixing

Melt mixing is a technique employed in the industry owing to its cost and speed efficiency. Since no solvents are needed, this process is used in the polymer industry to produce nanocomposites in an environment friendly manner. The general principle incorporates the dispersion of fillers in the polymer matrix in the molten state by applying a shear force. There is a chemical modification of the filler, and compatibilizers are used to enhance the filler–matrix interactions [16].

The melt mixing method has been used for the formation of polymer/clay nanocomposites and there are several studies focused on the polymer nanocomposites made up of MMT added to thermoplastics. The layered MMT is added to the polymer, and the mixture is heated above the polymer's softening point. The polymer chains penetrate inside the clay layers forming an intercalated or exfoliated nanocomposite [17]. This method was first used for the preparation of polystyrene (PS)/clay nanocomposites [18] and then expanded to other polymers such as polyolefin [19], nylon 6 [20], polylactide [21], polyethylene terephthalate [22], and polyvinyl chloride [23]. To melt-mix the hydrophobic polymer matrix (polyolefin) with clay platelets, it is needed to modify the surface of clay using surfactants to reduce the affinity difference between the hydrophilic clay and hydrophobic matrix [17].

2.2.4 Solution Intercalation

This method involves solvents in which polymer is soluble for the swelling and dispersion of nanoclay particles. The polymer is mixed into the clay suspension and is adsorbed on the clay platelets. Usually, water-soluble polymers are used for this method. However, the method can also be applied to polymer soluble in non-aqueous systems. Once the nanocomposite is formed, the solution is evaporated, which leads to physical changes such as weight loss, reduction in the thickness accompanied by the reorientation of the polymer chains [24]. Compared with the melt mixing method, the solution intercalation method is complex and not environment friendly due to the use of solvents.

2.2.5 Electrospinning

Nanoparticles, when added to polymers, produce nanocomposites with improved mechanical strength, resistance to wear, and thermal stability. Limited information exists regarding the impact of nanoparticles on the polymer spinning behavior. The structure and morphology of the electrospun fibers are dictated by the synergistic effects of physical parameters [25]. The electrospinning process is the balance of parameters that are not limited to conditions such as relative humidity, polymer weight, distance between capillary tip and collector plate, feed rate of solution, and solution composition [26]. The addition of nanoparticles in the electrospun fibers has been reported to influence polymer properties, electrospinning conditions, and morphology of the electrospun fibers. The use of different metal oxide nanoparticles (TiO_2, In_2O_3, Fe_2O_3) is found to affect viscosity, voltage, surface morphology, and diameter of the fibers, thereby leading to the formation of nanocomposites with potential water treatment applications such as nanofiltration and ion exchange [27].

Electrospinning is one of the versatile techniques that utilize high electrostatic forces for fiber production. Among different electrospun fibers, nanoparticle-spun fibers have exhibited potential applications. Nanoparticles such as nanorods and nanowires get aligned within the fibers and reduce the Gibb's free energy [28]. The nanoparticles are either stabilized on the surface or within the fibers, thus overcoming the disadvantages of conventional self-assembly methods. This technique does not require any surface functionalization process; just a suitable solvent is required in which nanoparticles can be uniformly dispersed and the solvent in which polymer can dissolve [29]. Since inorganic nanoparticles have high electron density than polymers, they could be easily encapsulated within the polymer fibers by the electrospinning technique.

2.2.6 Click Chemistry

Reactions of click chemistry have been extended from small molecules to the field of polymers. Click reactions have a wide scope, are feasible to perform with the use of readily available reagents, and are insensitive to oxygen and water [30]. Click chemistry approaches comprising copper-catalyzed azide-alkyne cylcoaddition (CuAAC), thiol-ene, and thiol-yne have been used for the functionalization of graphene with brushes of short chain polyethylene (PE) and analyzing the effect of chemistry used on the final nanocomposites of PE-modified graphene, with high-density polyethylene (HDPE) [31].

The main challenge in the synthesis of nanocomposites is the homogenous dispersion of nanoparticles in the polymer matrix as nanoparticles have a strong tendency to aggregate. This challenge has diverted the attention of researchers to click chemistry to achieve excellent filler dispersion in the polymer matrix. Click chemistry is based on the Huisgen cycloaddition of azide moiety with alkyne moiety to the surface of matrix as well as filler. Nanocomposites synthesized using this approach have been reported to be used as chemiresistive sensors for the detection of H_2O_2 vapor with rapid response and recovery at room temperature [32].

2.3 Polymer-Based Metal Oxide Nanocomposites

Polymers are regarded as the best hosting matrices for composites because of their long-term stability and good processability. Metal oxide nanoparticles have optical, magnetic, catalytic, and electronic properties that are different from their bulk counterparts. The combination of potential properties of polymers and metal oxide nanoparticles leads to the formation of nanocomposites with synergistically improved properties, which are exploited at the commercial scale.

The key features (light weight, ease of fabrication, durability, low cost) of some of the common polymers such as polyolefins, nylons, and polyesters have led to their widespread use. Despite the aforementioned features, the use of polymers is limited because of poor mechanical, thermal, and electrical properties as compared to metals and ceramics. But when they are combined with nanoparticles, there is not only an enhancement in their properties but also new functionalities are introduced [33]. This has led to the wide use of nanocomposites in different fields as military equipment, safety, automotive, aerospace, electronics, and optical devices.

One of the important aspects in the designing of nanocomposites is the dispersion of a specific nanoparticle in the polymer matrix to optimize the desired property of the hybrid. A considerable amount of work has been done for the spatial distribution of nanoparticles by controlling the nanoparticle–polymer matrix miscibility [34]. With the availability of new functional nanoparticles with finite aspect ratio (L/D), it is quite interesting to predict not only the electrical percolation threshold (ϕ_c) but also the properties of networks over the percolation threshold [35]. This is important to understand on account of enhancing the electrical properties of nanocomposites [36]. The following polymer/metal oxide nanocomposites will be discussed in brief to shed light on the advancements that have taken place till now:

- Polymer–iron oxide-based nanocomposites
- Polymer–zinc oxide-based nanocomposites
- Polymer–silica-based nanocomposites
- Polymer–titanium oxide-based nanocomposites

2.3.1 Polymer–Iron Oxide-Based Nanocomposites

In the recent years, due to their superparamagnetic nature, iron oxide nanoparticles have found wide applications in the biomedical field. They are used in magnetic resonance imaging (MRI), drug delivery, targeted magnetic hyperthermia as well as used as catalysts. Despite having potential applications, iron oxide nanoparticles suffer certain limitations such as toxicity issues. Bare nanoparticles could cause damage to cells by interfering with the cell cycle at high concentrations. They may aggregate with serum proteins if used in vivo [37]. Therefore, surface modification of nanoparticles may overcome these issues, and work has been initiated in this field.

Coating the surface with polymers stabilizes nanoparticles and prevents aggregation. Incorporation of magnetic nanoparticles in the polymer distinguishes between Néel and Brown relaxation. These are processes by which magnetic nanoparticles can be heated in a magnetic field, and their distribution within the polymer can be determined. Néel relaxation reorients the magnetic moment of particle to keep it aligned with the magnetic field. Thus, temperature is increased as the anisotropy barrier is crossed. Néel relaxation time (τ_N) is given by the following equation [38]:

$$\tau_N = \tau_0 \, e^{(KV/k_b T)} \tag{2.4}$$

where τ_0 (=10^{-9} s) is the exponential prefactor, K (=8 kJ/m^3) is the anisotropy constant of magnetite, V is the volume of the particle core [m^3], k_b is the Boltzmann constant [J/K], and T is the temperature [K].

Amphiphilic block copolymers have been reported to be excellent templates for nanoparticles and provide new properties to the hybrid of iron oxide nanoparticles and polymers. The incorporation of iron oxide nanoparticles into the polymeric aggregates involves two approaches: (i) metal ions are bound covalently or adsorbed on the polymer aggregates, followed by conversion into nanoparticles via chemical reactions [39]; (ii) nanoparticles are synthesized separately and then co-assembled in the presence of polymer matrix to form nanocomposites [40]. This approach has been widely employed for the synthesis of iron oxide nanoparticles. Karagoz et al. used triblock polymeric chains, poly(oligoethylene glycol methacrylate)-block-(methacrylic acid)-block-poly(styrene) (POEGMA-b-PMAA-b-PST) to fabricate iron oxide nanoparticles using simple and versatile polymerization-induced self-assembly (PISA) approach. The carboxylic groups present in the polymeric chains assisted in the complexation of Fe^{2+} and Fe^{3+} mixture. The formation of nanoparticles took place within the polymer by the alkaline co-precipitation of Fe^{2+} and Fe^{3+} salts. The nanoparticles were stable and could be used as MRI contrast agents. The concentration of iron oxide nanoparticles within the polymer can be varied by adjusting the ratio of iron and carboxylic acid groups [41].

A new strategy for the fabrication of nanocomposites is the encapsulation of nanoparticles in the matrix of biodegradable polymers by allowing the use of nanocomposites in a wide range of biological applications. Chitosan is the natural abundant polymer composed of randomly distributed β-(1→4) linked D-glucosamine and N-acetyl-D-glucosamine. Since iron oxide has antimicrobial activities, chitosan–iron oxide coated graphene oxide nanocomposite hydrogel is synthesized by the coprecipitation method and reported in literature. Iron oxide nanoparticles are coated on the surface of graphene oxide (GO) in a single step at room temperature. The hydrogel films exhibit significant antibacterial activity against gram-positive and gram-negative bacteria. Glycerol plays a prominent role in the fabrication of chitosan–iron oxide coated graphene oxide hydrogel films. A crosslinking occurs by electrostatic interaction as well as hydrogen bonding between the $-NH^{3+}$ group of chitosan and the –OH group of glycerol. The self-healing ability of the hydrogel films network results from the strong hydrogen bonding interaction [42]. Fe_3O_4/Chitosan nanocomposites have also been constructed for targeting cancer where the average diameter of iron oxide nanoparticles is 10 nm. Chitosan is used as a polymeric shell around nanoparticles due to its biocompatibility, biodegradability (in vivo susceptibility to lysosomes), and non-toxic character. The drug release profile of chitosan ensures the drug delivery into the acidic environment of the cancer tissue. The nanocomposite loaded with anticancer drug Gemcitabine displayed a pH-responsive drug delivery and was reported to be a potential candidate for cancer treatment because of dual possibilities: (i) the nanocomposite specifically delivered drug at the tumor site in appropriate concentration, and (ii) selective temperature increase in the cancer mass following exposition to an alternative magnetic gradient [43].

2.3.2 Polymer–Zinc Oxide-Based Nanocomposites

ZnO is a multifunctional inorganic material with a wide band gap of 3.37 eV at room temperature and large exciton binding energy of 60 MeV. At nanoscale, it exhibits many promising properties, thus exploring applications such as gas sensors, ultraviolet lasers, optoelectronic devices, surface acoustic wave devices, and solar cells. It is widely blended with polymer to form nanocomposites. Polyaniline (PANI) is one of the conducting polymers, which is distinguished by the ease of synthesis and high environmental synthesis. PANI/ZnO nanocomposites can be synthesized by the in situ polymerization method where individual redox properties of ZnO and PANI are maintained in the nanocomposite (Fig. 2.3). The electrical characteristic (I–V) of the nanocomposite exhibits a build-up of space charge between the interface of Al/ZnO-PANI and also a rectifying behavior with an I_F/I_R value of 241 where I_F and I_R are the forward and reverse current, respectively. This value indicates the diode formation between nanocomposites with Al [44].

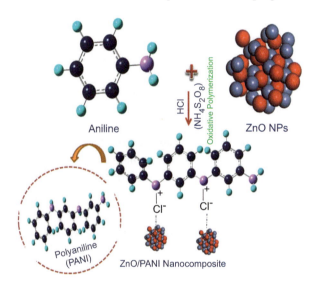

Figure 2.3 Synthesis of PANI/ZnO nanocomposite.

Kos et al. synthesized highly transparent and UV-absorbing PMMA/ZnO nanocomposites by dispersing ZnO nanoparticles homogenously in the PMMA (polymethyl methacrylate) matrix for optical applications using A-b-(AB) diblock copolymer poly (methyl methacrylate)-block-poly[(methyl methacrylate)-co-(zinc methacrylate acetate)], PMMA-b-P(MMA-co-ZnMAAc). Here two things were achieved: first, self-assembling of block copolymers, and second, ZnO nanoparticles were synthesized within the polymer matrix (in situ synthesis) via reversible addition–fragmentation chain transfer (RAFT) polymerization [45].

Polyaryletherketone (PAEK) belongs to the family of semi-crystalline thermoplastic polymers with high temperature stability and mechanical strength. In the literature, work has been reported where different weight percentages of ZnO nanoparticles are added into the PAEK matrix using the ball milling method. It was noticed that the properties of nanocomposites varied with the volume fraction of ZnO nanoparticles, which is given by the following equation:

$$V_f = W_f / [W_f + W_m(\rho_f/\rho_m)] \tag{2.5}$$

where V_f is the volume fraction, W_f is the weight fraction, W_m is the weight fraction of the PAEK matrix, ρ_f is the density of ZnO nanoparticles, and ρ_m is the density of polymer matrix. The dielectric constant and thermal stability of the nanocomposites were found to increase with the increasing content of ZnO nanoparticles in the PAEK matrix [46]. ZnO nanoparticles have also been dispersed in waterborne polyurethanes, which are a new generation of polyurethane polymers. They are of particular interest in environmental pollution, health and safety risks. The incorporation of ZnO nanoparticles in the polyurethane matrix increases the glass transition temperature, which is associated with hydrogen bonding, van der Waals forces, and electrostatic interaction between the nanoparticles and the polymer matrix [47].

2.3.3 Polymer–Silica-Based Nanocomposites

The synthesis, characterization, and application of polymer-silica based nanocomposites have become an expanding field of research. There are, in general, three ways to synthesize silica-polymer based nanocomposites: (i) silica nanoparticles are directly incorporated into the monomer and then polymerization takes place; (ii) silica nanoparticles are blended into the monomer via in situ polymerization; and (iii) silica precursors such as alkoxysilane containing polymers are used in the sol–gel process [48].

One of the challenging tasks in the fabrication of nanocomposites is the homogenous dispersion of nanoparticles in the polymer matrix as there is a tendency of nanoparticles to agglomerate. Thus, nanocomposites are formed where a number of loosened nanoparticle clusters are present within the polymer matrix, and thus, nanocomposites exhibit properties that are worse than the individual polymers. To overcome the aggregation of nanoparticles within the matrix, an irradiation grafting method is applied for the surface modification of nanoparticles, and then modified nanoparticles are mechanically mixed with the polymer [49]. One of the strategies followed to improve the dispersibility of silica nanoparticles within the polymer is the grafting of nanoparticles on amphiphilic and thickening ASE (alkali swellable emulsion) polymers. This enhances the colloidal stability of nanoparticles in the polymer matrices. This strategy has an advantage of decreasing the negative impact of nanoparticles (toxicity) on the environment as the nanoparticles are covalently attached to the polymer. Classical acrylate thickeners, also known as ASE, are an important group of materials mainly comprising methacrylic (MA) or acrylic (AA) acid and ethyl acrylate (EA). They combine the properties of being soluble in basic aqueous solutions due to the presence of carboxylic groups from MA or AA monomers and existence of crosslinking between the polymer chains that increase the viscosity of the aqueous solution [50]. Another approach that has been used is the swelling of preformed polymer particles with desired pore structure in tetraethoxysilane (TEOS) as silica gel precursor. The swelling process allows the filling of pores with TEOS, which penetrates into the spaces between the polymer chains. This process leads to the formation of spherically shaped polymer–silica nanocomposite beads after the transformation of the inorganic precursor in an aqueous solution of desired pH. This is an efficient route for the synthesis of polymer/metal oxide nanocomposites [51].

The thermal, fire retardant, mechanical properties and water resistance of the polymer film improve on incorporating silica nanoparticles in the polymer matrix. Soap-free emulsion polymerization leads to the formation of PAA-functionalized P(St-BA) latex particles. On the addition of an ethanol solution containing TEOS into PAA-functionalized P(St-BA) latex, silica nanoparticles are formed by the hydrolysis of TEOS catalyzed by ammonia and adsorb on the PAA-functionalized P(St-BA) particles, thereby producing raspberry-like polymer/SiO_2 nanocomposites. The weight percentage of silica to be loaded can be controlled by varying the amount of TEOS and ammonia [52].

2.3.4 Polymer–Titanium Oxide-Based Nanocomposites

Among the different semiconductor materials such as ZnO, $SrTiO_3$, CeO_2, WO_3, Fe_2O_3, Bi_2O_3, GaN, CdS, ZnS, CdS, and ZnSe, TiO_2 is widely used as a photocatalytic material. TiO_2 is used as filler in the polymer matrix as it forms strong interactions with the polymeric chains due to crosslinking and leads to improved and enhanced properties. One of the key points in encapsulating the nanoparticles in polymers is the control over their nucleation by terminating their growth, and thus preventing aggregation process. Inverted emulsion polymerization method has been used for the synthesis of PANI–TiO_2 nanocomposites. This method consists of aqueous solution of monomer, which is emulsified in an organic solvent and an initiator is used for the polymerization process. As compared to bulk polymerization, emulsion polymerization has significantly less thermal and viscosity problems since the reaction is carried out in heterogeneous systems. A chemical interaction takes place at the interface of PANI and TiO_2 nanoparticles. The mechanism involves electrostatic interaction between the nanoparticles, which are electronegative in acidic medium, and anilinium cations. These cations have a strong possibility of adsorbing on the surface of TiO_2 nanoparticles. Since these nanocomposites have improved electrical properties, they can find their potential at industrial scale as charge-storage materials and solar cells [53].

Block copolymers (BC) are used as an alternative for semiconductor patterning applications since they can act as templates for defining integrated circuit elements due to their ability to self-assemble. Amphiphilic polystyrene-b-poly(ethylene oxide) (SEO) block copolymers are extensively studied as templating agents. These polymers consist of a hydrophilic poly(ethylene oxide) (PEO) block, which adsorbs and interacts strongly with the nanoparticles, as well as a hydrophobic polystyrene (PS) block, which builds the matrix. It has been studied that TiO_2 nanoparticles synthesized by the sol–gel process and encapsulated in polystyrene-b-poly(ethylene oxide) (SEO) block retain their conductive properties [54].

The hydrolysis and condensation of titanium tetra-alkoxides in alcohol media lead to the formation of three-dimensionally interconnected poly(titanium oxide) gels, which are of great interest since they swell up in liquid media. Unique optical properties are exhibited by them due to ultraviolet (UV) induced transitions (Ti^{4+}, Ti^{3+}) as TiO_2 and $TiO_2.nH_2O$. Due to the instability of their properties in air, it is important to stabilize these gels by forming nanocomposites. The method is based on combining the process of hydrolytic polycondensation of titanium isopropoxide in the medium of hydroxyethylmethacrylate (HEMA) vinyl monomer with subsequent polymerization of the latter, which results in the formation of a solid material. The nanocomposites obtained by this method have an edge over the nanocomposites that are fabricated by incorporating TiO_2 nanoparticles in the polymer matrix [55]. The reactions involving hydrolysis and polycondensation are as follows:

Hydrolysis of titanium alkoxide

$$Ti\text{-}OR + H\text{-}OH \xrightarrow{HCl, H_2O} Ti\text{-}OH + ROH \quad (2.6)$$

(R = HEMA fragments)

Polycondensation

$$Ti\text{-}OR + HO\text{-}Ti \longrightarrow Ti\text{-}O\text{-}Ti + HOR \quad (2.7)$$

$$Ti\text{-}OH + HO\text{-}Ti \longrightarrow Ti\text{-}O\text{-}Ti + HOH \quad (2.8)$$

2.4 Role of Metal Oxide Nanoparticles in Enhancing the Properties of Nanocomposites

Metal oxide nanoparticles play a key role in enhancing the mechanical, electrical, and optical properties of nanocomposites, which are dependent on the nanoparticle–polymer matrix interactions and also interaction between the nanoparticles. The different types of forces such as attraction or repulsion can be controlled by controlling the weight fraction, volume fraction, surface modification of the particles, and nanoparticles size. The enhanced mechanical properties can be achieved by improving the interface between the nanoparticles and the polymer matrix. The strength of interaction at the nanoparticle–polymer interface determines the load transfer between the fillers, that is, nanoparticles and polymer matrix [56].

The advantage of using metal oxide nanoparticles as reinforcing agents in the polymer matrix is their size, which is smaller than the critical crack length, which is responsible for initiating failure in the nanocomposites. As a result, nanoparticles provide toughness and mechanical strength. They also significantly affect the glass transition temperature (T_g) of the polymers when incorporated by influencing the mobility of polymer chains due to bonding between the nanoparticles and the polymer, also the bridging of polymer chains between the nanoparticles. They also increase the optical and electrical properties of nanocomposites. This depends on the fact that the smaller the size of nanoparticles, the shorter the distance between them. This leads to the percolation at lower volume fraction resulting in higher electrical conductivity. The electrical conductivity also depends on the ordered states of the conducting polymer. One of the polymers, polyproplylene, has a soft lattice; therefore, its electronic and structural properties can be easily modified. Iron oxide nanoparticles serve as template for the formation of polypropylene matrix and leads to the enhancement of DC current, which is explained on the basis of variable range hopping (VRH) mechanism. This mechanism involves the transfer of charges between the nanoparticles and the polymer matrix [57].

The presence of micropollutants such as pesticides and pharmaceuticals in water has become a global concern because of their negative impact on humans and aquatic ecosystems. Insoluble polymers of β-cyclodextrins are an inexpensive source derived from the macrocycle of glucose. They can encapsulate micropollutants by forming well-defined host–guest complexes, but their small surface area is still a limitation [58]. The photocatalytic activity of these polymers can be enhanced by the use of nanoparticles. TiO_2 and ZnO nanoparticles, when embedded in cyclic polymers of β-cyclodextrin, cause the photocatalytic degradation of Rhodamine red dye, which is one of the organic pollutants in water. The mechanism of degradation of dye by the metal oxide (MO)-β-cyclodextrin (CD) nanocomposite can be explained on the basis that at the equilibrium stage, β-CD is linked to MO surface and Rhodamine dye enters the cavity of β-CD. Since, β-CD has more affinity for MO, it adsorbs on the surface of MO and captures the reactive sites, thereby forming MO/β-CD complex. Rhodamine red dye then interacts with this complex and is degraded. Hence, reaction between the dye and nanocomposite is a key for the photodegradation of the dye. The dye moves into the cavity of β-CD, which then adsorbs on the surface of MO. Thus, β-CD acts as a channel or bridge for the dye to get accumulated on the surface of metal oxide at higher concentrations, thereby leading to its effective degradation [59].

2.5 Applications of Nanocomposites

The incorporation of inorganic nanoparticles into the polymer matrices leads to a number of potential applications such as flame retardation, electrical conductivity, and biomedical applications. Hence, metal oxide polymer nanocomposites are emerging as new materials, thereby creating a new area of interest. A light has been shed on some of the applications in the subsequent sections (Fig. 2.4).

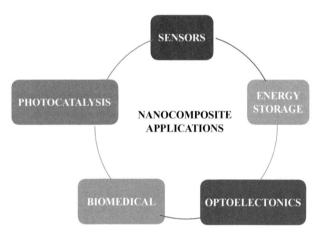

Figure 2.4 Applications of nanocomposites in different areas.

2.5.1 Sensors

For the detection of toxic pollutants and prevention of hazardous gas leaks from industries, gas sensor devices are used. Therefore, present research is focused on the fabrication of inexpensive and efficient gas-sensing devices that have high sensitivity and expedited response time. Nitrogen dioxide (NO_2) is one of the toxic gases and is an intermediate in the industrial synthesis of nitric acid and millions of tons are produced every year. It is a reddish-brown gas with sharp characteristic biting odor and is a major air pollutant. Hence, it is necessary to develop low-cost sensors that can detect NO_2 at low concentrations (5–100 ppm). Within the past few years, inorganic–organic hybrid nanocomposite materials have been devised as gas-sensing materials and have become prominent area of research. On combining metal oxide nanoparticles with polymer matrices, a new class of sensors with improved synergistic effects can be designed, which can tackle the monitoring of gas pollutants at the industrial level. Polypyrrole (PPy) is one of the conducting polymers that can be easily synthesized by electrochemical methods, and one of the advantages of using it is excellent environmental stability. It is used in electronic devices and also as chemical sensors. PPy/α-Fe_2O_3 hybrid nanocomposites with different weight percentages (10–50%) of camphor sulfonic acid (CSA) as a dopant have been synthesized using the solid-state synthesis method. The thin films of the hybrid nanocomposite are deposited on the glass substrate using the spin coating technique to sense different gases (Fig. 2.5). It is observed that among different gases, the nanocomposite films are most sensitive to NO_2 at room temperature with chemiresistive response of 64% at 100 ppm with fast response time of 148 s [60]. The response (S) of sensors is calculated by the following relation:

$$S(\%) = |R_a - R_g|/R_a \times 100\% \tag{2.9}$$

where R_a and R_g are the resistance values of the sensor films in fresh air and test gas, respectively. Response and recovery times of the sensor are defined as the time needed for 90% of total change in resistance upon exposure to test gas and fresh air, respectively.

The gas-sensing mechanism of the nanocomposite sensor is based on the resistance change that occurs when nanocomposite film is exposed to different gases as well as the number of adsorption sites available on the surface of the nanocomposite [61]. The gas response of a sensor is found to depend on the thickness of the film, porosity, size, and crystallinity of the nanoparticles as well as the nature and amount of dopant [62].

In one of the studies, dodecyl benzene sulfonic acid (DBSA) doped PPy-tungsten oxide (WO_3) hybrid nanocomposites have been designed for the detection of NO_2 gas at room temperature with 72% response at 100 ppm. Dopants are added to enhance the gas-sensing properties and, thus, play a crucial role in the fabrication of chemiresistive gas sensor. On exposure to gas (NO_2), there is a charge transfer between the gas molecules and PPy as WO_3 nanoparticles are well embedded in the polymer matrix. The gas molecules interact with the π-network of the nanocomposite, resulting in a decrease in sensor resistance. This confirms that the nanocomposite behaves as a p-type semiconductor and charge transfer is from PPy. The role of the dopant (DBSA) is to create additional active site on the surface of the nanocomposite [63].

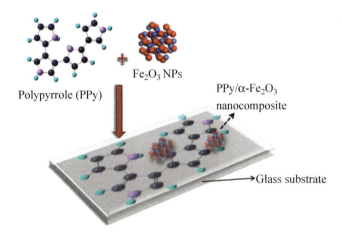

Figure 2.5 Schematic diagram of nanocomposite used as sensor.

Nanocomposites have emerged as an alternative for the detection of biomolecules as compared to the conventional techniques such as electrophoresis, fluorometry, chromatography, spectrophotometry, and chemiluminescence, which require extreme experimental conditions and complicated instrumentation. Dopamine (DA) is one of the very important biomolecule that play an important physiological role as an extracellular messenger for the central nervous, renal, and hormonal systems. The abnormal levels of DA could lead to schizophrenia, Parkinson's disease, and HIV infection. Ghanbari and Moloudi fabricated ZnO flower-like/polyaniline nanofiber/reduced graphene oxide nanocomposite (ZnO/PANI/RGO) electrodeposited on glassy carbon electrode (GCE) for the detection of dopamine and uric acid (UA). The detection limit for DA was found to be 0.8 nM, whereas for UA, the detection limit was 0.042 µM [64].

2.5.2 Energy Storage

Non-volatile memory devices based on organic/inorganic hybrid nanocomposites have emerged as promising candidates with potential applications as next-generation electronic and optoelectronic devices. For fabricating energy storage devices, electron donor and electron acceptor materials are used rather than semiconductor p–n junctions. The electron donor and acceptor phases are blended to form nanocomposites. The organic molecules, that is, polymers act as donors, whereas nanoparticles (inorganic) act as acceptors and are sandwiched between metal electrodes to form a non-volatile memory device.

Single-layer non-volatile memory devices are formed by solution method where there is single monolayer of polymer with nanoparticles embedded in. This type of nanocomposite is then sandwiched between two metal electrodes. The inorganic nanoparticles, ZnO, CuO, CdSe, etc., are dispersed randomly in the polymer matrix [poly(*N*-vinylcarbazole] and poly[2-methoxy-5-(2-ethylhexoxy)-1,4-phenylene]. The nanocomposite films are formed on the substrate using the spin coating technique. In these devices, the memory effect is strongly correlated with the presence of inorganic nanoparticles. They have applicability as flexible memory device in portable equipment [65].

Organic field-effect transistor (OFET) type memory devices are considered to be the next-generation potential memory devices owing to their high portability, flexibility, easily integrating structure, non-destructive read-out characteristics, and single device structure. A distinct charge-storage layer is incorporated for electrical programming function such as ferroelectric materials, nanofloating gate dielectric, or polymer-based electret. Since discrete floating gate elements act as effective charge trapping sites, they are promising candidates for high-performance memory devices. Nanofloating gate memory devices (NFGM) comprising a composite of hole-trapping polymer, poly[9-(4-vinylphenyl) carbazole] (PVPK), and

ZnO nanoparticles have been fabricated and found to have improved memory performance [66].

Due to energy crisis at the global level, the focus is on using renewable sources of energy to meet the present energy demands. Renewable sources also require the support of energy storage devices such as lithium ion batteries and supercapacitors that act as promising candidates because of their higher energy and power densities [67]. Electrochemical capacitors (ECs) are advanced storage systems that have attracted attention due to their unique features such as high power density, fast charge–discharge process, and long life cycles. Conductive polymers, metal oxide nanoparticles, and carbon materials are the three main categories that are used in the fabrication of ECs. Polypyrrole (PPy)/nanowire manganese oxide (NwMnO$_2$) nanocomposites have shown supercapacitance behavior studied by classical and modern electrochemical techniques. PPy and NwMnO$_2$ show specific capacitance values of 109 and 203 F/g, respectively. The presence of nanowires in the PPy matrix increases the capacitance by twofold [68]. This is studied using cyclic voltammetry (CV), which gives information about the nature of various electrodes. CVs of PPy and PPy/NwMnO$_2$ electrode exhibit more charge for the composite than PPy. Specific capacitance (SC) of the electrode can be calculated by:

$$C = I/mv \qquad (2.10)$$

where I is the current, m is the mass of the active material, and v is the potential rate scan.

The enhanced capacitance of the nanocomposite is contributed by (i) PPy nature duo to dope–undope of counter ions, and (ii) pseudo-capacitive behavior of NwMnO$_2$ due to the electrochemical reaction of MnO$_2$ in acidic media.

2.5.3 Optoelectronics

The nanocomposite material should take advantage of both the blended materials, that is, polymers and inorganic nanoparticles. Polymers have large band gap values along with interesting electrical conductivity that makes them useful in electronic devices such as organic light-emitting diodes (OLEDs) or organic photovoltaic cells (OPVs). The inorganic nanoparticles act as guest by enhancing a particular characteristic and stability of the organic material (polymer). The incorporation of nanoparticles in the polymer not only enhances the mechanical properties of the polymer but also provides a resistance against degradation by acting as an energy absorber.

The basic structure of OLED consists of four layers [69]:

1. Transparent anode (indium tin oxide, ITO) deposited on glass or plastic substrate.
2. Hole-transport layer (HTL), poly(ethylenedioxythiophene)-poly(styrene sulfonate), or PEDOT:PSS, facilitates the transport of hole injection from anode to active layer.
3. Active layer (polymer).
4. Cathode.

The external quantum efficiency of an optoelectronic device is defined as the ratio between the number of collected photons and the number of injected charges and is given by:

$$\eta_e = \frac{P/h\nu}{I/e} \qquad (2.11)$$

where P is the optical power emitted into free space, $h\nu$ is the photon energy, I is the current flowing through the diode, and e is the electronic charge.

The efficiency of the OLED, which depends on the number of increased recombinations, is improved by using nanocomposite (nanoparticles + polymer) in the active layer (Fig. 2.6). The nanoparticles in the active layer come in contact with anode, which increases the charge injection. As a result, the measured current is higher in a device using nanocomposite. Nanocomposites of poly(phenylene vinylene) (PPV) and SiO_2/TiO_2 have been used in the fabrication of optoelectronic devices [70]. The nanocomposites of TiO_2 and poly[2-methoxy-5-(2-ethylhexyloxy)-1,4-(1-cyanovinylene-1,4-phenylene)] (MEH-CNPPV) have been used in light-emitting diodes. Due to the surface modification, the device depicts improved electroluminescence at elevated voltage [71]. Polyaniline (PANI)/ZnO nanocomposites with varying concentration of ZnO have been synthesized by direct oxidation and in situ polymerization methods. These nanocomposites find potential application in solar cells [72].

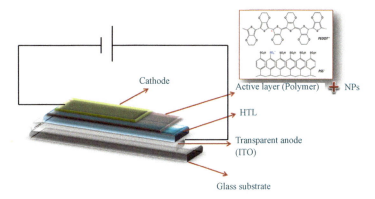

Figure 2.6 Diagram of OLED with active layer containing nanocomposite (polymer + NPs).

2.5.4 Biomedical

Polymer-based systems are being extensively used as therapeutic carriers as well as bioimaging agents. The polymer system has four components: (i) the polymeric component offering solubility and biocompatibility, (ii) a chemical group (contrast agent) used for imaging, (iii) therapeutic component (photosensitizer) carrying drug, and (iv) functional groups (antibodies) for specific cell targeting. Engineered magnetic nanoparticles and their oxides are considered to be one of the promising biomedical tools because of their small size and inherent ability to interact with external magnetic field. Polymer-based magnetic nanoparticles have acted as a new platform for simultaneous diagnostics and targeted drug delivery [73]. A mesoporous nanocomposite prepared by grafting fluorescent polymethacrylic acid and folic acid onto $Fe_3O_4@mSiO_2$ nanoparticles was found to be selective in targeting cancer and drug delivery. Folic acid was added to improve the biorecognition ability. Water solubility and biocompatibility were enhanced by conjugating the polymer with strong fluorescent emissions via the molecular replacement method. The nanocomposite had excellent drug loading efficiency (105 ± 8 mg of drug/mg of drug carrier) and showed favorable biocompatibility (cell viability above 85% at high concentration) and dispersibility under physiological conditions [74].

Nanocomposites are also used in wound dressings. Cryogels of polyvinyl alcohol (PVA) have been synthesized by the freeze thaw method. This process involves the solidification of PVA and avoids the chemical crosslinking. The physical crosslinking during the successive thawing cycles is based on the existence of regular pendant hydroxyl groups present in PVA that are capable of forming crystallites by strong inter-chain hydrogen bonding. The physical crosslinking brings interesting features to polymers such as bioactivity, non-toxicity, non-carcinogenicity, mechanical strength, elasticity, biocompatibility, and porosity. Thus, cryogels have emerged as promising materials for fabricating macro-porous structures. ZnO nanoparticles are dispersed in the cryogel network by in situ polymerization. It is noted that swelling and deswelling process depends on the chemical composition of the nanocomposites, number of freezing thaw cycles, as well as pH and temperature of the swelling medium. These nanocomposites exhibit excellent antibacterial activities against gram-positive and gram-negative bacteria, thereby advocating their use in medical applications such as wound dressing materials [75]. Recent advances involve nanocomposites of polymer brushes/inorganic nanoparticles. Polymer brushes consist of ultrathin layers of polymer tethered to other ends of polymer chains, which are in close proximity of each other. These can stabilize the nanoparticles and, hence, affect the function of nanocomposites [14].

2.5.5 Photocatalysis

Marine biofouling is the accumulation or adsorption of microorganisms, plants, or algae on the wetted surfaces and is a worldwide problem affecting maritime industries. It retards the speed of ships, accelerates corrosion, and increases the fuel consumption of ships. Traditional measures are self-polishing antifouling agents that work by the gradual erosion and release of toxic biocides such as copper. But the drawback of these compounds is the harmful effects on non-target organisms. Therefore, there is a need for non-toxic antifouling agents. Chitosan is a natural polymer with antimicrobial and antifungal properties. Chitosan/ZnO nanocomposites have been developed with antifouling properties. The coatings of nanocomposite show anti-diatom activity against *Navicula* sp. and activity against marine bacterium *Pseudoalteromonas nigrifaciens* [76].

Environmental pollution due to uranium has raised concerns, and efforts are carried out to remove uranium ions from contaminated drinking water. In this regard, polyacrylonitrile (PAN)/AgX/ZnO nanocomposites have been synthesized. Ion exchange method is used to load ZnO nanoparticles in AgX nanozeolite followed by the calcination process. This nancomposite is found to have excellent adsorption selectivity toward uranium ions because of their effective interaction with the nanocomposite [77]. In one of the studies, polypyrrole/TiO$_2$ nanocomposites have been reported to be efficient photocatalysts using density functional theory (DFT). In this study, titanium dioxide (Ti$_{16}$O$_{32}$) was interacted with a range of pyrrole (Py) oligomers to predict optimum composition of nPy-TiO$_2$ composite with suitable band structure for efficient photocatalytic properties. It was revealed that the nanocomposite has narrow band gap and better visible light absorption capability due to better interaction between the nanoparticles and polymer. A strong intermolecular interaction energy of the simulated nanocomposite in the range of −41 to −72 kcal/mol confirmed the existence of covalent and electrostatic types of bonding [78]. Experimentally, polypyrrole (PPy)/TiO$_2$ nanocomposites synthesized by in situ polymerization had high photocatalytic activity under simulated solar light. The nanocomposites caused the degradation of Rhodamine red dye. PPy plays a role of photosensitizer in the photocatalytic processes. When nanocomposite is illuminated by the simulated solar light, the electrons from the PPy are excited from the highest occupied molecular orbital (HOMO) to the lowest unoccupied molecular orbital (LUMO). Since the conduction band (CB) of TiO$_2$ is lower than the LUMO of PPy, electrons are injected into the CB of TiO$_2$, thereby creating holes in the HOMO of PPy. Some of the electrons present in the valance band (VB) of TiO$_2$ jump to CB, while some move to the HOMO of PPy combining with the holes. As a result of this movement, the number of electrons and holes increases and, thus, the electron–hole separation efficiency increases. The photogenerated electrons react with oxygen to form superoxide radicals and photogenerated holes react with OH$^-$ or H$_2$O to form hydroxyl radicals. These generated radicals are powerful in degrading the Rhodamine red dye [79]. Polyaniline/CoFe$_2$O$_4$ nanocomposites prepared by in situ polymerization with different weights of $CoFe_2O_4$ (CF-NPs) have exhibited photocatalytic activity against methyl orange (MO) dye due to the regeneration of reactive oxygen species (Fig. 2.7) [80].

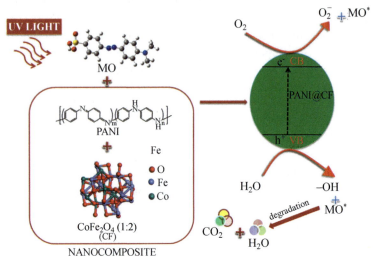

Figure 2.7 Schematic representation of degradation of MO dye in the presence of nanocomposite.

2.6 Commercial Opportunities for Metal Oxide/Polymer Nanocomposites

The polymer nanocomposite market, in terms of value, is expected to reach above $5100 million by 2020, growing at a significant compound annual growth rate (CAGR) from 2014 to 2019. The polymer nanocomposite market is moderately fragmented, where 3D System (USA), Foster Corporation (USA), Industrial Nanotech (USA), Hybrid Plastics Inc. (USA), Inframat Corporation (UK), InMat Inc. (USA), and Nanocor Incorporated (USA) have captured a majority of the market share in production and supply. The market trend for polymer nanocomposites has been divided based on the type of nanoparticles (carbon nanotubes, metal oxide, nanofiber, nanoclay, graphene), polymer type (thermosetting, thermoplastic), applications, and region (North America, Asia Pacific, Europe, RoW).

Some of the commercial applications of nanocomposites have been summarized in Table 2.1.

Table 2.1　Potential commercial applications of nanocomposites

Nanocomposites	Application	Stage
Silica nanoparticles/ Perfluorinated polymers	Fuel cells	Commercial prototype
Fluorine-doped TiO_2 nanoparticles/ORMOCER®s or Nafion	PEM membranes	Pilot commercial development
SiO_2/ORMOCERs	Solar anti-reflective coating	Commercial development
$SiO_2/ZrO_2/TiO_2$/ORMOCERs	Solar collectors	Commercial prototype
SiO_2/ORMOCERs	Dental	Commercial
ZrO_2/SiO_2/Dimethylacrylate	Dental polishing	Commercial

2.7　Conclusion and Future Prospects

Advances in the field of hybrid organic–inorganic materials represent a multidisciplinary area where academic and application-driven research has been extensively carried out in the last few years. At present, many functional hybrid nanocomposites with different shapes, sizes, properties, and composition have led to the generation of integrated and miniaturized devices. Nanocomposites, especially polymer/metal oxide, have emerged as potential candidates with application spanning over wide areas of science and technology (sensing, energy, optics, electrical, smart coatings, biomedicine, etc.).

Many of the fabricated nanocomposites have paved their way into industrial applications and are commercialized by being in the market and some of them are close to enter into the market. The commercial use of nanocomposites is mainly associated with automotive industry, construction, textiles, and packaging. They are paving their way into energy-related devices to handle the present energy crisis. The worldwide market for nanocomposites has been estimated to be in million pounds. Some of the leading companies are proactively working to expand as well as launch new polymer nanocomposite products in the market. These companies are DuPont, Nanophase Technologies Corporation, Inframat Corporation, Nanocor Inc., Evonik Industries, and The Arkema Group.

In 2015, the world polymer nanocomposite market was estimated at $5276 million and is projected to grow at a CAGR of 10.9% during 2016–22. The growing demand of nanocomposites in the automotive industry is the driving force for the polymer nanocomposite market. Apart from the automotive industry, nanocomposites are also used in the construction industry for repair and rehabilitation of buildings and bridges. The packaging industry is one of the fastest growing with great demand of nanocomposites owing to their antimicrobial properties. Pixelligent is one of the leading companies that use nanocomposites for OLED light extraction. They are specialized in synthesizing ZrO_2 nanocrystals and then use them in polymer systems to fabricate polymer nanocomposites.

With growing research in the field of nanocomposites, efforts are being carried out both at academic and industrial levels to find environment friendly, reliable, inexpensive, recyclable, and energy-efficient strategies for the production of nanocomposites, thereby bringing harmony between nature and human innovation. Natural biodegradable polymers and biocompatible nanoparticles are used for the emergence of nanocomposites as smart materials, and this has already driven active research in this area. The extensive research is bridging the gap between the different domains of science and moving toward biology by combining the physical and chemical disciplines. Experiments are done to comprehend at the molecular level and have full control over the functionalities and applications of hybrid nanocomposites for their development at the industrial level.

References

1. Patel, V. and Y. Mahajan, Polymer nanocomposites: Emerging growth driver for the global automotive industry, in *Handbook of Polymernanocomposites. Processing, Performance and Application: Volume A: Layered Silicates*, J. K. Pandey, K. R. Reddy, A. K. Mohanty, and M. Misra (Eds.), 2014, Springer Berlin Heidelberg: Berlin, Heidelberg. pp. 511–538.

2. Okada, A. and A. Usuki, *Twenty-Year Review of Polymer-Clay Nanocomposites at Toyota Central R&D Labs., Inc.* 2007, SAE International.

3. Camargo, P. H. C., K. G. Satyanarayana, and F. Wypych, Nanocomposites: Synthesis, structure, properties and new application opportunities. *Materials Research*, 2009, **12**: pp. 1–39.

4. Hassanabadi, H. M. and D. Rodrigue, Effect of particle size and shape on the reinforcing efficiency of nanoparticles in polymer nanocomposites. *Macromolecular Materials and Engineering*, 2014, **299**(10): pp. 1220–1231.

5. Kao, J., et al., Toward functional nanocomposites: Taking the best of nanoparticles, polymers, and small molecules. *Chemical Society Reviews*, 2013, **42**(7): pp. 2654–2678.

6. Mezzenga, R. and J. Ruokolainen, Nanocomposites: Nanoparticles in the right place. *Nature Materials*, 2009, **8**(12): pp. 926–928.

7. Hassan, T. A., V. K. Rangari, and S. Jeelani, Value-added biopolymer nanocomposites from waste eggshell-based $CaCO_3$ nanoparticles as fillers. *ACS Sustainable Chemistry & Engineering*, 2014, **2**(4): pp. 706–717.

8. Turova, N. Y., *The Chemistry of Metal Alkoxides*. 2002: Springer US.

9. Krasia-Christoforou, T., Organic–inorganic polymer hybrids: Synthetic strategies and applications, in *Hybrid and Hierarchical Composite Materials*, C.-S. Kim, C. Randow, and T. Sano (Eds.), 2015, Springer International Publishing: Cham. pp. 11–63.

10. Liyanage, A. U. and M. M. Lerner, Template preparation of $NiPS_3$ polymer nanocomposites. *RSC Advances*, 2012, **2**(2): pp. 474–479.

11. Raman, N., S. Sudharsan, and K. Pothiraj, Synthesis and structural reactivity of inorganic–organic hybrid nanocomposites: A review. *Journal of Saudi Chemical Society*, 2012, **16**(4): pp. 339–352.

12. Caseri, W. R., In situ synthesis of polymer-embedded nanostructures, in *Nanocomposites*, 2013, John Wiley & Sons, Inc. pp. 45–72.

13. Reid, D. L., et al., In situ synthesis of polyurethane-TiO_2 nanocomposite and performance in solid propellants. *Journal of Materials Chemistry A*, 2014, **2**(7): pp. 2313–2322.

14. Nie, G., et al., Nanocomposites of polymer brush and inorganic nanoparticles: Preparation, characterization and application. *Polymer Chemistry*, 2016, **7**(4): pp. 753–769.

15. Kim, J.-Y., et al., In situ chemical synthesis of ruthenium oxide/reduced graphene oxide nanocomposites for electrochemical capacitor applications. *Nanoscale*, 2013, **5**(15): pp. 6804–6811.

16. Papageorgiou, D. G., I. A. Kinloch, and R. J. Young, Graphene/elastomer nanocomposites. *Carbon*, 2015, **95**: pp. 460–484.

17. Cui, Y., et al., Gas barrier properties of polymer/clay nanocomposites. *RSC Advances*, 2015, **5**(78): pp. 63669–63690.

18. Vaia, R. A., H. Ishii, and E. P. Giannelis, Synthesis and properties of two-dimensional nanostructures by direct intercalation of polymer melts in layered silicates. *Chemistry of Materials*, 1993, **5**(12): pp. 1694–1696.

19. Sarkar, M., et al., Polypropylene-clay composite prepared from Indian bentonite. *Bulletin of Materials Science*, 2008, **31**(1): pp. 23–28.

20. Fornes, T. D., et al., Nylon 6 nanocomposites: The effect of matrix molecular weight. *Polymer*, 2001, **42**(25): pp. 09929–09940.

21. Sinha Ray, S., et al., New polylactide/layered silicate nanocomposites. 1. Preparation, characterization, and properties. *Macromolecules*, 2002, **35**(8): pp. 3104–3110.

22. Davis, C. H., et al., Effects of melt-processing conditions on the quality of poly(ethylene terephthalate) montmorillonite clay nanocomposites. *Journal of Polymer Science Part B: Polymer Physics*, 2002, **40**(23): pp. 2661–2666.

23. Awad, W. H., et al., Material properties of nanoclay PVC composites. *Polymer*, 2009, **50**(8): pp. 1857–1867.

24. Zeng, Q. H., et al., Clay-based polymer nanocomposites: Research and commercial development. *Journal of Nanoscience and Nanotechnology*, 2005, **5**(10): pp. 1574–1592.

25. Deitzel, J. M., et al., The effect of processing variables on the morphology of electrospun nanofibers and textiles. *Polymer*, 2001, **42**(1): pp. 261–272.

26. Casper, C. L., et al., Controlling surface morphology of electrospun polystyrene fibers: Effect of humidity and molecular weight in the electrospinning process. macromolecules, 2004, **37**(2): pp. 573–578.

27. von Reitzenstein, N. H., et al., Morphology, structure, and properties of metal oxide/polymer nanocomposite electrospun mats. *Journal of Applied Polymer Science*, 2016, **133**(33).

28. Zhang, C.-L., et al., Controlled assemblies of gold nanorods in PVA nanofiber matrix as flexible free-standing SERS substrates by electrospinning. *Small*, 2012, **8**(5): pp. 648–653.

29. Zhang, C.-L. and S.-H. Yu, Nanoparticles meet electrospinning: Recent advances and future prospects. *Chemical Society Reviews*, 2014, **43**(13): pp. 4423-4448.

30. Lowe, A. B., Thiol-ene "click" reactions and recent applications in polymer and materials synthesis. *Polymer Chemistry*, 2010, **1**(1): pp. 17-36.

31. Castelaín, M., et al., Effect of click-chemistry approaches for graphene modification on the electrical, thermal, and mechanical properties of polyethylene/graphene nanocomposites. *Macromolecules*, 2013, **46**(22): pp. 8980-8987.

32. Mazumdar, P., S. Rattan, and M. Mukherjee, Polymer nanocomposites using click chemistry: Novel materials for hydrogen peroxide vapor sensors. *RSC Advances*, 2015, **5**(85): pp. 69573-69582.

33. Jeon, I.-Y. and J.-B. Baek, Nanocomposites derived from polymers and inorganic nanoparticles. *Materials*, 2010, **3**(6): pp. 3654.

34. Kumar, S. K., et al., Nanocomposites with polymer grafted nanoparticles. *Macromolecules*, 2013, **46**(9): pp. 3199-3214.

35. White, S. I., et al., Electrical percolation behavior in silver nanowire-polystyrene composites: Simulation and experiment. *Advanced Functional Materials*, 2010, **20**(16): pp. 2709-2716.

36. Hore, M. J. A. and R. J. Composto, Functional polymer nanocomposites enhanced by nanorods. *Macromolecules*, 2014, **47**(3): pp. 875-887.

37. Laurent, S., et al., Superparamagnetic iron oxide nanoparticles for delivery of therapeutic agents: Opportunities and challenges. *Expert Opinion on Drug Delivery*, 2014, **11**(9): pp. 1449-1470.

38. Rovers, S. A., et al., Influence of distribution on the heating of superparamagnetic iron oxide nanoparticles in poly(methyl methacrylate) in an alternating magnetic field. *The Journal of Physical Chemistry C*, 2010, **114**(18): pp. 8144-8149.

39. Suh, S. K., et al., Synthesis of nonspherical superparamagnetic particles: In situ coprecipitation of magnetic nanoparticles in microgels prepared by stop-flow lithography. *Journal of the American Chemical Society*, 2012, **134**(17): pp. 7337-7343.

40. Luo, Q., R. J. Hickey, and S.-J. Park, Controlling the location of nanoparticles in colloidal assemblies of amphiphilic polymers by tuning nanoparticle surface chemistry. *ACS Macro Letters*, 2013, **2**(2): pp. 107-111.

41. Karagoz, B., et al., An efficient and highly versatile synthetic route to prepare iron oxide nanoparticles/nanocomposites with tunable morphologies. *Langmuir*, 2014, **30**(34): pp. 10493–10502.

42. Konwar, A., et al., Chitosan–iron oxide coated graphene oxide nanocomposite hydrogel: A robust and soft antimicrobial biofilm. *ACS Applied Materials & Interfaces*, 2016, **8**(32): pp. 20625–20634.

43. Arias, J. L., L. H. Reddy, and P. Couvreur, Fe_3O_4/chitosan nanocomposite for magnetic drug targeting to cancer. *Journal of Materials Chemistry*, 2012, **22**(15): pp. 7622–7632.

44. Alvi, F., et al., Evaluating the chemio-physio properties of novel zinc oxide-polyaniline nanocomposite polymer films. *Polymer Journal*, 2010, **42**(12): pp. 935–940.

45. Kos, T., et al., Zinc-containing block copolymer as a precursor for the in situ formation of nano ZnO and PMMA/ZnO nanocomposites. *Macromolecules*, 2013, **46**(17): pp. 6942–6948.

46. Divij, V. and R. K. Goyal, Thermal and dielectric properties of high performance polymer/ZnO nanocomposites. *IOP Conference Series: Materials Science and Engineering*, 2014, **64**(1): pp. 012016.

47. Awad, S., et al., Free volumes, glass transitions, and cross-links in zinc oxide/waterborne polyurethane nanocomposites. *Macromolecules*, 2011, **44**(1): pp. 29–38.

48. Zou, H., S. Wu, and J. Shen, Polymer/Silica nanocomposites: Preparation, characterization, properties, and applications. *Chemical Reviews*, 2008, **108**(9): pp. 3893–3957.

49. Wu, C. L., et al., Silica nanoparticles filled polypropylene: Effects of particle surface treatment, matrix ductility and particle species on mechanical performance of the composites. *Composites Science and Technology*, 2005, **65**(3-4): pp. 635–645.

50. Zenerino, A., et al., Homogeneous dispersion of SiO_2 nanoparticles in a hydrosoluble polymeric network. *Reactive and Functional Polymers*, 2013, **73**(8): pp. 1065–1071.

51. Krasucka, P., et al., Polymer–silica composites and silicas produced by high-temperature degradation of organic component. *Thermochimica Acta*, 2015, **615**: pp. 43–50.

52. Zhou, X., H. Shao, and H. Liu, Preparation and characterization of film-forming raspberry-like polymer/silica nanocomposites via soap-free emulsion polymerization and the sol–gel process. *Colloid and Polymer Science*, 2013, **291**(5): pp. 1181–1190.

53. Karim, M. R., et al., Conducting polyaniline-titanium dioxide nanocomposites prepared by inverted emulsion polymerization. *Polymer Composites*, 2010, **31**(1): pp. 83–88.

54. Gutierrez, J., et al., Conductive properties of inorganic and organic TiO_2/polystyrene-block-poly(ethylene oxide) nanocomposites. *The Journal of Physical Chemistry C*, 2009, **113**(20): pp. 8601–8605.

55. Salomatina, E. V., et al., Synthesis, structure, and properties of organic-inorganic nanocomposites containing poly(titanium oxide). *Journal of Materials Chemistry C*, 2013, **1**(39): pp. 6375–6385.

56. Islam, M. S., R. Masoodi, and H. Rostami, The effect of nanoparticles percentage on mechanical behavior of silica-epoxy nanocomposites. *Journal of Nanoscience*, 2013, **2013**: pp. 10.

57. Guo, Z., et al., Fabrication and characterization of iron oxide nanoparticles filled polypyrrole nanocomposites. *Journal of Nanoparticle Research*, 2009, **11**(6): pp. 1441–1452.

58. Alsbaiee, A., et al., Rapid removal of organic micropollutants from water by a porous β-cyclodextrin polymer. *Nature*, 2016, **529**(7585): pp. 190–194.

59. Rajalakshmi, S., et al., Enhanced photocatalytic activity of metal oxides/β-cyclodextrin nanocomposites for decoloration of Rhodamine B dye under solar light irradiation. *Applied Water Science*, 2014: pp. 1–13.

60. Navale, S. T., et al., Camphor sulfonic acid doped PPy/[small alpha]-Fe_2O_3 hybrid nanocomposites as NO_2 sensors. *RSC Advances*, 2014, **4**(53): pp. 27998–28004.

61. Han, C.-H., et al., Synthesis of Pd or Pt/titanate nanotube and its application to catalytic type hydrogen gas sensor. *Sensors and Actuators B: Chemical*, 2007, **128**(1): pp. 320–325.

62. Hong, W.-K., et al., Tunable electronic transport characteristics of surface-architecture-controlled ZnO nanowire field effect transistors. *Nano Letters*, 2008, **8**(3): pp. 950–956.

63. Mane, A. T., S. T. Navale, and V. B. Patil, Room temperature NO_2 gas sensing properties of DBSA doped PPy–WO_3 hybrid nanocomposite sensor. *Organic Electronics*, 2015, **19**: pp. 15–25.

64. Ghanbari, K. and M. Moloudi, Flower-like ZnO decorated polyaniline/reduced graphene oxide nanocomposites for simultaneous determination of dopamine and uric acid. *Analytical Biochemistry*, 2016, **512**: pp. 91–102.

65. Kim, T. W., et al., Electrical memory devices based on inorganic/organic nanocomposites. *NPG Asia Materials*, 2012, **4**: pp. e18.

66. Shih, C.-C., et al., High performance transparent transistor memory devices using nano-floating gate of polymer/ZnO nanocomposites. *Scientific Reports*, 2016, **6**: pp. 20129.

67. Mai, Y., F. Zhang, and X. Feng, Polymer-directed synthesis of metal oxide-containing nanomaterials for electrochemical energy storage. *Nanoscale*, 2014, **6**(1): pp. 106–121.

68. Shayeh, J. S., et al., Advanced studies of coupled conductive polymer/metal oxide nano wire composite as an efficient supercapacitor by common and fast fourier electrochemical methods. *Journal of Molecular Liquids*, 2016, **220**: pp. 489–494.

69. Nguyen, T.-P., Polymer-based nanocomposites for organic optoelectronic devices. A review. *Surface and Coatings Technology*, 2011, **206**(4): pp. 742–752.

70. Yang, S. H., et al., Optical and electrical investigations of poly(p-phenylene vinylene)/silicon oxide and poly(p-phenylene vinylene)/titanium oxide nanocomposites. *Thin Solid Films*, 2005, **471**(1–2): pp. 230–235.

71. Singh, P., et al., Studies on morphological and optoelectronic properties of MEH-CN-PPV:TiO_2 nanocomposites. *Materials Chemistry and Physics*, 2012, **133**(1): pp. 317–323.

72. Singh, R. and R. B. Choudhary, Optical absorbance and ohmic behavior of PANI and PANI/ZnO nanocomposites for solar cell application. *Optik: International Journal for Light and Electron Optics*, 2016, **127**(23): pp. 11398–11405.

73. Krasia-Christoforou, T. and T. K. Georgiou, Polymeric theranostics: Using polymer-based systems for simultaneous imaging and therapy. *Journal of Materials Chemistry B*, 2013, **1**(24): pp. 3002–3025.

74. Chen, D., et al., Modification of magnetic silica/iron oxide nanocomposites with fluorescent polymethacrylic acid for cancer targeting and drug delivery. *Journal of Materials Chemistry*, 2010, **20**(31): pp. 6422–6429.

75. Chaturvedi, A., et al., Evaluation of poly(vinyl alcohol) based cryogel-zinc oxide nanocomposites for possible applications as wound dressing materials. *Material Science and Engneering C*, 2016, **65**: pp. 408–418.

76. Al-Naamani, L., et al., Chitosan-zinc oxide nanocomposite coatings for the prevention of marine biofouling. *Chemosphere*, 2016, **168**: pp. 408–417.

77. Shakur, H. R., et al., Highly selective and effective removal of uranium from contaminated drinking water using a novel PAN/AgX/ZnO nanocomposite. *Microporous and Mesoporous Materials*, 2016, **234**: pp. 257–266.
78. Ullah, H., A. A. Tahir, and T. K. Mallick, Polypyrrole/TiO_2 composites for the application of photocatalysis. *Sensors and Actuators B: Chemical*, 2017, **241**: pp. 1161–1169.
79. Gao, F., et al., Preparation of polypyrrole/TiO_2 nanocomposites with enhanced photocatalytic performance. *Particuology*, 2016, **26**: pp. 73–78.
80. Khan, J. A., et al., Synthesis and characterization of structural, optical, thermal and dielectric properties of polyaniline/$CoFe_2O_4$ nanocomposites with special reference to photocatalytic activity. *Spectrochima Acta Part A: Molecular and Biomolecular Spectroscopy*, 2013, **109**: pp. 313–321.

Chapter 3

Biomedical Insights of Lipid- and Protein-Based Biocomposites

Aasim Majeed, Raoof Ahmad Najar, Shruti Chaudhary,
Sapna Thakur, Amandeep Singh, and Pankaj Bhardwaj
Molecular Genetics Laboratory, Centre for Plant Sciences, School of Basic and Applied Sciences, Central University of Punjab, Bathinda 151001, India
majeedaasim@gmail.com

Because of biodegradability, biocompatibility, and environment friendly nature, biomaterials are gaining prodigious and stupendous attention of researchers. A myriad of biomaterials such as cellulose, starch, gelatin, fibrin, chitosan, chitin, and collagen are employed to generate composites, hydrogels, and films, which possess enhanced properties. Proteins and lipids are equally used to achieve this goal. Although protein- and lipid-based composites find their major applications in food and packaging industries, cosmetic, automobile, and glass industries, their utility in the field of medicine cannot be ignored. In the field of medicine, protein- and lipid-based composites play an important role in tissue engineering, cancer therapy, drug delivery, anti-infection, wound healing, skin, and dental protection.

Biocomposites: Biomedical and Environmental Applications
Edited by Shakeel Ahmed, Saiqa Ikram, Suvardhan Kanchi, and Krishna Bisetty
Copyright © 2018 Pan Stanford Publishing Pte. Ltd.
ISBN 978-981-4774-38-3 (Hardcover), 978-1-315-11080-6 (eBook)
www.panstanford.com

This chapter focuses on the general concept and biomedical applications of these composites.

3.1 Introduction

A composite material is constituted of two or more components. These constituents bear different chemical, physical, or biological properties. Blending of these constituents generates a composite with entirely new set of properties, which neither of these individual components possess. The resulting composite offers advantageous properties for specific utility. When either of the components is of biological origin, the composites are termed biocomposites. When we look back in time, we find that people knowingly or unknowingly prepared composites for their specific use. The composites made from mud and straw for construction purposes were used by humans since prehistoric times and are still used in rural areas in some countries. In the modern times, concrete, a composite of stones and cement, has replaced the mud and straw type of composite. There are two phases in the composite: matrix, or the continuous phase, and the filler, or the dispersing phase. A compatibilizer can also be added for additional advantage [1]. Stiffness and strength of a composite depend on the reinforcing component, while the continuous phase helps in transferring the weight and maintaining the position of the dispersed phase [2]. The type of matrix varies in different composites. It can be metal, ceramic, or polymer based. Polymer-based composite is gaining fame over others rapidly. The dispersed phase can be particles or fibers of both macro- and nanoscale [1]. Biocomposites and nanocomposites form the most important class of polymer-based composites because of their unique attributes. Polymer-based composites have lesser weight, lower processability costs, greater corrosion, and fatigue resistance than metal-based composites [2].

Glass-fiber-reinforced resin and petroleum-based composites, although have revolutionized the industries for past decades, certain environmental and health concerns raised by their continuous use have shifted the trend toward a more environment friendly and healthy system [3]. Further rapid and continuous use of petroleum-based composites is draining away its reserves, thereby posing a threat of permanent loss of petroleum reserves. So a dire need is felt to replace such composites with more environment friendly and renewable source based composites, which smoothly paves way to sustainable development. Composites of biological origin can solve this problem to a great extent. The biological materials can act both as matrix as well as dispersed phase. Cellulose fibers, starch, hemp, cotton, and jute fibers have excellent reinforcing properties and have been widely used as the dispersed phased in different composites. Vegetable oils, starch, and proteins can act as matrix phase [4].

3.2 Protein-Based Biocomposites

Biomaterials are emerging as a preferred choice due to their environment friendly nature, so the polymers from biological origin are an excellent alternative to hazardous materials such as petroleum. Recent research focuses on the use of cellulose, gelatin, collagen, etc., for the improvement of biomaterials. Proteins are the polymers of amino acids having peptide linkage and form a substantial portion of living organisms. The property that makes proteins unique in comparison to other polymers is their sequence-specific structure, thereby rendering them more complex. The cohesive nature of proteins and their property to form matrix draws attention of researchers toward its potential as a biomaterial. Further, protein molecules can be modified due to their diverse functional groups, which allows researchers to play with them at relative ease [5]. Amino acids (building blocks of proteins) are optically active; they possess a wide range of chemical properties and are electrically reactive. These attributes of amino acids make proteins desirable candidate for improvement and refinement of biomaterials. Side chains of proteins largely determine properties such as reactivity, charge, and solubility of proteins. The side chains offer special attributes to proteins, and accordingly, proteins are classified as either acidic or basic, polar, or non-polar, aliphatic or aromatic and charged or uncharged [6]. Further, the sequence and composition of amino acids of proteins also determine their physiochemical and functional attributes.

Inside living organisms, proteins are synthesized from mRNA molecules through a complex process called translation, in which the sequence specificity of proteins is determined by codons (a triplet of ribonucleotides that codes for a specific amino acid) of mRNA. The mRNA molecules, in turn, are transcribed from genes present in DNA. This pathway of flow of information from DNA to mRNA to proteins is commonly called the central dogma in biological science (Fig. 3.1). The translation of mRNA results into a polypeptide having a linear sequence of amino acids linked by peptide bonds, which constitutes the primary structure of proteins. Hydrogen bonds can form in polypeptide chains, which then interact in diverse manners to yield a second level of hierarchical structure called secondary structure. Among the various secondary structures, α-helix and β-sheet are most common. The folding of the secondary structure into a three-dimensional structure yields a tertiary structure. Finally, in its quaternary structure, different polypeptides interact with each other to form a complex of different subunits.

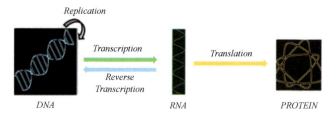

Figure 3.1 Schematic diagram of the central dogma.

A wide variety of proteins from both plant and animal origin have the potential to be used as biomaterials, such as soy protein, corn protein, collagen, and keratin. During the processing of cereal grains, plant proteins are produced as coproducts. Among the various plant proteins, soy protein from soybean; gluten, gliadin, and glutenin from wheat; zein and gluten from maize attract the attention of researchers. Plant proteins, in general, have low mechanical strength and are highly sensitive to moisture when compared with animal proteins [5]. They possess comparatively less molecular weight although with higher charge. So for general purposes, where moisture and mechanical strength are not key considerations, they can be fairly utilized [6]. Similarly, keratin from chicken feather, casein, collagen and proteins from meat, bones, and blood are the key proteins of animal origin that are employed for generating biomaterials. Both plant and animal proteins are used for tissue engineering. In order to improve the properties of proteins and minimize brittleness, plasticization is employed [7]. Plasticizers such as glycerol, water, and palmitic acid interfere with hydrogen bonding and electrostatic interactions of protein polypeptides to modify them to generate protein plastics [8, 9].

Proteins are sensitive to moisture or wet environment, pH and temperature and also degrade at a faster rate. To solve this problem, proteins are blended with other materials to confer them stability. The resulting composite possesses desirable properties that none of the individual components own. Proteins could be blended with other polymers such as poly(butylene adipate-co-therephthalate) (PBAT), poly(lactic acid), and poly(butylene succinate) (PBS), either by the melt process, where through thermal processing, dispersions of protein and the polymer are prepared, or through solvent blending, where both protein and polymer are dispersed together in a common solvent. The blends of these biodegradable polymers retain their biodegradability. Since proteins are fast degrading, their blending with slow-degrading polymers such as PLA confers intermediate degrading attribute to the resulting composite [5]. The interaction between protein and the polymer at their interfaces is important for composite formation. A compatibilizer enhances their interfacial adhesiveness. Using maleic anhydride as a compatibilizer, soy protein and PBAT exhibit enhanced phase interaction [10]. Synthetic elastomers, when blended with keratin protein, exhibit desired properties of enhanced mechanical strength and reduced flammability [11].

Natural fibers such as hemp, jute, and corn stalk can also be used to generate protein biocomposites having reinforced properties. Such protein composites retain biodegradability, have acceptable mechanical properties, and bear low cost [12]. Soy protein plastic exhibits the properties of comparatively higher moisture absorption and lower strength, which limits its utility. Using hemp fiber as a reinforcing material and biodegradable plastics such as poly(ester amide) and nylon 6, a blend with soy protein yields a biocomposite with enhanced properties for the automobile industry [12]. Keratin fibers enhance the thermal stability and storage modulus of poly(methyl methacrylate) matrix [13]. A 260% and 285% increase in tensile modulus and flexural strength, respectively, is achieved when ramie fiber is added to plasticized soy protein [14]. At the cost of slight decrease in tensile strength, the tensile modulus increases by 606% on blending banana fiber and plasticized soy protein [15]. Natural fibers could improve the impact strength and heat deflection temperature (HDT) of the protein composites. Using hemp fibers, up to 40% increase in impact strength and 23–35°C increase in HDT of soy protein plastics are achieved [12].

Natural polymers can be reinforced by particles to improve mechanical properties. Size, shape, and distribution of these particles have a large impact on the resulting composites. Particles as small as nanoscale range can be used to reinforce proteins. Apart from particulates of soybean husk, wood floor, and rice hull, protein reinforcement with nanoparticles to generate a unique blend, called protein nanocomposites, is getting more attention [5]. Casting and compounding methods enable us to load nanoparticles such as cellulose nanocrystals and nanoclay over protein plastics and films to generate protein-based nanocomposites [16–18]. Generally successful composite formation between protein and nanoparticles depends on interaction between them, so proper dispersion of particles in the matrix and higher degree of intercalation by protein matrix are desired. Proportion of filler is important for tensile strength, which generally increases with increase in filler concentration. However, increase in filler proportion beyond maximum optimal level leads to reduced mechanical properties owing to their poor distribution in the protein matrix. Improved mechanical properties, resistance to moisture and temperature are observed when soy protein is blended with clay (montmorillonite) [19]. Much increase in tensile strength and modulus is achieved by incorporating cellulose whiskers in soy protein matrix [20]. Wheat gluten displays cohesiveness and elasticity so has excellent film-forming properties [21]. Using hydroxyethyl cellulose as filling agent, the matrix of wheat gluten yields a biocomposite through plasticization by glycerol and matrix crosslinking by thermal modeling at 120°C. The resulting composite possesses improved Young's modulus and tensile strength accompanied by reduction in glass transition temperature [22]. Further, a similar increase in both tensile strength and Young's modulus although with increase in glass transition temperature is observed when methylcellulose is used as filler [23]. Soy proteins are used to make glues because of their adhesive properties. However, their adhesiveness declines to such extent under drying and wetting that leads to their rejection by industries. Calcium carbonate nanoparticles after blending with soy proteins yield a nanocomposite that retains adhesive properties even after drying and wetting, so can be utilized as wood glue [24]. Nanocomposite of multi-walled carbon nanotubes and matrix of soy proteins are found to possess higher water resistance [17].

3.2.1 Medical Applications of Protein-Based Composites

Biocomposites have a wide range of applications in almost all major fields, ranging from industrial to medical sphere, and have revolutionized textile, cosmetic, automobile, paper, and medicinal industries. Although cellulose- and chitosan-based biocomposites are of prime importance in the medical field, protein- and lipid-based biocomposites are now in the focus of researchers to be used as biomaterials in medicine. Cellulose-based composites are used in generating constructs for bone tissue engineering, cartilage tissue engineering, ligament and tendon substitute, drug delivery, wound healing, and antibacterial [25–29]. Chitosan-based biocomposites also find their application in wound healing [30], tissue engineering [31], bone tissue engineering [32], and drug delivery [33]. Scaffolds for tissue engineering based on starch biocomposites are utilized in bone tissue engineering [34, 35]. Further, wound healing [36] is yet another important application of starch-based composites. Apart from cellulose-, chitosan-, and starch-based biocomposites, lipid- and protein-based biocomposites have been successfully tested in tissue engineering, drug delivery, wound dressing, dental and antimicrobial applications and have given promising results (Fig. 3.2). The medical applications of protein- and lipid-based biocomposites are dealt in detail below.

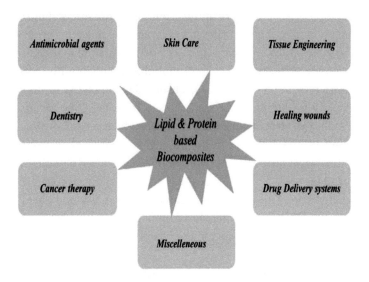

Figure 3.2 Biomedical role of lipid- and protein-based biocomposites.

3.2.1.1 Tissue engineering

In tissue engineering, nature and properties of scaffolds for cell attachment are crucial. Among the various scaffolds, electrospun fiber scaffolds mimic extracellular matrix and have greater surface-to-volume ratio to provide greater surface for attachment of cells. They find their application in neural, cardiovascular, musculoskeletal, and stem cell tissue engineering. A composite can be formed by encapsulating a protein into these fibers to provide additional properties. Peripheral nerve regeneration over large gaps is much difficult probably due to the formation of insufficient extracellular matrix [37] and lack of neurotrophic signals from distal nerve end [38]. The treatment involves grafting, which is limited by donor nerve availability. Use of synthetic nerve is another choice; however, it is successful only over small gaps. However, if the gap can be filled by extracellular matrix and neurotrophic signal is incorporated, the degree of success can be enhanced. Human glial cell-derived neurotrophic factor (GDNF) is a potent neurotrophic signal that promotes nerve fiber myelination and Schwann cell proliferation [39]. GDNF protein when encapsulated in the matrix of a biodegradable fiber of caprolactone and ethyl ethylene phosphate

(PCLEEP) generates an aligned protein–polymer composite, which shows sustained release of GNDF up to a few months in rats having peripheral nerve injury. Protein-encapsulated fiber offered synergistic in vivo peripheral nerve regeneration ability to the composite, so it is well suited for in vivo tissue engineering experiments [40]. Similar encapsulation of human beta-nerve growth factor (NGF) in PCLEEP electrospun fibers showed sustained release of the protein up to three months, thereby confirming its use as a scaffold in tissue engineering [41].

Bone tissue engineering requires a scaffold that shares similar architecture and composition with bone matrix. A 3D scaffold having pores is desired. Nanocomposite scaffold of gelatin and amorphous calcium phosphate prepared by double diffusion technique shows even dispersion of minerals in the gelatin matrix and 82% porosity. After implantation of the scaffold into the body, the precursor minerals are converted to hydroxyapatite, a biocompatible mineral mimicking bone minerals, thereby highlighting its feasibility as scaffold for bone tissue engineering and repair [42]. Likewise, a composite of engineered spider silk protein [eADF4 (C16)] and polyesters such as poly(butylene terephthalate) (PBT) or poly[butylene terephthalate-co-poly(alkylene glycol) terephthalate] (PBTAT) is effective in bone tissue engineering. The spider silk protein, due to their carboxylic residues, enhances their mineralization with calcium phosphate and calcium carbonate loaded on the composite film [43]. A nanocomposite of hydroxyapatite and gelatin with 82% porosity and mechanical parameters similar to spongy bones shows efficient attachment, migration, and penetration of cultured osteoblast-like cells into its pores, thereby proving its feasibility in bone tissue engineering [44]. Similarly, nanocomposites of gelatin and hydroxyapatite showed increased attachment and proliferation of MG63 osteoblastic cells, enhanced osteocalcin, and alkaline phosphatase activity, which validate its use in bone tissue engineering [45]. Since hydroxyapatite has composition and mechanical properties similar to bone besides possessing biocompatibility and osteoconductivity, researchers have tried to create artificial bones from this biomaterial. Engineering of bioartifical bone tissues may help in combating bone defects and also provide solution to limitations posed by donor morbidity and size limitations. Nano-hydroxyapatite/collagen (nHAC) is a promising bone regeneration material due to its structural similarity with bone matrix. Calcium sulfate hemihydrate (CSH) is biocompatible and possess rapid setting properties, so has been widely utilized as a scaffold in bone repair [46]. A composite of nHAC and CSH displays synergistic bone repair ability in rabbit femoral condyle defects. The resulting composite is biocompatible and possesses the property to accelerate the initiation of a new bone. rhBMP-2 (a bone morphogenetic protein) is proven to initiate bone regeneration during fractures [47]. The nHAC/CSH composite loaded with rhBMP-2 is more bioactive than the non-loaded composites. Release of calcium ions into the bone defect site from CSH may stimulate osteoblast differentiation. BMP induces mesenchymal cell proliferation and differentiation. All these factors accelerate bone regeneration. Further rhBMP-2 induces osteoinductivity. The composite is injectable and thus can act as a better substitute for hard tissues in bone tissue engineering [48].

Nanofibrous bone scaffolds were produced by electrospun technique from gelatin, polycaprolactone, and hydroxyapatite. The 3D structure of the resulting composite provides flexibility for enhanced attachment, penetration, and proliferation of osteoblast cells for bone tissue regeneration in the scaffold pores [49]. In an attempt to elucidate the response of buffalo embryonic stem cells to the scaffolds of chitosan and gelatin composite, the researchers observed enhanced cell proliferation and spreading while regaining their pluripotency, thereby showing that the chitosan gelatin composite can be effectively used in tissue engineering, which involves embryonic cells [50]. A composite of polydioxanone and fibrinogen is generated by the electrospinning technique and loaded with bladder smooth muscle cells. The latter successfully migrate through the composite and produce collagen, implying its potential in urological tissue engineering [51]. After incorporation of fibrin and chondrocytes into the scaffold of PLGA [poly(lactic-co-glycolic acid)], hybrid biomaterial resulted in enhanced cell proliferation and cartilage tissue formation in rabbit articular chondrocytes, suggesting its suitability in chondrogenesis [52]. A fibrin glue created from fibrinogen and thrombin after incorporation with calcium ceramics yielded a biocomposite that showed bone forming character in paravertebral muscles of sheep, implying its feasibility in filling bone cavities [53].

3.2.1.2 Cancer therapy

A patented nanomedicine comprising protein–protein composite is claimed to combat various diseases, including cancer. Here one protein delivers one therapeutic molecule and other protein delivers the second therapeutic molecule. In this way, a single entity can be used to carry different therapeutic agents. This composite is advantageous where drug resistance needs to be overcome through multi-drug therapy [54]. One of the main drugs for treating bone cancer is doxorubicin, but it imposes cardiotoxicity when administered through circulatory route. In order to make its use safer for bone cancer patients, a collagen-based composite was generated where glutaraldehyde acts as a crosslinking agent for both the gelatin matrix and doxorubicin to confer stability and sustained drug release ability to the conjugate. Further, the composite can be implanted locally, so it overcomes the danger of cardiovascular side effects [55]. Targeting an anticancer drug to appropriate site other than normal cells is highly desired and a challenging task yet to be achieved with absolute success. However, if an antigen on the surface of cancer cells is targeted through the drug-delivery system, relatively more specificity can be achieved. Drug-loaded gelatin microspheres conjugated with anti-bovine serum antibody target only cancer cells and have low cytotoxicity, so they can be effectively used in bladder cancer [56]. The composite of collagen and hydroxyapatite loaded with cisplatin drug is found effective on G292 osteosarcoma cells in terms of cytotoxicity, anti-proliferative ability, and anti-invasive property. So they can be used in treating bone cancers locally [57]. A similar composite of collagen and hydroxyapatite, although loaded with paclitaxel, showed satisfying result on metastatic MDA-MB-231 cancer cells [58].

Bone cancer may involve surgical removal of the bone tumor and filling the gap. All cancer cells need to be removed during surgery. The disease can relapse even if only a few cells are left. A composite of collagen and hydroxyapatite conjugated with magnetite and generated through the coprecipitation method can be used to fill the gap after surgery. The area can then be specifically exposed to alternating magnetic field, which causes apoptosis of the unremoved cancer cells [59]. In this way, a complete removal of cancer cells is achieved for better success of the surgery. Bovine blood fibrinogen and Adriamycin hydrochloride solutions in distilled water, upon mixing and homogenization with cottonseed oil, resulted into an emulsion, which formed microspheres on cooling. These composite microspheres, after testing against Ehrlich ascites carcinoma in mice, showed controlled release of the anticancer drug, Adriamycin over 7 days. Further, the delivery system showed good biocompatibility and the lifespan of the tumor-bearing mice was increased [60]. A mixture of olive oil, docetaxel, and fibrinogen resulted into the formation of micronized droplets, which on administration to mice having fibrin(ogen)-rich ascites, a form of tumor in mammary, increased the life of the mice up to 29 days [61].

3.2.1.3 Wound healing

Delay in healing of chronic wound occurs due to slower tissue formation and action of local proteinases. Wound dressings that provide an appropriate environment for tissue regeneration would be desirable for faster wound healing. Addition of oxidized regenerated cellulose in powder form to collagen suspension in acetic acid results into the formation of a composite sponge after thermal crosslinking. This sponge accelerates wound healing by promoting proliferation and migration of fibroblasts in diabetic mouse models. Increased proliferation and migration was also observed in human dermal fibroblasts. This biomaterial can, thus, be used to achieve quick wound closure [62]. At the site of wound, there occurs a local increase in metalloproteases in the tissue matrix that causes wound chronicity. Addition of protease inhibitors in wound dressings can be effective for enhanced wound healing. Promogran matrix, Ethicon contains OCR/collagen matrix loaded with protease inhibitor. Administration of Ethicon to 33 patients showed that in 18 patients, there occurred acceleration in wound healing than the rest of the patients [63]. A composite of fibrin and gelatin copolymerized with 2-hydroxyethyl methacrylate (HEMA) exhibits enhanced skin wound healing. Here the wound contraction was rapid, which emphasizes that the scaffold has the ability to remodel skin and also possesses re-epithelialization tendency by providing suitable environment at the site of wound [64]. Through the freeze drying method, a composite of isabgol and silk fibroin is prepared, which displays good porosity and provides sufficient supply of gas and nutrients to the cells. Further, the composites are biodegradable and cytocompatible and also enhance the attachment and proliferation of NIH 3T3 fibroblast cells, thereby causing rapid wound contraction, quick re-epithelialization, and tissue regeneration in wounds of rats [65]. Crosslinking of soya protein and sago starch with glutaraldehyde yielded a composite that can be used as wound dressing. This composite absorbs excess fluid and provides appropriate moisture for wound healing and causes rapid wound contraction. Here skin remodeling and re-epithelialization at the wound site in rats are attributed to the migration of keratinocytes [66]. To prevent the infection of burn wounds, proper dressing is needed. Reduction of inflammation at the site of wound is a key consideration when designing wound-dressing material. In an attempt to achieve reduced inflammation, prevent infection, and accelerate healing of wounds, a composite sheet was prepared from *Macrotyloma uniflorum* plant extract (MPE), collagen derived from fish scale, and fibrin. Biochemical and molecular analysis revealed that expression of nitric oxide synthase and cyclo-oxygenase-2 was repressed, thereby reducing inflammation. Further, the healing response was quick due to enhancement of collagen synthesis, vascular endothelial growth factor, transforming growth factor, and epidermal growth factor along with downregulation of matrix metalloproteinases [67]. Minor wounds are healed up automatically, but when wounds are severe, repair is hampered and there is a danger of sepsis. Effective and adequate dressing is required for prevention of septic infection along with rapid healing and tissue regeneration. Both chitosan and gelatin have been proven to possess healing properties. In an attempt to synergize the healing property of chitosan and gelatin into a single entity, a composite film of chitosan and gelatin shows accelerated and enhanced wound-healing ability than the individual components. The resulting composite possesses increased water-absorbing capacity, which proved advantageous to soak the wound fluid to keep it dry inside for better healing. The increased water-absorbing capacity is attributed to gelatin. Further, the tensile strength and wound-contracting ability of the composite were higher than chitosan and gelatin alone [68].

3.3 Lipid-Based Biocomposites

Lipids are naturally occurring organic molecules that form one of the main groups of biomolecules apart from carbohydrates, amino acids, and nucleic acids. They function as both structural building blocks and energy reserves. They act as permeability barriers of cells and subcellular organs by forming a lipid bilayer. They are readily soluble in organic solvents such as toluene and chloroform and are insoluble in water. Much structural variation exists among lipids. Structurally, they can be fatty acids, fats and oils, waxes, phospholipids, prostaglandins, thromboxanes, leukotrianes, terpenes, steroids, and lipid-soluble vitamins. The structural details and complex biosynthesis of these lipid classes are beyond the scope of this chapter. The primary building blocks of most biological membranes are formed of phospholipids [69]. They also act as signaling molecules in both plants and animals. Various classes such as glycerophospholipids and shingolipids play a crucial role in signal transduction [70]. Their signaling response occurs when they confront various environmental stresses such as salinity, drought temperature, and pathogen attack [71].

A wide variety of composites of lipids have been prepared and utilized for different purposes. Lipid-based composites can act as protective coating of food materials. Such composites can be formed by blending pure lipids with proteins, cellulose, or starch either through emulsion technique where lipids are directly mixed with film-forming solution or through generation of a bilayer where a lipid layer is added to the already formed film. Lipids such as palmitic acid, stearic acid, lecithin as well as bee wax form composite films with cellulose ether, carrageenan, starch, etc. [72]. Further, several additives such as emulsifiers, tanning agents, antioxidants and antibacterial substances, salts, acids, and alkalis are incorporated into the composite films to provide improved functionality [73]. Composites of cassava starch, sodium bicarbonate, and lipids such as bee wax, corn oil, and coconut oil confer increased shelf life to orange up to 10 days, while retaining physiological and biochemical properties of the fruits [74]. Lipids can form composites with proteins also. A composite film of wheat gluten matrix and bee wax showed enhanced moisture barrier ability although its opaque nature and disintegration in water put it at a disadvantage. However, using diacetyl tartaric acid ester of monoglycerides instead of bee wax increased transparency and strength [75]. Many biological experiments involve the transfer of genes. Different transfer systems are utilized depending on the objective and the material involved. However, the traditional gene transfer techniques are not precise in transferring a gene to a specific site on a scaffold. Surface-mediated gene transfer technique offers solution to this problem. Using a DNA–lipid–apatite composite layer derived from polyamidoamine dendron-bearing lipid, enhanced gene transfer rates are observed in the presence of serum than traditional particle-based systems. Further, such layers were area specific in the sense that only those cells were transformed that adhered to the surface of the layer. This high rate of gene transfer and area specificity can prove beneficial in tissue engineering experiments [76]. A myriad of industrial and other applications of lipid-based composites exist; however, due to the specificity of the chapter, they are not described here. In the field of medicine, lipid-based composites play a substantial role in solving different medical ailments and are discussed as follows:

3.3.1 Medical Applications of Lipid-Based Composites

Lipid-based biocomposites also play a significant role in biomedical industry and health. Lipids are hydrophobic in nature, so they can easily penetrate lipophilic barriers such as plasma membrane. Lipid-based biocomposites are, thus, primarily focused at delivering substances across the cell membrane at much relative ease. Besides other industrial uses, lipid biocomposites find their application in drug delivery, cancer therapy, skin protection, and dental and antimicrobial application. A detailed account of medical applications of lipid-based biocomposites is as follows:

3.3.1.1 Drug delivery

The discovery and identification of new drugs to cure various ailments move at a brisk pace. The challenge that researchers face is to elucidate their effective delivery systems. Among the myriad of delivery options, lipid-based drug-delivery systems have the advantage of increased solubility and bioavailability, reduced food effects, and variability in absorption. Also the inhibitory role of lipid-based systems over certain biological processes such as drug efflux and drug metabolism offers them further advantage over other delivery platforms. *Plasmodium falciparum*, a malaria-causing pathogen, is responsible for numerous deaths of humans around the globe. Since there is no vaccine available to cure the disease, drug therapy is the primary way to treat it. Although several drugs are available to target this disease, their poor oral bioavailability, erratic absorption, and shorter half-life cause a major setback to their treatment efficacy. Tafenoquine, besides possessing greater potential to combat this disease, has poor aqueous solubility, thereby reducing its oral bioavailability and also affect its treatment dose. However, its higher dose application to patients having glucose-6 phosphate dehydrogenase deficiency resulted in hemolysis and gastrointestinal disorders [77, 78]. A huge number of people around the world suffer from glucose-6 phosphate dehydrogenase deficiency [79]. To the aqueous solution of 1% w/v polyvinyl alcohol and 0.2% w/v sodium oleate in 1:1 ratio, dropwise addition of ethanol solution of Tafenoquine and citronella oil followed by addition of Tween 80 and then incubating the mixture at 60°C for 5 min resulted in the formation of a microemulsion composite having citronella oil as the lipid phase. This microemulsion composite substantially improves both solubility and oral bioavailability of the Tafenoquine drug. Treatment efficacy increases in comparison to non-emulsion drug as pathogen infection reduces to 4–10 fold in microemulsion drug treatment in mice. Further toxicity in glucose-6 phosphate dehydrogenase-deficient patients is reduced [80]. Using carbon dioxide as antisolvent, a hybrid composite of G44/14 and G50/13 commercial lipids, Eudragit RS100 and Eudragit RL100 polymers plus silica microparticles and Naproxen (a hydrophobic drug) was prepared through a batch mode process, which show enhanced drug release property [81]. Fenofibrate, a lipophilic drug, has poor water solubility and bioavailability. This drug, after incorporation into a hybrid composite, aminoclay-lipid through antisolvent precipitation method followed by prompt freeze drying, shows enhanced solubility and oral bioavailability in rats [82].

By the melt emulsion ultrasonic technique, the model drug Resina Draconis is incorporated into solid lipid nanoparticles (SLNs). Dispersion of these nanoparticles in a matrix of thermosensitive hydrogel resulted in the formation of a composite that is feasible for ophthalmic drug delivery. Further, the composite is nonirritant, shows steady state drug release, and has deeper corneal penetration [83]. Similarly, SLNs and nanostructured lipid carriers prepared through hot oil in water microemulsion technique showed enhanced delivery potential and bioavailability for the ophthalmic drug, acyclovir. However, the penetration power of the SLN-based system is reduced [84]. Likewise, the composite containing the lipid matrix of stearic acid and compritol and Poloxamer-188 and sodium taurocholate as surfactant and co-surfactant, respectively, has good ocular delivery potential [85]. In order to screen a suitable sugar ester that could act as emulsifier/stabilizer for efficient and controlled release of clotrimazole model drug through SLNs and nanostructured lipid carriers, sucrose ester D-1216 turned to be the best for both. Although both showed faster drug delivery, nanostructured lipid carriers have greater stability [86]. The delivery of drugs to the brain is hampered by the blood–brain barrier. However, due to their lipophilic nature, SLNs can cross the barrier. On conjugation of lactoferrin to SLNs, drug delivery to brain is enhanced. Further, the delivery system is biocompatible and exhibits much stability [87]. Similarly, SLNs, on conjugation with p-aminophenyl-α-D-mannopyranoside, exhibit enhanced ability to augment the delivery of the model drug docetaxel to brain [88].

3.3.1.2 Cancer therapy

Cancer is one of the most dreadful diseases in the world. The adverse effects of the current therapeutic systems have prompted researchers to design new, efficient, and less invasive therapy systems. Gold nanoparticles possess unique chemical, optical, and electronic properties than their elemental form [89]. The strong light absorption of gold nanoparticles, the conversion and dissipation of the absorbed light into heat render gold nanoparticles an excellent photothermal agent [90], so they have attracted the focus of researchers in clinical applications. In order to enhance the anticancer effect of docetaxel and lower its adverse effects, nanogold-based composites were employed and tested. Through seed-mediated and citrate-stabilized techniques, gold nanorods and gold nanoparticles were generated followed by coating with thermosensitive phospholipids and loading of docetaxel to generate lipid-coated gold nanocomposites. In vitro study showed significantly higher cytotoxic effect of the drug-loaded nanocomposite at equal concentration than free docetaxel in breast cancer cell line MCF-7 and melanoma cell line B16F10. Further, the uptake of the nanocomposite by the cancer cells is enhanced. The nanocomposite, therefore, possesses efficient anticancer effect, so it can be a promising therapy in cancer treatment [91]. Targeting non-specific cells and penetration inefficiency are the major setbacks that impede the chemotherapic drug delivery to cancer cells via nanoparticles. To address this issue, SLNs loaded with docetaxel on conjugation with adenosine showed sustained release of the drug and improved efficiency in targeting the drug to breast cancer cell line MCF-7 and prostate cancer cell line DU-145, both of which overexpress adenosine receptor at their surfaces. Here, adenosine mediates the internalization of the drug complex [92].

3.3.1.3 Antimicrobial application

Listeria monocytogenes is a gram-positive pathogenic bacteria that causes listeriosis in which infections primarily occur in the central nervous system, causing meningitis and other brain disorders, especially in newborn babies and pregnant women. The use of biomaterial as antimicrobial agents is environment friendly and low health risk strategy. Essential oils such as cinnamaldehyde possess excellent antimicrobial activity. A biocomposite of starch and lipid, on the incorporation of emulsion of the antimicrobial cinnamaldehyde, shows high toxicity to *L. monocytogenes*. Hence, this composite can be used to treat listeriosis [93]. During pathogenic infection, controlled release of the antibiotic drug is preferred to combat the infection. Antibiotic-loaded nanoparticles are gaining interest in this aspect. SLNs were prepared from a microemulsion of stearic acid, lecithin, sodium taurocholate, water, and ciprofloxacin. Such a nanoparticle-based system prolongs the release of the ciprofloxacin to combat eye and skin infections. For eye infections, this formulation is particularly advantageous because normally in other formulations, there occurs prompt release of the drug causing a very high initial drug concentration followed by sudden decline in concentration. To combat this, frequent administration of the drug is needed, which can cause toxicity. Also due to fluid and blinking reflexes of the eye, there is low drug absorption. Solid lipid nanoparticle-based formulations offer solution to both these problems by their enhanced penetration and gradual drug release and can also combat lung infections [94]. Solid lipid microparticles were embedded in the drug-loaded spongy matrix of chitosan and alginate to generate a composite that possesses the ability of controlled release of the drug, lidocaine HCl. Such composites are effective in wound healing as they counter microbes at the injury site [95].

3.3.1.4 Skin protection

Due to the declining ozone layer in the stratosphere, more UV radiations are now reaching the earth's surface. Besides damage to plants and property, UV radiations cause ailments in humans, particularly skin-related diseases. So effective sunscreen creams need to be designed to combat increased UV exposure for better protection of skin. SLNs have emerged as novel agents that can act as physical blocking agents to ultraviolet radiations, thus can be used as an effective ingredient in sunscreen systems for enhanced skin protection. Incorporation of SLNs into molecular sunscreens showed positively synergistic effect in skin protection [96]. Further, solid lipid nanoparticle-based dispersions systems show gradual release of UV-protecting agents in the sunscreens and also increase their photo-stability [97]. 2-hydroxy-4-methoxybenzophenone, upon incorporation into solid lipid nanoparticle dispersion, exhibited threefold increase in photoprotective effect against UV radiations. The formulation also exhibited dense film formation on the skin to synergistically protect it [98]. Similarly, 3,4,5-trimethoxybenzoylchitin (TMBC), a UV-protective agent, after loading with SLNs, showed enhanced protective effect, which is further enhanced when tocopherol was added [99]. The outer dead layer of skin is referred to as stratum corneum. The primary constituents of stratum corneum include cholesterol and its esters, fatty acids especially palmitic acid and stearic acid. These fatty acids are easily removed by surfactants from the skin, which necessitates their replenishing [100]. Cosmetic and dermatologic products, therefore, should contain stratum corneum fatty acids for providing better hydration. SLNs have occlusive property, which can enhance skin hydration [101]. Silver nanoparticles are antimicrobial. Blending of SLNs of stearic and palmitic acid and silver nanoparticles yields a nanocomposite that exhibits the synergistic property of skin hydration and antimicrobial action. This nanocomposite can thus form an effective ingredient in skin protective creams [102]. Likewise, dermatological cream of oil/water nanoemulsions containing ceramide 3B plus the orthodox stratum corneum fatty acids such as palmitic, stearic acid, and cholesterol shows enhanced skin hydration and elasticity [103].

3.3.1.5 Dental application

Bacterial growth in the dental caries results in the formation of acids that cause demineralization of enamel and dentin. 2-Methacryloyloxyethyl phosphorylcholine (MPC) contains a phospholipid choline at its side chains and possesses the property of repelling the proteins that are produced by bacteria during infection for adhesion to teeth [104]. Inclusion of MPC into the dental composite greatly reduces the film formation due to reduced protein adsorption to the teeth, which hampers attachment of bacteria, thereby protecting teeth from decay [105]. C10-LAla/pts and C12-L-Ala/pts, synthetic amphiphilic lipids, when dissolved in MMA/TBB resin, provide antibacterial property to the blend with C12-L-Ala/pts conferring higher antimicrobial activity than C10-LAla/pts. The amphiphilic lipids significantly reduce the bond strength of MMA/TBB resin with bovine dentin as well as enamel. Such resins are used in direct pulp capping or as direct adhesive in dental applications [106]. Using compritol as a lipid and pluronic F68 as surfactant, SLNs were generated by the solvent emulsion evaporation method. Diplofenac diethylamine was then incorporated into these nanoparticles. The drug-loaded SLNs were further incorporated into transmucosal patch. This composite is useful for local delivery at the gingival site immediately after dental surgery. Diplofenac release is controlled and prolonged. Further, the composite is effective in pain management and gastric irritation after dental surgery [107].

3.3.1.6 Miscellaneous

Anemia is an iron deficiency disease usually found in children and women. The cure includes iron supplement as ferrous sulfate. The currently available iron supplement tablets results in constipation and blood stool. Further, the variability in bioavailability and absorption of the iron puts them at additional disadvantage. To overcome such risks, SLNs were prepared from a composite mixture of compritol, lecithin, poloxamer, and dicetylphosphate. These SLNs were further incorporated with iron in the form of ferrous sulfate. The iron-loaded SLNs showed enhanced bioavailability and entrapment. So they can be safely used as carriers of iron [108].

3.4 Conclusion

Biocomposites have tremendous potential in industrial, textile, agriculture, and medicinal fields. Besides, protein and lipid biocomposites have left a landmark impact in the medical field. Both protein and lipid biocomposites have proven to be very effective in drug-delivery systems and have produced fascinating results regarding their biocompatibility, biodegradability, and in sustained drug release to overcome the adverse effects of drug overdose. Moreover, cell migration, attachment, and proliferation in tissue engineering, drug targeting to specific sites to ensure site-specific treatment strengthen their applicability. Further refinement and advancement are required to produce protein- and lipid-based composites that employ the diverse array of both proteins and lipids present in nature rather than focusing on only a few of them that are used currently. This would broaden their scope in medical and other fields.

References

1. Barton, J., Niemczyk, A., Czaja, K., and Sacher-Majewska, B. (2006). Polymer composites, biocomposites and nanocomposites. Production, composition, properties and application fields. *CHEMIK Nauka-technika-rynek*, **1**(68), pp. 280–287.
2. Mitra, B. C. (2014). Environment friendly composite materials: Biocomposites and green composites. *Defence Science Journal*, **64**(3), pp. 244–261.
3. Hanselka, H. (1998). Fiber composites of raw renewable materials for the ecological lightweight design. *Materialwissenschaft und Werkstofftechnik*, **29**(6), pp. 300–311.
4. Fowler, P. A., Hughes, J. M., and Elias, R. M. (2006). Biocomposites: Technology, environmental credentials and market forces. *Journal of the Science of Food and Agriculture*, **86**(12), pp. 1781–1789.
5. Mekonnen, T. H., Misra, M., and Mohanty, A. K. (2015). Processing, performance and applications plant and animal protein-based blends

and their biocomposites, in *Biocomposites Design and Mechanical Performance*, pp. 201–235. Elsevier Lt.

6. Reddy, N. and Yang, Y. (2011). Potential of plant proteins for medical applications. *Trends in Biotechnology*, **29**(10), pp. 490–498.

7. Hernandez-Izquierdo, V. M. and Krochta, J. M. (2008). Thermoplastic processing of proteins for film formation: A review. *Journal of Food Science*, **73**(2), pp. R30–R39.

8. Sothornvit, R. and Krochta, J. M. (2001). Plasticizer effect on mechanical properties of β-lactoglobulin films. *Journal of Food Engineering*, **50**(3), pp. 149–155.

9. Mekonnen, T., Mussone, P., Khalil, H., and Bressler, D. (2013). Progress in bio-based plastics and plasticizing modifications. *Journal of Materials Chemistry A*, **1**(43), pp. 13379–13398.

10. Chen, F. and Zhang, J. (2010). In-situ poly(butylene adipate-co-terephthalate)/soy protein concentrate composites: Effects of compatibilization and composition on properties. *Polymer*, **51**, pp. 1812–1819.

11. Janowska, G., Kucharska-Jastrzabek, A., Prochon, M., and Przepiorkowska, A. (2013). Thermal properties and combustibility of elastomer-protein composites. Part II. Composites. *Thermal Analysis and Calorimetry*, **113**, pp. 933–938.

12. Mohanty, A. K., Tummala, P., Liu, W., Misra, M., Mulukutla, P. V., and Drzal, L. T. (2005). Injection molded biocomposites from soy protein based bioplastic and short industrial hemp fiber. *Journal of Polymers and the Environment*, **13**(3), pp. 279–285.

13. Martínez-Hernández, A. L., Velasco-Santos, C., De-Icaza, M., and Castano, V. M. (2007). Dynamical–mechanical and thermal analysis of polymeric composites reinforced with keratin biofibers from chicken feathers. *Composites Part B: Engineering*, **38**(3), pp. 405–410.

14. Lodha, P. and Netravali, A. N. (2005). Characterization of Phytagel® modified soy protein isolate resin and unidirectional flax yarn reinforced "green" composites. *Polymer Composites*, **26**(5): pp. 647–659.

15. Kumar, R., Choudhary, V., Mishra, S., and Varma, I. (2008). Banana fiber-reinforced biodegradable soy protein composites. *Frontiers of Chemistry in China*, **3**(3), pp. 243–250.

16. Chen, F. and Zhang, J. (2010). In-situ poly(butylene adipate-co-terephthalate)/soy protein concentrate composites: Effects of

compatibilization and composition on properties. *Polymer*, **51**, pp. 1812–1819.

17. Zheng, H., Ai, F., Wei, M., Huang, J., and Chang, P. R. (2007). Thermoplastic soy protein nanocomposites reinforced by carbon nanotubes. *Macromolecular Materials and Engineering*, **292**(6), pp. 780–788.

18. Lu, Y., Weng, L., and Zhang, L. (2004). Morphology and properties of soy protein isolate thermoplastics reinforced with chitin whiskers. *Biomacromolecules*, **5**(3), pp. 1046–1051.

19. Echeverria, I., Eisenberg, P., and Mauri, A. N. (2014). Nanocomposites films based on soy proteins and montmorillonite processed by casting. *Journal of Membrane Science*, **449**, pp. 15–26.

20. Wang, Y., Cao, X., and Zhang, L. (2006). Effect of cellulose whiskers on properties of soy protein thermoplastics. *Macromolecular Bioscience*, **6**(7), pp. 524–531.

21. Payne, P. I. and Corfield, K. G. (1979). Subunits composition of wheat glutenin proteins isolated by gel filtration in a dissociating medium. *Planata*, **14**, pp. 83–88.

22. Song, Y., Zheng, Q., and Cheng, L. (2008). Green biocomposites from wheat gluten and hydroxyethyl cellulose: Processing and properties. *Industrial Crops and Products*, **28**(1), pp. 56–62.

23. Song, Y. and Zheng, Q. (2009). Structure and properties of methylcellulose microfiber reinforced wheat gluten based green composites. *Industrial Crops and Products*, **29**(2–3), pp. 446–454.

24. Liu, D., Chen, H., Chang, P. R., Wu, Q., Li, K., and Guan, L. (2010). Biomimetic soy protein nanocomposites with calcium carbonate crystalline arrays for use as wood adhesive. *Bioresource Technology*, **101**(15), pp. 6235–6241.

25. Ul-Islam, M., Khan, T., and Park, J. K. (2012). Nanoreinforced bacterial cellulose–montmorillonite composites for biomedical applications. *Carbohydrate Polymers*, **89**(4), pp. 1189–1197.

26. Millon, L. E. and Wan, W. K. (2006). The polyvinyl alcohol-bacterial cellulose system as a new nanocomposite for biomedical applications. *Journal of Biomedical Materials Research Part B: Applied Biomaterials*, **79**(2), pp. 245–253.

27. Miao, J., Pangule, R. C., Paskaleva, E. E., Hwang, E. E., Kane, R. S., Linhardt, R. J., and Dordick, J. S. (2011). Lysostaphin-functionalized cellulose fibers with antistaphylococcal activity for wound healing applications. *Biomaterials*, **32**(36), pp. 9557–9567.

28. Jiang, L., Li, Y., Wang, X., Zhang, L., Wen, J., and Gong, M. (2008). Preparation and properties of nano-hydroxyapatite/chitosan/carboxymethyl cellulose composite scaffold. *Carbohydrate Polymers*, **74**(3), pp. 680–684.
29. Wan, Y. Z., Huang, Y., Yuan, C. D., Raman, S., Zhu, Y., Jiang, H. J., and Gao, C. (2007). Biomimetic synthesis of hydroxyapatite/bacterial cellulose nanocomposites for biomedical applications. *Materials Science and Engineering: C*, **27**(4), pp. 855–864.
30. Ahmed, S. and Ikram, S. (2016). Chitosan based scaffolds and their applications in wound healing. *Achievements in the Life Sciences*, **10**(1), pp. 27–37.
31. Croisier, F. and Jérôme, C. (2013). Chitosan-based biomaterials for tissue engineering. *European Polymer Journal*, **49**(4), pp. 780–792.
32. Li, Z., Ramay, H. R., Hauch, K. D., Xiao, D., and Zhang, M. (2005). Chitosan–alginate hybrid scaffolds for bone tissue engineering. *Biomaterials*, **26**(18), pp. 3919–3928.
33. Chavda, H. and Patel, C. (2010). Chitosan superporous hydrogel composite-based floating drug delivery system: A newer formulation approach. *Journal of Pharmacy and Bioallied Sciences*, **2**(2), pp. 124.
34. Rodrigues, A. and Emeje, M. (2012). Recent applications of starch derivatives in nanodrug delivery. *Carbohydrate Polymers*, **87**(2), pp. 987–994.
35. Nasri-Nasrabadi, B., Mehrasa, M., Rafienia, M., Bonakdar, S., Behzad, T., and Gavanji, S. (2014). Porous starch/cellulose nanofibers composite prepared by salt leaching technique for tissue engineering. *Carbohydrate Polymers*, **108**, pp. 232–238.
36. Torres, F. G., Commeaux, S., and Troncoso, O. P. (2013). Starch-based biomaterials for wound-dressing applications. *Starch-Stärke*, **65**(7–8), pp. 543–551.
37. Ceballos, D., Navarro, X., Dubey, N., Wendelschafer-Crabb, G., Kennedy, W. R., and Tranquillo, R. T. (1999). Magnetically aligned collagen gel filling a collagen nerve guide improves peripheral nerve regeneration. *Experimental Neurology*, **158**(2), pp. 290–300.
38. Wang, S., Cai, Q., Hou, J., Bei, J., Zhang, T., Yang, J., and Wan, Y. (2003). Acceleration effect of basic fibroblast growth factor on the regeneration of peripheral nerve through a 15-mm gap. *Journal of Biomedical Materials Research Part A*, **66**(3), pp. 522–531.
39. Höke, A., Ho, T., Crawford, T. O., LeBel, C., Hilt, D., and Griffin, J. W. (2003). Glial cell line-derived neurotrophic factor alters axon schwann

cell units and promotes myelination in unmyelinated nerve fibers. *The Journal of Neuroscience*, **23**(2), pp. 561–567.

40. Chew, S. Y., Mi, R., Hoke, A., and Leong, K. W. (2007). Aligned protein–polymer composite fibers enhance nerve regeneration: A potential tissue-engineering platform. *Advanced Functional Materials*, **17**(8), pp. 1288–1296.

41. Chew, S. Y., Wen, J., Yim, E. K. F., and Leong, K. W. (2005). Sustained release of proteins from electrospun biodegradable fibers. *Biomacromolecules*, **6**(4), pp. 2017–2024.

42. Azami, M., Moosavifar, M. J., Baheiraei, N., Moztarzadeh, F., and Ai, J. (2012). Preparation of a biomimetic nanocomposite scaffold for bone tissue engineering via mineralization of gelatin hydrogel and study of mineral transformation in simulated body fluid. *Journal of Biomedical Materials Research Part A*, **100**(5), pp. 1347–1355.

43. Hardy, J. G., Torres-Rendon, J. G., Leal-Egaña, A., Walther, A., Schlaad, H., Cölfen, H., and Scheibel, T. R. (2016). Biomineralization of engineered spider silk protein-based composite materials for bone tissue engineering. *Materials*, **9**(7) pp. 560.

44. Azami, M., Samadikuchaksaraei, A., and Poursamar, S. A. (2010). Synthesis and characterization of a laminated hydroxyapatite/gelatin nanocomposite scaffold with controlled pore structure for bone tissue engineering. *International Journal of Artificial Organs*, **33**(2), pp. 86.

45. Kim, H.-W., Kim, H.-E., and Salih, V. (2005). Stimulation of osteoblast responses to biomimetic nanocomposites of gelatin–hydroxyapatite for tissue engineering scaffolds. *Biomaterials*, **26**(25), pp. 5221–5230.

46. Sidqui, M., Collin, P., Vitte, C., and Forest, N. (1995). Osteoblast adherence and resorption activity of isolated osteoclasts on calcium sulphate hemihydrate. *Biomaterials*, **16**(17), pp. 1327–1332.

47. Jones, A. L., Bucholz, R. W., Bosse, M. J., Mirza, S. K., Lyon, T. R., Webb, L. X., Pollak, A. N., Golden, J. D., and Valentin-Opran, A. (2006). Recombinant human BMP-2 and allograft compared with autogenous bone graft for reconstruction of diaphyseal tibial fractures with cortical defects. *The Journal of Bone and Joint Surgery, American Volume*, **88**(7), pp. 1431–1441.

48. Liu, J., Mao, K., Liu, Z., Wang, X., Cui, F., Guo, W., Mao, K., and Yang, S. (2013). Injectable biocomposites for bone healing in rabbit femoral condyle defects. *PloS One*, **8**(10), pp. e75668.

49. Venugopal, J. R., Low, S., Choon, A. T., Kumar, A. B., and Ramakrishna, S. (2008). Nanobioengineered electrospun composite nanofibers and

osteoblasts for bone regeneration. *Artificial Organs,* **32**(5), pp. 388–397.

50. Thein-Han, W. W., Saikhun, J., Pholpramoo, C., Misra, R. D. K., and Kitiyanant, Y. (2009). Chitosan–gelatin scaffolds for tissue engineering: Physico-chemical properties and biological response of buffalo embryonic stem cells and transfectant of GFP–buffalo embryonic stem cells. *Acta Biomaterialia,* **5**(9), pp. 3453–3466.

51. McManus, M. C., Sell, S. A., Bowen, W. C., Koo, H. P., Simpson, D. G., and Bowlin, G. L. (2008). Electrospun fibrinogen-polydioxanone composite matrix: Potential for in situ urologic tissue engineering. *Journal of Engineered Fibers and Fabrics,* **3**(2), pp. 12–21.

52. Sha'Ban, M., Kim, S. H., Idrus, R. B. H., and Khang, G. (2008). Fibrin and poly(lactic-co-glycolic acid) hybrid scaffold promotes early chondrogenesis of articular chondrocytes: An in vitro study. *Journal of Orthopaedic Surgery and Research,* **3**(1), pp. 1.

53. Le Nihouannen, D., Saffarzadeh, A., Aguado, E., Goyenvalle, E., Gauthier, O., Moreau, F., Pilet, P., Spaethe, R., Daculsi, G., and Layrolle, P. (2007). Osteogenic properties of calcium phosphate ceramics and fibrin glue based composites. *Journal of Materials Science: Materials in Medicine,* **18**(2), pp. 225–235.

54. Manzoor, K., Archana, R., and Shantikumar, V. N. (2014). A core-shell nanostructure on the basis of proteins with corresponding therapeutic agents. Google patents, NO. WO2014002108 A1.

55. Fan, H. and Dash, A. K. (2001). Effect of cross-linking on the in vitro release kinetics of doxorubicin from gelatin implants. *International Journal of Pharmaceutics,* **213**(1), pp. 103–116.

56. Muvaffak, A., Gurhan, I., Gunduz, U., and Hasirci, N. (2005). Preparation and characterization of a biodegradable drug targeting system for anticancer drug delivery: Microsphere-antibody conjugate. *Journal of Drug Targeting,* **13**(3), pp. 151–159.

57. Andronescu, E., Ficai, A., Albu, M. G., Mitran, V., Sonmez, M., Ficai, D., Ion, R., and Cimpean, A. (2013). Collagen-hydroxyapatite/cisplatin drugs for locoregional treatment of bone cancer. *Technology in Cancer Research & Treatment,* **12**(4), pp. 275–284.

58. Watanabe, K., Nishio, Y., Makiura, R., Nakahira, A., and Kojima, C. (2013). Paclitaxel-loaded hydroxyapatite/collagen hybrid gels as drug delivery systems for metastatic cancer cells. *International Journal of Pharmaceutics,* **446**(1), pp. 81–86.

59. Andronescu, E., Ficai, M., Voicu, G., Ficai, D., Maganu, M., and Ficai, A. (2010). Synthesis and characterization of collagen/hydroxyapatite: Magnetite composite material for bone cancer treatment. *Journal of Materials Science: Materials in Medicine,* **21**(7), pp. 2237–2242.
60. Myzaki, S., Hashiguchi, N., Yokoyuchi, C., and Takada, M. (1986). Preparation and evaluation in vitro and in vivo of fibrinogen microspheres containing adriamycin. *Chemical and Pharmaceutical Bulletin,* **34**(8), pp. 3384–3393.
61. Einhaus, C. M., Retzinger, A. C., Perrotta, A. O., Dentler, M. D., Jakate, A. S., Desai, P. B., and Retzinger, G. S. (2004). Fibrinogen-coated droplets of olive oil for delivery of docetaxel to a fibrin(ogen)-rich ascites form of a murine mammary tumor. *Clinical Cancer Research,* **10**(20), pp. 7001–7010.
62. Hart, J., Silcock, D., Gunnigle, S., Cullen, B., Light, N. D., and Watt, P. W. (2006). The role of oxidised regenerated cellulose/collagen in wound repair: Effects in vitro on fibroblast biology and in vivo in a model of compromised healing. *The International Journal of Biochemistry & Cell Biology,* **34**(12), pp. 1557–1570.
63. Lobmann, R., Zemlin, C., Motzkau, M., Reschke, K., and Lehnert, H. (2006). Expression of matrix metalloproteinases and growth factors in diabetic foot wounds treated with a protease absorbent dressing. *Journal of Diabetes and Its Complications,* **20**(5), pp. 329–335.
64. Noorjahan, S. E. and Sastry, T. P. (2004). An in vivo study of hydrogels based on physiologically clotted fibrin–gelatin composites as wound-dressing materials. *Journal of Biomedical Materials Research Part B: Applied Biomaterials,* **71**(2), pp. 305–312.
65. Ponrasu, T., Vishal, P., Kannan, R., Suguna, L., and Muthuvijayan, V. (2016). Isabgol–silk fibroin 3D composite scaffolds as an effective dermal substitute for cutaneous wound healing in rats. *RSC Advances,* **6**(77), pp. 73617–73626.
66. Ramnath, V., Sekar, S., Sankar, S., Sastry, T. P. and Mandal, A. B. (2012). In vivo evaluation of composite wound dressing material containing soya protein and sago starch. *International Journal of Pharmacy and Pharmaceutical Sciences,* **4**, pp. 414–419.
67. Muthukumar, T., Anbarasu, K., Prakash, D., and Sastry, T. P. (2014). Effect of growth factors and pro-inflammatory cytokines by the collagen biocomposite dressing material containing *Macrotyloma uniflorum* plant extract: In vivo wound healing. *Colloids and Surfaces B: Biointerfaces,* **121**, pp. 178–188.

68. Hima Bindu, T. V. L., Vidyavathi, M., Kavitha, K., Sastry, T. P., and Suresh Kumar, R. V. (2010). Preparation and evaluation of chitosan-gelatin composite films for wound healing activity. *Trends in Biomaterials and Artificial Organs*, **24**(3), pp. 123–130.
69. Dowhan, W. and Bogdanov, M. (2002). Functional roles of lipids in membranes. *New Comprehensive Biochemistry*, **36**, pp. 1–35.
70. Fernandis, A. Z. and Wenk, M. R. (2007). Membrane lipids as signaling molecules. *Current Opinion in Lipidology*, **18**(2), pp. 121–128.
71. Okazaki, Y. and Saito, K. (2014). Roles of lipids as signaling molecules and mitigators during stress response in plants. *The Plant Journal*, **79**(4), pp. 584–596.
72. Wu, Y., Weller, C. L., Hamouz, F., Cuppett, S. L., and Schnepf, M. (2002). Development and application of multicomponent edible coatings and films: A review. *Advances in Food and Nutrition Research*, **44**, pp. 347–394.
73. Debeaufort, F. and Voilley, A. (2009). Lipid-based edible films and coatings, in *Edible Films and Coatings for Food Applications*, pp. 135–168. Springer, New York.
74. Wijewardane, R. M. N. A. (2013). Development of polysaccharide-lipid based composite wax formulation to enhance the storage quality of orange. *International Journal of Agricultural Technology*, **9**(2), pp. 349–356.
75. Gontard, N., Duchez, C., Cuq, J.-L., and Guilbert, S. (1994). Edible composite films of wheat gluten and lipids: Water vapour permeability and other properties. *International Journal of Food Science & Technology*, **29**(1), pp. 39–50.
76. Oyane, A., Yazaki, Y., Araki, H., Sogo, Y., Ito, A., Yamazaki, A., and Tsurushima, H. (2012). Fabrication of a DNA-lipid-apatite composite layer for efficient sand area-specific gene transfer. *Journal of Materials Science: Materials in Medicine*, **23**(4), pp. 1011–1019.
77. Shanks, G. D., Oloo, A. J., Aleman, G. M., Ohrt, C., Klotz, F. W., Braitman, D., Horton, J., and Brueckner, R. A. (2001). New primaquine analogue, tafenoquine (WR 238605), for prophylaxis against *Plasmodium falciparum* malaria. *Clinical Infectious Diseases*, **33**(12), pp. 1968–1974.
78. Cappellini, M. D. and Fiorelli, G. (2008). Glucose-6-phosphate dehydrogenase deficiency. *Lancet*, **371**, pp. 64–74.
79. Nkhoma, E. T., Poole, C., Vannappagari, V., Hall, S. A., and Beutler, E. (2009). The global prevalence of glucose-6-phosphate dehydrogenase

deficiency: A systematic review and meta-analysis. *Blood Cells, Molecules and Diseases,* **42**(3), pp. 267–278.

80. Melariri, P., Kalombo, L., Nkuna, P., Dube, A., Hayeshi, R., Ogutu, B., and Gibhard, L. (2015). Oral lipid-based nanoformulation of tafenoquine enhanced bioavailability and blood stage antimalarial efficacy and led to a reduction in human red blood cell loss in mice. *International Journal of Nanomedicine,* **10**, pp. 1493.

81. Murillo-Cremaes, N., Subra-Paternault, P., Domingo, C., and Roig, A. (2014). Preparation and study of naproxen in silica and lipid/polymer hybrid composites. *RSC Advances,* **4**(14), pp. 7084–7093.

82. Yang, L., Shao, Y., and Han, H.-K. (2016). Aminoclay–lipid hybrid composite as a novel drug carrier of fenofibrate for the enhancement of drug release and oral absorption. *International Journal of Nanomedicine,* **11**, pp. 1067.

83. Hao, J., Wang, X., Bi, Y., Teng, Y., Wang, J., Li, F., Li, Q., Zhang, J., Guo, F., and Liu, J. (2014). Fabrication of a composite system combining solid lipid nanoparticles and thermosensitive hydrogel for challenging ophthalmic drug delivery. *Colloids and Surfaces B: Biointerfaces,* **114**, pp. 111–120.

84. Seyfoddin, A. and Al-Kassas, R. (2013). Development of solid lipid nanoparticles and nanostructured lipid carriers for improving ocular delivery of acyclovir. *Drug Development and Industrial Pharmacy,* **39**(4), pp. 508–519.

85. Kalam, M. A., Sultana, Y., Ali, A., Aqil, M., Mishra, A. K., and Chuttani, K. (2010). Preparation, characterization, and evaluation of gatifloxacin loaded solid lipid nanoparticles as colloidal ocular drug delivery system. *Journal of Drug Targeting,* **18**(3), pp. 191–204.

86. Das, S., Ng, W. K., and Tan, R. B. H. (2014). Sucrose ester stabilized solid lipid nanoparticles and nanostructured lipid carriers: I. Effect of formulation variables on the physicochemical properties, drug release and stability of clotrimazole-loaded nanoparticles. *Nanotechnology,* **25**(10), pp. 105101.

87. Singh, I., Swami, R., Pooja, D., Jeengar, M. K., Khan, W., and Sistla, R. (2016). Lactoferrin bioconjugated solid lipid nanoparticles: A new drug delivery system for potential brain targeting. *Journal of Drug Targeting,* **24**(3), pp. 212–223.

88. Singh, I., Swami, R., Jeengar, M. K., Khan, W., and Sistla, R. (2015). *p*-Aminophenyl-α-D-mannopyranoside engineered lipidic nanoparticles for effective delivery of docetaxel to brain. *Chemistry and Physics of Lipids,* **188**, pp. 1–9.

89. Shaw, C. P., Fernig, D. G., and Lévy, R. (2011). Gold nanoparticles as advanced building blocks for nanoscale self-assembled systems. *Journal of Materials Chemistry*, **21**(33), pp. 12181–12187.

90. Tong, L., Wei, Q., Wei, A., and Cheng, J. X. (2009). Gold nanorods as contrast agents for biological imaging: Optical properties, surface conjugation and photothermal effects. *Photochemistry and Photobiology*, **85**(1), pp. 21–32.

91. Kang, J. H. and Ko, Y. T. (2015). Lipid-coated gold nanocomposites for enhanced cancer therapy. *International Journal of Nanomedicine*, **10**, pp. 33.

92. Swami, R., Indu, S., Manish, K. J., Wahid, K., and Ramakrishna, S. (2015). Adenosine conjugated lipidic nanoparticles for enhanced tumor targeting. *International Journal of Pharmaceutics*, **486**(1), pp. 287–296.

93. Bilbao-Sáinz, C., Chiou, B.-S., de Campos, A., Du, W.-X., Wood, D. F., Klamczynski, A. P., Glenn, G. M., and Orts, W. J. (2012). Starch–lipid composites containing cinnamaldehyde. *Starch-Stärke*, **64**(3), pp. 219–228.

94. Jain, D. and Banerjee, R. (2008). Comparison of ciprofloxacin hydrochloride-loaded protein, lipid, and chitosan nanoparticles for drug delivery. *Journal of Biomedical Materials Research Part B: Applied Biomaterials*, **86**(1), pp. 105–112.

95. Albertini, B., Di Sabatino, M., Calonghi, N., Rodriguez, L., and Passerini, N. (2013). Novel multifunctional platforms for potential treatment of cutaneous wounds: Development and in vitro characterization. *International Journal of Pharmaceutics*, **440**(2), pp. 238–249.

96. zur Mühlen, A., Schwarz, C., and Mehnert, W. (1998). Solid lipid nanoparticles (SLN) for controlled drug delivery–drug release and release mechanism. *European Journal of Pharmaceutics and Biopharmaceutics*, **45**(2), pp. 149–155.

97. Potard, G., Laugel, C., Schaefer, H., and Marty, J.-P. (2000). The stripping technique: In vitro absorption and penetration of five UV filters on excised fresh human skin. *Skin Pharmacology and Physiology*, **13**(6), pp. 336–344.

98. Wissing, S. A. and Müller, R. H. (2001). Solid lipid nanoparticles (SLN): A novel carrier for UV blockers. *Die Pharmazie*, **56**(10), pp. 783–786.

99. Song, C. and Liu, S. (2005). A new healthy sunscreen system for human: Solid lipid nanoparticles as carrier for 3, 4, 5-trimethoxybenzoylchitin

and the improvement by adding Vitamin E. *International Journal of Biological Macromolecules,* **36**(1), pp. 116–119.

100. Ananthapadmanabhan, K. P., Mukherjee, S., and Chandar, P. (2013). Stratum corneum fatty acids: Their critical role in preserving barrier integrity during cleansing. *International Journal of Cosmetic Science,* **35**(4), pp. 337–345.

101. Müller, R. H., Radtke, M., and Wissing, S. A. (2002). Solid lipid nanoparticles (SLN) and nanostructured lipid carriers (NLC) in cosmetic and dermatological preparations. *Advanced Drug Delivery Reviews,* **54**, pp. S131–S155

102. Swarnavalli, G. C. J., Dinakaran, S., and Divya, S. (2016). Preparation and characterization of nanosized Ag/SLN composite and its viability for improved occlusion. *Applied Nanoscience,* **6**(7), pp. 1065–1072.

103. Yilmaz, E. and Borchert, H. H. (2006). Effect of lipid-containing, positively charged nanoemulsions on skin hydration, elasticity and erythema: An in vivo study. *International Journal of Pharmaceutics,* **307**(2), pp. 232–238.

104. Sibarani, J., Takai, M., and Ishihara, K. (2007). Surface modification on microfluidic devices with 2-methacryloyloxyethyl phosphorylcholine polymers for reducing unfavorable protein adsorption. *Colloids and Surfaces B: Biointerfaces,* **54**(1), pp. 88–93.

105. Zhang, N., Chen, C., Melo, M. A. S., Bai, Y.-X., Cheng, L., and Xu, H. H. K. (2015). A novel protein-repellent dental composite containing 2-methacryloyloxyethyl phosphorylcholine. *International Journal of Oral Science,* **7**(2), pp. 103–109.

106. Kazuno, T., Fukushima, T., Hayakawa, T., Inoue, Y., Ogura, R., Kaminishi, H., and Miyazaki, K. (2005). Antibacterial activities and bonding of MMA/TBB resin containing amphiphilic lipids. *Dental Materials Journal,* **24**(2), pp. 244–250.

107. Malviyaa, N., Somisettyb, K., and Vemulab, K. (2015). Design and development of a novel transmucosal patch embedded with diclofenac diethylamine loaded solid lipid nanoparticles. *Journal of Young Pharmacists,* **7**(1), pp. 45.

108. Hosny, K. M., Banjar, Z. M., Hariri, A. H., and Hassan, A. H. (2015). Solid lipid nanoparticles loaded with iron to overcome barriers for treatment of iron deficiency anemia. *Drug Design, Development and Therapy,* **9**, pp. 313.

Chapter 4

Biocomposites for Hyperthermia Applications

Tomy J. Gutiérrez
Thermoplastic Composite Materials (CoMP) Group, Institute of Research in Materials Science and Technology (INTEMA), Faculty of Engineering, National University of Mar del Plata (UNMdP) and National Council of Scientific and Technical Research (CONICET), Colón 10850, Mar del Plata 7600, Buenos Aires, Argentina
tomy.gutierrez@fi.mdp.edu.ar, tomy_gutierrez@yahoo.es

Currently, cancer is one of the main causes of death worldwide. In this sense, many researches in the area of oncology are conducted. However, many of treatments have generalized secondary effects on patients, due to effectuation of drugs on other healthy organs, which also reduces the effect of drug on the cancer. As an alternative, composite biomaterials have been mainly developed from magnetic nanoparticles—biopolymers or magnetic nanoparticles—hydroxyapatite with the aim of directing and releasing the drug under the application of a magnetic field in the place where the cancer is located (hyperthermia). In this chapter, the recent advances in biocomposites for hyperthermia applications will be analyzed.

Biocomposites: Biomedical and Environmental Applications
Edited by Shakeel Ahmed, Saiqa Ikram, Suvardhan Kanchi, and Krishna Bisetty
Copyright © 2018 Pan Stanford Publishing Pte. Ltd.
ISBN 978-981-4774-38-3 (Hardcover), 978-1-315-11080-6 (eBook)
www.panstanford.com

4.1 Introduction

Hyperthermia has attracted considerable attention as a method for the treatment of malignant tumors. In addition, hyperthermia is regarded as a novel cancer treatment with low invasion and low side effects. Hyperthermia using magnetic particles was proposed in the 1950s by Gilchrist et al. [1] and is currently under development [2]. Compared with radiotherapy and chemotherapy, hyperthermia is a novel cancer treatment, which is an efficient complement that artificially elevates target tissue temperatures and causes minimal side effects to other organs; besides that, it is of low invasion [3]. The efficiency of this type of thermotherapy has been demonstrated on several types of cancers, including brain cancer, prostate cancer, and breast cancer [3].

Hyperthermia is a treatment where cancer cells in the tumors are killed by heat irradiation. The technique consists of targeting magnetic nanoparticles (MNPs) toward tumor tissue followed by the application of an external alternating magnetic field (AMF) that induces two heating mechanisms: (1) hysteresis loss for ferromagnetic particles and/or (2) Néel and Brownian relaxation for superparamagnetic particles and on a magnetic field through targeting [4], which in turn leads to heating the tissue containing these MNPs (Fig. 4.1) [2, 5, 6]. The temperature in tumor tissue is increased in the range of 41–46°C [7], which causes necrosis of cancer cells (cell processes up to apoptosis), "but does not damage surrounding normal tissue." Among this direct effect, tumor-specific immune responses, including heat-shock protein expression, have been observed during in vivo and in vitro experiments, demonstrating the potential of this therapy to act not only locally, but also at distant sites, including metastatic cancer cells [8].

Two kinds of heating treatments are currently distinguished: (1) hyperthermia performed in the range of 41–46°C to stimulate the immune response for non-specific immunotherapy and (2) thermoablation using the temperature range of 46–56°C aiming to initiate cell necrosis, coagulation, or carbonization for tumor destruction [3, 9].

The characteristic temperature of tumor cell thermoablation is very close to that of normal cell; therefore, temperature control is necessary. MNPs can play a role as nanoscale mediators converting the electromagnetic energy into heat when exposed to an external electrical or magnetic field when injected as particle dispersion. Inductive hyperthermia (with MNPs) seems currently more useful because body tissues susceptibility is very low and they cannot be the sources of heat in a magnetic field [10].

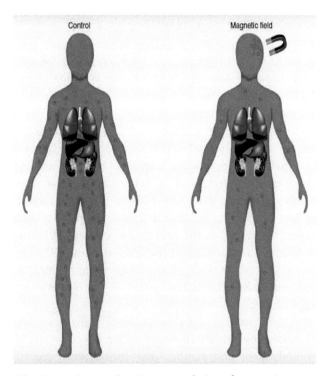

Figure 4.1 Magnetic targeting. No accumulation of magnetic nanoparticles (MNPs) occurs in the absence of a magnetic field, whereas under the influence of this field, MNPs alone or in combination with therapeutic cargo accumulate at a destined site. This includes the brain. Targeting efficiency of MNPs can be further improved by modifying the MNP surface using cell-specific targeting moieties, for instance, transferrin for brain targeting.

However, MNPs, as a rule, are toxic for living organisms. Therefore, magnetic particles should be coatings or encapsulated into biocompatible materials during or after the synthesis in order to prevent changes from the initial state, the formation of large aggregates, and the biodegradation due to the interaction with the biological system.

For in vivo biomedical applications, MNPs should be non-toxic, non-immunogenic, and small enough to remain in circulation after injection and to pass through the capillary system of organs and tissues, avoiding embolism of blood vessels. These MNPs should also have a high magnetization, so that their motion in the blood could be controlled by varying a magnetic field and they could be delivered to the site of the diseased tissue [11].

In this context, composite materials from iron oxide/biomaterials or iron oxide/hydroxyapatite are typically used in this field (hyperthermia) [12]. Although at physiological temperature, nickel and cobalt oxide composites also have ferromagnetic properties for hyperthermia applications [13].

Iron oxides such as magnetite (Fe_3O_4) or γ-hematite (γ-Fe_2O_3) structure are commonly used as thermoseeds for the hyperthermia due to their biodegradable nature, biocompatibility, and superparamagnetic effect, that is, they achieve heat generation in alternative magnetic fields [14–17]. Fe_3O_4 is widespread in the environment, despite the fact that it is thermodynamically unstable with respect to γ-Fe_2O_3 in the presence of oxygen [18]. Therefore, the lack of long-term stability of the properties of MNPs has made researchers to study γ-Fe_2O_3. The disadvantage of slightly lower bulk saturation magnetization of Fe_2O_3 [19, 20] is compensated by its higher stability.

On the other hand, Fe_3O_4 microspheres have also been developed [21-23], since they exhibit an embolization effect by blocking the blood vessels near the tumors and consequently shutting off nutrition supply to the cancer cells.

Now well, iron oxide particles are used in the nanoscale (iron nanoparticles, INPs) for hyperthermia application. It has been observed that at a diameter range of 6–30 nm of the INPs, many of their special properties can be modified, for example, the superparamagnetism properties and high saturation field (the external field needed for saturation magnetization) [24–26].

INPs usually present superparamagnetic behavior due to their small volume, meaning that the thermal energy may be enough to change spontaneously the magnetization within each INP. In other words, the magnetic moment of each INP will be able to rotate randomly (in reference to the orientation of the INP) just because of the temperature influence. For this reason, in the absence of an electromagnetic field, the net magnetic moment of a system containing INPs will be zero at high enough temperatures [27].

However, in the presence of a field, there will be a net statistical alignment of magnetic moments, analogous to what happens to paramagnetic materials, except that now the magnetic moment is not that of a single atom but of the MNPs containing various atoms, which can be up to 10^4 times larger than for a paramagnetic material [27].

Additionally, these properties allow the in vivo real-time monitoring of MNP distribution [28, 29]. Nonetheless, the nanosized magnetite particles tend to aggregate because of their high specific area and strong interparticle interaction, which limit their utilization [30]. In order to ensure stability and non-toxicity under physiological conditions, as well as to allow for functionalization and targeting, these materials must be coatings or encapsulated, which ideally would have a high affinity for the iron oxide core, and be non-immunogenic, non-antigenic, and prevent opsonization by plasma proteins [31]. These coatings or encapsulated include liposomes, lipids, dendrimers, proteins, polyethylene glycol, polysaccharides, polyacrylamide, bisphosphonates, silicon dioxide [32], noble metals (Au and Ag) [33], and titanium dioxide [31], which have resulted in the development of composite materials from INPs and biopolymers.

In addition, the poor solubility and stability in water at physiological pH of INPs could be prevented by coating them with a water-soluble polymer [34, 35]. For example, biocompatible polymers have been used as coated, since they can be bound to drugs, antibodies, enzymes, proteins, or nucleotides and can be directed to an organ, tissue, or tumor using an external magnetic field. However, there are some studies showing that a non-polar coating constituted of fatty acids could improve the antitumor effect of MNPs [36].

4.2 Synthesis of Iron Nanoparticles

The performance of INPs is dependent on the chemical and physical characteristics of the MNPs and their surfaces, which largely depend on the method of synthesis chosen for their preparation [37]. The control of particle size, shape, and distribution and the crystallinity and colloidal and magnetic properties, such as saturation magnetization and susceptibility, are of crucial importance. Therefore, the method of synthesis will allow the tailoring of the size and surface chemistry of MNPs to meet specific demands for physical and biological applications [37].

The INPs can be synthesized by various methods: coprecipitation, hydrothermal, laser pyrolysis, sol–gel, and biopolymer-inducing method or sonochemical synthesis [26, 38–45]. The first two methods are the most used.

4.2.1 Coprecipitation

The most efficient and facile method is coprecipitation using soluble salts in water (e.g., chloride, nitrate) [40, 41], and magnetite is prepared by one of two procedures:

1. Controlled oxidation of Fe^{2+} aqueous solution in an alkaline medium, to produce Fe^{2+} and Fe^{3+} with a molar ratio of 1:2 [42]; in this case, because controlled oxidation of Fe^{2+} is very difficult to obtain, only Fe_3O_4 results;
2. Addition of high pH alkaline solution to the aqueous mixture of Fe^{2+} and Fe^{3+} with a molar ratio of 1:2 [43–48]:

$$Fe^{2+} + 2Fe^{3+} + 8OH^- \rightarrow Fe_3O_4 + 4H_2O \quad (4.1)$$

This reaction takes place at pH = 9–14, under a non-oxidizing oxygen-free environment. If oxygen is present, the Fe_3O_4 can be oxidized to $Fe(OH)_3$:

$$Fe_3O_4 + 1/2O_2 + 4H_2O \rightarrow 3Fe(OH)_3 \quad (4.2)$$

Also, in air conditions, FeO from Fe_3O_4 gets oxidized, forming an Fe_2O_3 pure phase:

$$2(FeO \cdot Fe_2O_3) + 1/2O_2 \rightarrow 3Fe_2O_3 \quad (4.3)$$

So due to the oxidation process in air, it is not possible to obtain the pure magnetite. To avoid this inconvenience, the reaction can be conducted in inert nitrogen atmosphere [49, 50]. Also distilled water degassed with N_2 can be used for the preparation of an aqueous solution. After precipitation, magnetite can be calcinated in an N_2 atmosphere.

By coprecipitation in highly basic aqueous medium, the magnetite nanoparticles (NPs) acquire negative charges on their surfaces, so their agglomeration is prevented by repulsion phenomena.

Negativity of the magnetite surfaces increases with the alkalinity of the aqueous medium.

The experimental parameters affect this process, which involves the formation of intermediate hydroxyl species, such as temperature, pH, and concentration of the cations and nature of the base; these parameters have been studied in order to vary the average MNP size in the range from 3 to 20 nm. It is noteworthy that the pH is a critical parameter in affecting both the MNP size (by increasing the pH, the repulsion among primary MNPs is induced and smaller magnetite MNPs are obtained) and the stability of the MNP dispersion. In particular, thanks to the surface electrostatic repulsion, stable ionic ferrofluids can be obtained in a wide range of pH. The coprecipitation approach offers a wide range of advantages, including the use of cheap chemicals and mild reaction conditions; the possibility to perform direct synthesis in water; the ease of scale-up; and the production of highly concentrated ferrofluids thanks to the high density of surface hydroxyls. Most important, the synthetic route is extremely flexible when it comes to the modulation of the core and surface properties. Conversion to maghemite is easily obtained by the chemical oxidation of the magnetite colloids, and substituted ferrites can be prepared by alkalinization of aqueous mixtures of a ferric salt and a salt of a divalent metal under boiling conditions [51]. Likewise, thanks to the high density of reactive sites, surface modification can be easily performed by direct incorporation of additives, which is particularly useful for large-scale production as it is the case of the carbonate method [52]. A general limitation of the hydrolytic approach lies in the large number of parameters, which have to be carefully monitored in order to control the synthetic outcome, which deals with the complex aqueous chemistry and rich phase diagram of iron oxide phases.

As a major drawback of hydrolytic routes lies in the limited control of the MNP size distribution, synthesis in confined environments such as microemulsions has been proposed. In particular, reverse micelles have been used to carry out the classic coprecipitation reaction [53] and the hydrolysis of metal-surfactant complexes [54] in water-in-oil emulsions. The parameters, which affect the MNP size, are the microstructure and composition of the microemulsion (both the surfactant most commonly sodium bis(2-ethylhexyl) sulfosuccinate (AOT), cetyl trimethylammonium bromide (CTAB), dodecylsulfonate (DS) and the hydrocarbon, which constitutes the continuous phase such as hexane, heptane, octane), the temperature, and the kind of counterion. Reverse micelles have been successfully used as a means to mediate the formation of iron oxide MNPs as well as substituted ferrites with improved size distribution in the 4–12 nm range (typical size of the water-in-oil droplets of the microemulsion) [55–58].

In addition to improving the magnetic properties of the produced MNPs, the coprecipitation method can be performed under hydrothermal conditions [53]. Hydrothermal routes have also been used for hydrolytic procedures starting from iron complexes, such as the ageing in aqueous acidic/basic solution of iron polyolates followed by digestion in autoclave at 80–150°C for several days [54]. In this synthetic approach, the reaction conditions, such as solvent, temperature, and time, usually have important effects on the synthetic outcome. The MNP size in crystallization is controlled mainly through the rate processes of nucleation and particle growth, which compete with each other.

4.2.2 Hydrothermal Method

Hydrothermal method is used to obtain many fine metal oxide particles with various shapes and morphologies, which have an important influence on their properties. This method uses a pressure higher than 1 atm and low synthesis temperature (100–500°C), without subsequent heat treatments, with different plateaus. Advantages of this method are no organic reagents to be used, relative cost-effectiveness, high particle crystallinity with possibility of controlling efficiently the size and desired morphology (e.g., nanorods, nanowires, nanotubes, nanobelts, necklace and hollow nanospheres), dispersion characteristics (e.g., monodispersed), high yield of easily obtained products [59–65]. Also, this method uses the water-soluble salts. Generally, the reaction takes place in alkaline medium and N_2 atmosphere. Also for the preparation of an aqueous solution, the distilled water degassed with N_2 (for half or one hour) and surfactants or templates could be used for obtaining the mesoporous magnetite.

4.3 Magnetite: Tumor Treatment Using External Magnetic Field

Metal-based nanoscale particles possess unique optoelectronic or magnetic properties that make them highly promising as imaging agents in cancer therapy research [66–72]. Being inspired by physiologically existing nanomachines, NPs are designed to safely reach their target and specifically release their cargo at the site of the disease, thus increasing the drug's tissue bioavailability. The site-specific delivery of therapeutics to tumors is accomplished by both active and passive mechanisms.

With their unique structural properties of high surface-to-volume ratio and hollow structure, nanomaterials can carry an extremely high drug payload [15, 73, 74]. Nanomaterials with specific optical or magnetic characteristics may also be regulated by radiation or magnetic field for the controlled release of drug molecules [75, 76].

NPs have the advantage of targeting cancer by simply being accumulated and entrapped in tumors (passive targeting). The phenomenon is called the enhanced permeation and retention (EPR) effect, caused by leaky angiogenetic vessels and poor lymphatic drainage and has been used to explain why macromolecules and NPs are found at higher ratios in tumors compared to normal tissues [77]. Exploitation of the EPR effect requires careful size selection of NPs that allows NPs to extravasate leaky tumor vasculature and to be retained in the tumor due to insufficient lymphatic drainage [78]. NPs between 100 and 200 nm have been shown to accumulate in tumors by the EPR effect. The retention of large molecules such as NPs is typically higher than small molecules, which can more easily diffuse back into vasculature. In addition to appropriate size, NPs must achieve an optimum concentration gradient, for a sustained period of at least 6 h, which will allow for a long circulation time [76].

4.4 In Vivo Studies Demonstrating the Anticancer Effect of Magnetic Nanocarriers

Kawai et al. [79] demonstrated that hyperthermia using magnetic cationic liposomes (MCLs) is an effective therapy for prostate cancer, by acting directly to kill the rat prostate cancer cells in vivo by heating at 45°C, but also indirectly, by inducing an immune response. MCLs have a positive surface charge and generate heat in an AMF due to hysteresis losses. The tumor regression and the presence of CD3, CD4, and CD8 immunocytes were observed in the hyperthermic group. HSP70 also appeared in the viable area at its boundary with the necrotic area. Induction of antitumor immunity by intracellular hyperthermia using MCLs was also demonstrated on rat solid T-9 glioma tissues. On the treatment side, the tumor tissue disappeared completely in many rats exposed to the AMF (118 kHz, 384 Oe) for 30 min given thrice at 24 h intervals. The tumor tissue on the opposite side also disappeared completely, even though MCLs were not injected into the right solid tumors. To examine whether a long-lasting and tumor-specific immunity could be generated, the rats that had been cured by the hyperthermia treatment were rechallenged with T-9 cells 3 months later. After a period of transient growth, all tumors disappeared. Furthermore, immunocytochemical assay revealed that the immune response induced by the hyperthermia treatment was mediated by both $CD8^+$ and $CD4^+$ T cells and accompanied by a marked augmentation of tumor-selective cytotoxic T-lymphocyte activity. These results suggest that the magnetic particles are potentially effective tools for hyperthermic treatment of solid tumors, because in addition to killing of the tumor cells by heat, a host immune response is induced [80].

Ito et al. [81] constructed anti-HER2 immuno-liposomes containing magnetite NPs, which act as tumor-targeting vehicles, combining anti-HER2 antibody therapy with hyperthermia. The magnetite NP-loaded anti-HER2 immuno-liposomes exerted HER2-mediated antiproliferative effects on SKBr3 breast cancer cells in vitro. Moreover, 60% of magnetite NPs were incorporated into SKBr3, and the cells were then heated at 42.5°C under an AMF, resulting in strong cytotoxic effects. These results suggest that this novel therapeutic tool is applicable to treatment of HER2-overexpressing cancer [81].

The dextran magnetite was incorporated in liposomes in order to obtain thermosensitive magneto-liposomes, which proved to exhibit antitumoral effect on AH60C rat tumors, after injection of 15 mg iron/cm^3 and further exposure to 500 kHz electromagnetic field generated by inductive heating. Inside tumor, an increase in temperature to 42°C was obtained for 7 min, without affecting the tissues surrounding the tumor. The tumor cells disappeared completely in the treated animals, and the survival rates were significantly higher than in the control group [82].

4.5 In Vitro Studies Demonstrating the Improvement in Intake Rate of Anticancer Agents Loaded into Nanoparticles in Different Tumor Cells

Hu et al. [83] synthesized tamoxifen-loaded magnetite/poly(L-lactic acid) composite nanoparticles (TMCN) with an average size of approximately 200 nm, and studied there in vitro anticancer activity against MCF-7 breast cancer cells. The superparamagnetic property (saturation magnetization value of approximately 7 emu/g) of the TMCN is provided by Fe_3O_4 NPs of approximately 6 nm encapsulated in the poly(L-lactic acid) matrix. The uptake of TMCN and tamoxifen by MCF-7 was estimated from the intracellular iron concentration. After 4 h incubation of MCF-7 tumor cells with TMCN, significant changes in the cell morphology were discernible from phase contrast microscopy and approximately 80% of these cells were killed after incubation for 4 days with TMCN [83].

Temperature-sensitive poly(*N*-isopropylacrylamide-acrylamide-allylamine)-coated iron oxide MNPs (TPMNPs) prepared by free radical polymerization of monomers on the surface of silane-coupled INPs were cytocompatible and effectively taken up by advanced thyroid cancer (ATC) cells in a dose-dependent manner. An external magnetic field significantly increased NP uptake, especially when cells were exposed to physiological flow conditions. Drug loading and release studies using doxorubicin confirmed the temperature-responsive release of drugs from NPs. In addition, doxorubicin-loaded NPs significantly killed ATC cells when compared to free doxorubicin. These in vitro results indicate that TPMNPs have potential as targeted and controlled drug carriers for thyroid cancer treatment [84].

Sun and Liang [85] compared the antitumor activity between cisplatin (CDDP)-loaded liposomes and NPs in vitro, demonstrating that nanocarriers with similar pharmaceutical parameters can induce differences in cellular internalization and elimination, which influence the antitumor activity eventually. Compared with gelatin NP, liposome is preferable for cisplatin delivery [85].

At present, the research is focused on the design and engineering of new, scalable, and economic multifunctional (multiplex) systems, capable of identifying malignant cells by means of molecular detection, visualizing their location in the body by providing enhanced contrast in medical imaging techniques, killing diseased cells with minimal side effects through selective drug targeting, and monitoring treatment in real time [86]. The in vivo fate and functions of NPs depend on their interaction with the blood proteins-based research, and in this context, the MNPs coating strongly influences the cellular uptake rate of the MNPs.

4.6 Saturated Fatty Acids as Coatings for MNPs with Improved Properties as Anticancer Drugs Carriers

Saturated fatty acids (SFAs) account for 30–40% of the total fatty acids in animal tissues, distributed in palmitic acid (15–25%), stearic acid (10–20%), myristic acid (0.5–1%), and lauric acid (less than 0.5%). Palmitic and stearic acids are universally found in natural fats [87, 88]. Lauric acid is specifically abundant in copra (39–54%) and palmist oils (44–51%). Myristic acid and short-chain fatty acids (including butyric acid) represent each about 10% of fatty acids in milk fat. The body is also capable of synthesizing SFAs. The SFA C12:0 to C18:0 could be converted to the respective monounsaturated product through the action of Δ9-desaturase (stearoyl–CoA desaturase, SCD). Myristic and palmitic acids are involved in the proteins fatty acid acylation, processes called N-terminal myristoylation to the NH_2-terminal glycine and side-chain palmitoylation by posttranslational formation of a thioester linkage between the side-chain of cysteine and palmitic acid [89, 90].

Myristoylation induces the protein activation, the myristoyl moiety being involved in the mediation of protein subcellular localization, protein–protein interaction or protein–membrane interactions. About 0.5% of human proteins (structural proteins, components of intracellular signaling pathways, oncogenes, partially caspase degraded actin, gelsolin, protein kinases) [91–94], but also viral proteins could be myristoylated [95].

The association of the protein with the palmitoyl moiety is reversible and facilitates protein–membrane interactions and subcellular trafficking of proteins (e.g., the α subunit of many heterotrimeric G proteins) [96]. The SFA (C10:0–C18:0) could also elevate or activate the transcription factors (PGC-1β, SREBP family) and consequently increase the transcription of lipogenic target genes (*FAS*, SCD-1). Co-activation of the nuclear receptor LXR/RXR could promote VLDL secretion. Palmitate induced the recruitment of several transcription factors like NF-κB, HNF4, CEBPα, and PPARα [97]. SFAs (but also monounsaturated fatty acids) are known to bind hepatocyte nuclear factor 4 (HNF4). In liver cells, palmitate and oleate have been shown to inhibit the transcription of glucose-6-phosphatase gene [98].

SFAs, when linked to the lipid A moiety of lipopolysaccharides, or free, also indirectly induce NF-κB nuclear translocation, activation, and expression of COX-2, and other pro-inflammatory cytokines, through the recently described toll-like receptor 4-derived signaling pathways [99]. Butyric acid is an inhibitor of the histone deacetylase activity, with consequences for the structure of chromatin [100]. The inhibition of histone deacetylase could induce cellular differentiation, growth arrest, and apoptosis in a variety of cancer cells [101] by different mechanisms (NF-κB activation, influence on histones activity, ceramide de novo synthesis) [102–104]. A recent study of fatty acid biosynthesis in senescent cells showed that a profound modification of fatty acid biosynthesis and fatty acid desaturation occurred in the senescence process in cultured human fibroblasts [105].

It is commonly recognized that SFAs play a role in debilitating age-related illness such as type-2 diabetes and coronary heart disease. Elevated concentrations of palmitic acid are toxic to mitochondria and endoplasmic reticulum and can induce apoptosis without the involvement of reactive oxygen species. The fatty acid changes with aging are consistent with reduction in the activity of the stearoyl-CoA-desaturase 1 gene and consequent increases in palmitic and stearic acids relative to palmitoleic and oleic acid. The reduced activity of stearoyl-CoA-desaturase 1 is an outcome of *p53* activation that has an ongoing effect on mitochondrial function and cell function [106]. The stearic acid has been proved to have neutral effect on cholesterol, but could be pro-lipogenic, being a stimulating factor for VLDL–TAG [107, 108]. Rat studies have shown that lauric acid could be a precursor for ω3 fatty acid biosynthesis, as α-linolenic acid, by successive Δ6-desaturation, elongation, Δ5-desaturation, and two final elongations [109].

Thermally stable poly[aniline-co-sodium N-(1-one-butyric acid) aniline] (SPAnNa) coated MNPs of Fe_3O_4 were used as a praclitaxel (PTX) carrier, proving to be more stable at 37°C than free PTX (57 h versus 19 h at 37°C), with circulation time and a lower IC_{50} than free PTX in human prostate carcinoma cells PC3 and CWR22R, respectively. When the magnetic field was applied, an even lower IC_{50} was obtained [110].

Oleic acid-coated and pluronic-stabilized MNPs proved to assure an increased circulation time in mice and synergistic antiproliferative effects of doxorubicin and PTX when incorporated into these MNPs [111].

The NPs incorporating palmitoyl ascorbate have been proved to enhance the antitumor activity of ascorbate, which in high doses acts as a pro-oxidant in tissue fluids and delivers peroxide to tissues and fluids, which is then detoxified by erythrocytes and plasma catalase in normally perfused areas, but it could kill cancer cells in vitro [112].

4.7 Fabrication, Characterization, and In Vitro Assay of Antitumor Activity of Magnetite Coated with Non-polar Shell Without Using External Magnetic Field

It is well known that free ferrous iron (Fe^{2+}) can participate in the Fenton reaction, producing the highly toxic hydroxyl radical (•OH), that could favor the occurrence of malignant cells by inducing DNA lesions [113]. On the other side, cancer cells are generally deficient in the antioxidant enzymes present in normal cells [114], making them vulnerable to iron-mediated oxidative assault. Thus, the iron overload in tumor cells could become a successful therapeutic approach for the treatment of cancer [115]. There are only a few studies showing that the passive accumulation of INPs in tumor cells could exhibit an antitumor effect. For example, the injection of athymic nude mice bearing MCF-7 xenograft tumors with NPs containing the equivalent of total iron body stores decreased tumors and increased the animal's survival [115]. While MNPs localize to the tumors passively through the enhanced permeability and retention effect, a targeted formulation may further increase the effectiveness of the proposed therapy. Local delivery of the iron oxide through targeting by a magnetic field or through an adequate coating should be explored.

Fatty acids are used in the design of solid lipid NPs, which are a class of particulate drug carriers that remain in the solid state at room and body temperatures. They exhibit the advantage of physical stability with low toxicity and are increasingly used for the protection of labile drugs from degradation in the body and for controlled and sustained release [116, 117]. The application of lipid-based formulations for anticancer drug delivery has overcome many obstacles commonly seen in conventional cancer chemotherapy, such as limited specificity, high toxicity, and tendency of drug resistance [118, 119].

4.8 Biocomposites from Iron Nanoparticles— Biopolymers

For biomedical applications, iron oxide MNPs must be pre-coated with substances that assure their stability, biodegradability, and non-toxicity in the physiological medium in order to achieve combined properties of high magnetic saturation, biocompatibility, and interactive functions on the surface [120]. Size and surface properties of iron oxide NPs are two important factors that could dramatically affect the NP efficiency as well as their stability. MNPs are preferred to be superparamagnetic and have high magnetization property so that their movement in the blood can be controlled with external magnetic field and be immobilized close to the targeted tissue [121]. Surfactants are used to coat MNPs, since acts as a steric barrier to prevent aggregation caused by magnetic dipole–dipole attractions between particles and avoid opsonization [122].

In this context, polymeric coatings provide a means to tailor the surface properties of MNPs such as surface charge and chemical functionality [123]. The iron oxide core can be coated with polymers during the synthesis process and it must be a long chain.

Now well, there are a few reports where the MNPs have been coated with a biocompatible shell [124] or embedded in a polymer [125] to avoid aggregation and confer biocompatibility [126]. Recently, Soleymani et al. [127] have reported that polymer-coated $La_{0.73}Sr_{0.27}MnO_3$ NPs can have potential applications in cancer hyperthermia therapy and magnetically activated drug delivery. But challenges in current magnetic drug-delivery systems include unacceptable coincidental heating of healthy tissue, control of the drug release time as well as the released amount, cytotoxicity, and biocompatibility. Therefore, more extensive work in this direction is required.

According to a few other reports [128], the particles in the range of 10–100 nm appear to be ideal for biomedical use because they are small enough to penetrate very small capillaries within the body tissues for most effective distribution, ensuring adequate blood circulation times. Biswas et al. [129], in order to study the drug loading and release properties of the grown sample, loaded a test antibiotic, ciprofloxacin, into it. The controlled release profile of this drug loaded in the sample was investigated as a function of time in distilled water as reported in [130]. The main aim of this study was to see the loading and release capacity of the drug loaded in the grown polymer embedded with $La_{0.67}Sr_{0.33}MnO_3$ (LSMO) NPs and their influence on different microorganisms. From the measurement of DC magnetization, it was observed that the grown polymer embedded with the LSMO sample exhibited magnetic behavior similar to that of LSMO without any significant change in Curie temperature (T_C). It also preserved the hysteresis behavior of the parent sample with almost the same value of coercive field, but with lower magnetic moment. The drug loading and release experiments using ciprofloxacin showed that after 8 h, an amount of ≫90% from the drug loaded in the grown LSMO-embedded polymer was released. The minimum inhibitory concentration (MIC) value of ciprofloxacin loaded in the grown sample was studied for a few gram-positive and gram-negative bacteria. Good antibacterial activity was found against a gram-positive bacteria *Bacillus subtilis* and a gram-negative bacteria *Salmonella typhi*. The result is encouraging and as good as ordinary ciprofloxacin for some of the bacteria strains. Such samples may be used for magnetically activated drug delivery, which implies that when reaching the intended diseased site in the body, the drug carried by this composition can be released. It needs to be mentioned that the focus of this work is on the drug loading and release studies of this sample. Obviously, there are a few other challenges in releasing the drug in the targeted position with fewer side effects.

On the other hand, among the coating materials studied to date, chitosan has drawn considerable attention. Chitosan prevents the particles reacting with blood proteins and receptors [131]. Aziz et al. [132] studied magnetic INPs, which were synthesized by the coprecipitation method because of their potential for large-scale manufacturing, cost-effectiveness, ease of production, and hydrophilicity of nanocrystals [133].

For biomedical applications, chitosan-coated MNPs are generally synthesized by the in situ coating method, which is alkaline coprecipitation of Fe (II) and Fe (III) precursors in aqueous solutions of hydrophilic chitosan polymers. These polymers serve to limit the core growth of iron oxide during the preparation and to stabilize via steric repulsions when the NPs disperse in aqueous media [134]. The coprecipitation method involves the precipitation of iron salts in the presence of chitosan and trisodium phosphate, which act as a crosslinker. Trisodium phosphate crosslinks the adsorbed chitosan molecules to each other through the ionic interaction.

The work carried out by Aziz et al. [132] had the purpose of evaluating magnetic chitosan-coated INPs for biomedical application. The prepared biocomposite was characterized by several analyses for comparative study. The method used is more advantageous than previously published methods [135] because the process is simple and carried out under mild conditions without using hazardous organic solvents. The authors had expected that the NPs obtained had a better biocompatibility than covalently crosslinked chitosan [136, 137], as the chitosan was crosslinked with ionic interactions. The XRD pattern indicated crystalline structure of iron oxide NP and the coating with chitosan resulted in a noisy amorphous peak because chitosan raw material is essentially non-crystalline [138]. The crystallite size obtained from X-ray powder diffraction is about

13.4 nm, which successfully conforms to the biological application. The SEM image of chitosan-coated MNPs showed that the particles were spherical. The FTIR spectra confirmed the presence of metal–oxygen bond.

Lyubutin et al. [139] developed hollow microcapsules from biodegradable polyelectrolytes poly-L-lysine (PLL) and dextran sulfate (DS). These microcapsules were fabricated by the layer-by-layer adsorption technique. The capsule shells (PLL/DS)$_4$ were modified with the maghemite NPs by in situ synthesis. XRD, HRTEM, Raman, and Mössbauer spectroscopy data revealed that the INPs had the crystal structure of maghemite γ-Fe$_2$O$_3$. TEM images showed that an average diameter of the capsule was about 6.7 μm, while the average thickness of the capsule shell was 0.9 μm. The maghemite NPs formed in the capsule shell were rather monodisperse with the medium size of 7.5 nm, indicating a unique and efficient mechanism of formation of the microencapsulation. Furthermore, the most important data provided by Mössbauer spectroscopy reveal that approximately 80% of all maghemite NPs with the size of 7–9 nm had a marked superparamagnetic behavior, which was retained up to room temperature due to slow spin relaxation; this allows directing the microcapsules to a place determined with the presence of a magnetic field of a constant magnet. Additionally, the porous nature of the core and dissolution of CaCO$_3$ after layer-by-layer coating make it possible to absorb molecules that may remain trapped within the microcapsule. Therefore, mild conditions in the synthesis of MNPs incorporated in the microcapsules may enable encapsulating bioactive substances without loss of its biological activity. Moreover, because of the characteristics of the microcapsules obtained, it may suggest its application in the administration of drugs, emphasizing therapies for hyperthermia.

Zhou et al. [4] showed that thermoplastic magnetic bionanocomposite can be prepared from biocompatible dextran fatty acid ester and magnetite NPs with melting temperature slightly above human body temperature. The heating response of bionanocomposites to the application of high-frequency AMF depended on magnetite NPs content and geometry of the sample. With an optimal content of magnetite NPs between 1 and 2 wt.% and a thickness of at least 50 μm, heating above the melting temperature is possible. Thus, this is a proof of principle for a new approach toward a controlled release system triggered by remote magnetic heating. Advantages in comparison to conventional methods could be a limited tendency toward leaking and a fast response.

According to Zhu et al. [3], a way to increase the efficacy and reduce the toxicity of antitumor drugs is to deliver the drug directly to its target and maintain its concentration at the site for a sufficiently therapeutic time. Recent strategies to increase drug accumulation in a target solid tumor involve also the use of hydrogels from biopolymers. The widespread application of hydrogels in the biomedical field is due to their hydrated environment and tunable properties, which are similar to the native extracellular matrix. In situ forming systems are aqueous solutions before administration but in gel under physiological conditions. Such behavior endows the hydrogel with injectability and is most suited for localized and minimally invasive drug delivery, providing simultaneously the sustained release of the drug. Thermosensitive hydrogels based on chitosan and β-glycerophosphate are currently a promising candidate, since they present some fundamental properties such as biodegradability, biocompatibility, non-toxicity, and the non-inflammatory tendency. However, challenges still exist regarding the utilization of the application of hydrogels, such as their poor controllability, actuation, and response properties in drug delivery. Recently, magnetic hydrogels have emerged as a novel biocomposite due to their superparamagnetic and responsive properties.

Miyazaki et al. [12] developed carboxymethyldexran-Fe_3O_4 composites by an emulsion route to prepare sol–gel microspheres for the thermoseed. Microspheres were obtained by dehydration of the sol in water-in-oil emulsion. Sol–gel silica coating was then attempted using different catalysts for hydrolysis and polycondensation, since the microspheres released a lot of iron ions in aqueous condition. The silica coating used as an acidic catalyst was effective for the improvement of chemical durability in simulated body environment but not the coating using the basic one. Numerous spherical NPs were observed on the microspheres prepared by the basic catalyst. Therefore, it is assumed that the formed silica NPs on the carboxymethyldexran-Fe_3O_4 microspheres do not play a role as continuous protective layer.

4.9 Biocomposites from Iron Nanoparticles— Hydroxyapatite

In the field of biomaterials science, the development of new materials for effective repair of the bone is an important objective. Bone is a kind of composite material made up of 60–70% inorganic mineral crystals and 30–40% organic matrix consisting mostly of collagen protein fibers and the major mineral component of bone is hydroxyapatite (HA) in the form of tiny elongated crystal [140, 141]. HA with the chemical formula $Ca_{10}(PO_4)_4(OH)_6$ has been extensively used for hard tissue replacement and augmentation due to its biocompatibility and osteoconductive potential [142]. However, this material is difficult to shape into the specific forms required for bone substitution due to its hardness and brittleness. Combining biopolymer with minerals to give a biomaterial with the toughness and flexibility of the biopolymer and the strength and hardness of the mineral filler has its origin in nature, such as shell and crab. In virtue of this inspiration, composites of HA and bioorganic polymers that can overcome these problems have ignited great interest [143].

At present, HA has attracted much attention due to the prospects for use in hyperthermia treatment of cancer [144]. A number of methods have been proposed for the synthesis of biocompatible magnetic composites with HA and magnetic fillers, for example, spinel ferrites [145, 146], metallic iron [147], and hexagonal ferrites [148].

Markak and Clyne [149] proved that magneto mechanical could stimulate bone growth in a bonded array of ferromagnetic fibers. Takegami et al. [150] prepared ferromagnetic bone cement by blending magnetite powder and silica glass powder with resin, which could be used for local hyperthermia in the skeletal system. Also the magnetic therapy on the healing of bone fractures was studied by Baibekov and Khanapiyaev [151]. The preparation and application of magnetic polymer composites are of great interest for biomedical application [51]. For such applications, it is necessary that the composite should be biocompatible, non-toxic, and biodegradable.

Keshri et al. [152] reported about the synthesis and characteristic properties of NPs of LSMO and its biocomposite, obtained by mixing with HA. The synthesis pathway and some of the basic properties of LSMO manganite-based biocomposite were presented in this chapter. The NPs of LSMO were mixed with NPs of HA to make them biocompatible. XRD and FTIR results confirm the coexistence of both the phases. From the measurement of DC magnetization, it is observed that the LSMO–HA sample exhibits magnetic behavior similar to that of LSMO. However, such mixing causes lowering of the value of TC as well as of magnetization. Irreversibility in the temperature-dependent DC magnetization has been observed in ZFC and FC measurements. From the results of magnetization hysteresis loops, it can be understood that the admixture of HA preserved the magnetic behavior of the parent sample with slightly lower values of saturation field, coercive field, and magnetic moment. From TEM results, it is understood that in HA–LSMO composite, the NPs of LSMO are surrounded by HA particles and their size is 300–600 nm. Particles of such sizes might be proven advantageous as in vivo drug-delivery systems. However, for the uniform coating of HA around manganite NPs, more investigation in this direction is still required.

Tkachenko and Kamzin [2] developed a method for the synthesis of hybrid HA–ferrite (magnetic filler based on Fe_3O_4) ceramics with a higher magnetization than the values available in the literature and to investigate the structure of the synthesized hybrid ceramics, as well as the behavior of the material in an external magnetic field. In this sense, particles of the carbonated HA–ferrite composite were synthesized using a two-stage procedure. The first stage included the synthesis of ferrite particles by coprecipitation from $FeCl_2$ and $FeCl_3$ aqueous solutions and the synthesis of carbonated HA. The Mössbauer investigations demonstrated that ferrite particles consisted of magnetite (Fe_3O_4) and maghemite (γ-Fe_2O_3). The second stage included the synthesis of carbonated HA–ferrite composite particles by mixing of ferrite, $CaCO_3$, and H_3PO_4 particles, followed by annealing at a temperature of 1200°C. The formation of the HA–ferrite composite was confirmed by the X-ray diffraction analysis, investigation of the composition, and measurement of the magnetic properties. The saturation magnetizations of the ferrite in the HA–ferrite composites were found to be 46.4 and 48.0 emu/g for the ferrite components consisting of γ-Fe_2O_3 and Fe_3O_4, respectively.

Cui et al. [18] prepared novel superparamagnetic nanocomposites with various Fe_3O_4/HA/chitosan (CS) ratios, being prepared using in situ compositing method. Chitosan (CS), poly-β-(1,4)-2-amino-2-

deoxy-D-glucose, is the partly deacetylated product of chitin, which can be extracted from crustacean and insects. Their use in orthopedic application was suggested to provide temporary mechanical support for the regeneration of bone cell ingrowth owing to its good biocompatible, non-toxic, biodegradable, and inherent wound-healing characteristics [153]. In recent years, incorporation of CS with biominerals has aroused mounting interest for the preparation of biomaterials [154]. A critical obstacle in assembling and maintaining nanoscaled materials from NP clusters is the tendency of the latter to aggregate to reduce the energy associated with a high ratio of surface area to volume. The authors found that Fe_3O_4 and HA NPs with maximum sizes under 50 nm dispersed homogeneously in the nanocomposites obtained, and chemical bonds between inorganic materials and CS molecules were also formed.

Another method of treating oncological diseases is magnetic hyperthermia of malignant bone tumors using thermoseeds from composite materials of a bioactive matrix (bioglass or ceramics based on calcium phosphates) and ferrimagnetic nano- and microparticles [155]. Brushite ($CaHPO_4 \cdot H_2O$)-forming calcium phosphate bone cements have the advantage of being resorbable compared to HA-forming cements but suffer in application from their fast, water-consuming setting reaction and their low mechanical strength [6].

Matsumine et al. [156] proposed an Fe_3O_4-containing calcium phosphate-based cement for the hyperthermia of metastatic bone tumors in the femur, fibula, humerus, or tibia. They conducted clinical trials for hyperthermic treatment in 15 patients with metastatic bone lesions (HT group). The results were then compared with those for eight patients treated by palliative operation (Op group) and 22 patients treated by operations as well as radiotherapy (Op + RT group). The patients in the HT group showed better radiographic outcomes than those in the Op group and no significant differences from those in the Op + RT group. The Fe_3O_4-containing calcium phosphate-based cement is useful for hyperthermic treatment for metastatic bone tumors, but the mechanical strength of calcium phosphate cement is generally lower than that of polymethyl methacrylate (PMMA)-based cement, and hence, the Fe_3O_4-containing calcium phosphate cement is not ideal for hyperthermic treatment of bone tumors subjected to high load. To overcome this disadvantage of the Fe_3O_4-containing calcium phosphate cement,

PMMA cement containing Fe_3O_4 NPs has been proposed recently [12, 157, 158].

Beherei et al. [6] performed nano-brushite filler powder. The load of nano-brushite and γ-Fe_2O_3 powders onto a polymeric matrix in scaffolds for improving the bioactivity, biodegradation as well as the mechanical properties and anticancer effect was carried out. The characterization of the prepared biocomposites to verify the homogeneity between the two matrices and in vitro test were performed, to insure the formation of apatite layer onto the surface of the materials. The authors obtained a multifunctional scaffolds material in order to assure bone regeneration and anticancer effect. According to the in vitro behavior, the concentrations of Ca and P ions are inversely proportional with the ratios of Fe_2O_3. The scaffold materials that contained 5% γ-Fe_2O_3 cannot produce the necessary hyperthermia; the scaffold with higher content of the composite (e.g., 10% and 15%) can be successfully used as hyperthermia generator system, the activation time being of about 20–30 min (at 150 kHz).

4.10 Conclusion

Hyperthermia is a technology used in the fight against cancer, which is based on the magnetic behavior of biocomposites, mainly INPs. This technology has made it possible to reduce the side effects of conventional treatments such as chemotherapy, since it allows localized delivery of the drug. However, this technological tool still requires improvements in the future, since problems related to the surface characteristics of these biocomposites and the size of the biocomposites caused undesired physiological reactions. For this reason, the methods of preparation of these biocomposites as well as the coatings used and the characteristics of the cancer will determine the type of bionanocomposites that can act with better efficiency. In this context, this chapter sought to gather information recently on the subject with the purpose of increasing the number of publications in this scientific area. Specifically, INPs-biopolymers and INPs-hydroxyapatite were studied here.

Acknowledgments

The authors thank Consejo Nacional de Investigaciones Científicas y Técnicas (CONICET) (Postdoctoral fellowship internal PDTS-Resolution 2417) and Universidad Nacional de Mar del Plata (UNMdP) for the financial support, and Dr. Mirian Carmona-Rodríguez.

References

1. Gilchrist, R. K., Medal, R., Shorey, W. D., Hanselman, R. C., Parrott, J. C., and Taylor, C. B. (1957). Selective inductive heating of lymph nodes, *Ann. Surg.*, **146**(4), pp. 596.

2. Tkachenko, M. V. and Kamzin, A. S. (2016). Synthesis and properties of hybrid hydroxyapatite–ferrite (Fe_3O_4) particles for hyperthermia applications, *Phys. Solid State*, **58**(4), pp. 763–770.

3. Zhu, X., Zhang, H., Huang, H., Zhang, Y., Hou, L., and Zhang, Z. (2015). Functionalized graphene oxide-based thermosensitive hydrogel for magnetic hyperthermia therapy on tumors, *Nanotechnology*, **26**(36), pp. 365103.

4. Zhou, M., Liebert, T., Müller, R., Dellith, A., Gräfe, C., Clement, J. H., and Heinze, T. (2015). Magnetic biocomposites for remote melting, *Biomacromolecules*, **16**(8), pp. 2308–2315.

5. Safarik, I., Horska, K., and Safarikova, M. (2011). Magnetically responsive biocomposites for inorganic and organic xenobiotics removal. In: *Microbial Biosorption of Metals*, pp. 301–320. Springer, Netherlands.

6. Beherei, H. H., Abdel-Aal, M. S., Shaltout, A. A., and El-Magharby, A. (2012). Biophysiochemical characterization of anticancer nano-ceramic polymer scaffold for bone grafting, *Pharma. Chem.*, **4**(1), pp. 544–551.

7. Moroz, P., Jones, S. K., and Gray, B. N. (2001). Status of hyperthermia in the treatment of advanced liver cancer, *J. Surg. Oncol.*, **77**(4), pp. 259–269.

8. Kobayashi, T. (2011). Cancer hyperthermia using magnetic nanoparticles, *Biotechnol. J.*, **6**(11), pp. 1342–1347.

9. Novoselova, J. P., Safronov, A. P., Samatov, O. M., Beketov, I. V., Khurshid, H., Nemati, Z., Srikanth, H., Denisova, T. P., Andrade, R., and Kurlyandskaya, G. V. (2014). Laser target evaporation Fe_2O_3 nanoparticles for water-

based ferrofluids for biomedical applications, *IEEE Magn.*, **50**(11), pp. 1–4.

10. Mornet, S., Vasseur, S., Grasset, F., and Duguet, E. (2004). Magnetic nanoparticle design for medical diagnosis and therapy, *J. Mater. Chem.*, **14**(14), pp. 2161–2175.

11. Thorek, D. L., Chen, A. K., Czupryna, J., and Tsourkas, A. (2006). Superparamagnetic iron oxide nanoparticle probes for molecular imaging, *Ann. Biomed. Eng.*, **34**(1), pp. 23–38.

12. Miyazaki, T., Kawashita, M., and Ohtsuki, C. (2016). Ceramic-polymer composites for biomedical applications. In: *Handbook of Bioceramics and Biocomposites*, pp. 287–300. Springer International Publisher, Switzerland.

13. Klostergaard, J. and Seeney, C. E. (2012). Magnetic nanovectors for drug delivery, *Nanomedicine*, **1**, pp. 37–50.

14. Kawashita, M., Tanaka, M., Kokubo, T., Inoue, Y., Yao, T., Hamada, S., and Shinjo, T. (2005). Preparation of ferrimagnetic magnetite microspheres for in situ hyperthermic treatment of cancer, *Biomaterials*, **26**, pp. 2231–2238.

15. Grumezescu, A. M., Ilinca, E., Chifiriuc, C., Mihaiescu, D., Balaure, P., Traistaru, V., and Mihaiescu, G. (2011). Influence of magnetic MWCNTs on the antimicrobial activity of cephalosporins, *Biointerface Res. Appl. Chem.*, **1**(4), pp. 139–144.

16. Saviuc, C., Grumezescu, A. M., Holban, A., Bleotu, C., Chifiriuc, C., Balaure, P., and Lazar, V. (2011). Phenotypical studies of raw and nanosystem embedded *Eugenia carryophyllata* buds essential oil antibacterial activity on *Pseudomonas aeruginosa* and *Staphylococcus aureus* strains, *Biointerface Res. Appl. Chem.*, **1**(3), pp. 111–118.

17. Heidari, F., Bahrololoom, M. E., Vashaee, D., and Tayebi, L. (2015). In situ preparation of iron oxide nanoparticles in natural hydroxyapatite/chitosan matrix for bone tissue engineering application, *Ceram. Int.*, **41**(2), pp. 3094–3100.

18. Cui, W., Hu, Q., Wu, J., Li, B., and Shen, J. (2008). Preparation and characterization of magnetite/hydroxyapatite/chitosan nanocomposite by in situ compositing method, *J. Appl. Polym. Sci.*, **109**(4), pp. 2081–2088.

19. Kumar, A., Mohapatra, S., Fal-Miyar, V., Cerdeira, A., Garcia, J. A., Srikanth, H., Gass, J., and Kurlyandskaya, G. V. (2007). Magnetoimpedance biosensor for Fe_3O_4 nanoparticle intracellular uptake evaluation, *Appl. Phys. Lett.*, **91**(14), p. 143902.

20. Beketov, I. V., Safronov, A. P., Medvedev, A. I., Alonso, J., Kurlyandskaya, G. V., and Bhagat, S. M. (2012). Iron oxide nanoparticles fabricated by electric explosion of wire: Focus on magnetic nanofluids, *AIP Advances*, **2**(2), 022154.

21. Saviuc, C., Grumezescu, A. M., Holban, A., Chifiriuc, C., Mihaiescu, D., and Lazar, V. (2011). Hybrid nanostructured material for biomedical applications, *Biointerface Res. Appl. Chem.*, **1**(2), pp. 064–071.

22. Zhao, J., Sekikawa, H., Kawai, T., and Unuma, H. (2009). Ferrimagnetic magnetite hollow microspheres prepared via enzimatically precipitated iron hydroxide on a urease-bearing polymer template, *J. Ceram. Soc. Jpn.*, **117**, pp. 344–346.

23. Miyazaki, T., Miyaoka, A., Ishida, E., Li, Z., Kawashita, M., and Hiraoka, M. (2012). Preparation of ferromagnetic microcapsules for hyperthermia using water/oil emulsion as a reaction field, *Mater. Sci. Eng. C*, **32**, pp. 692–696.

24. Willard, M. A., Kurihara, L. K., Carpenter, E. E., Calvin, S., and Harris, V. G. (2004). Chemically prepared magnetic nanoparticles, *Int. Mater. Rev.*, **49**, pp. 125.

25. Ma, Z. Y., Guan, Y. P., Liu, X. Q., and Liu, H. Z. (2005). Covalent immobilization of albumin on micron-sized magnetic poly(methyl methacrylate-divinylbenzene-glycidyl methacrylate) microspheres prepared by modified suspension polymerization, *Polym. Adv. Technol.*, **16**, pp. 554–558.

26. Wang, Y., Li, B., Zhou, Y., and Jia, D. (2008). Chitosan-induced synthesis of magnetite nanoparticles via iron ions assembly, *Polym. Adv. Technol.*, **19**, pp. 1256–1261.

27. Colombo, M., Carregal-Romero, S., Casula, M. F., Gutiérrez, L., Morales, M. P., Böhm, I. B., Heverhagen, J. T., Prosperi, D., and Parak, W. J. (2012). Biological applications of magnetic nanoparticles, *Chem. Soc. Rev.*, **41**(11), pp. 4306–4334.

28. Alexiou, C., Arnold, W., Klein, R. J., Parak, F. G., Hulin, P., Bergemann, C., Erhardt, W., Wagenpfeil, S., and Lübbe, A. S. (2000). Locoregional cancer treatment with magnetic drug targeting, *Cancer Res.*, **60**, pp. 6641–6648.

29. Maeda, H., Wu, J., Sawa, T., Matsumura, Y., and Hori, K. (2000). Tumor vascular permeability and the EPR effect in macromolecular therapeutics: A review, *J. Control Rel.*, **65**, pp. 271–284.

30. Yang, X., Chen, L., Han, B., Yang, X., and Duan, H. (2010). Preparation of magnetite and tumor dual-targeting hollow polymer microspheres

with pH-sensitivity for anticancer drug-carriers, *Polymer*, **51**(12), pp. 2533–2539.

31. McCarthy, J. R. and Weissleder, R. (2008). Multifunctional magnetic nanoparticles for targeted imaging and therapy, *Adv. Drug. Deliv. Rev.*, **60**(11), pp. 1241–1251.

32. Dandamudi, S. and Campbell, R. B. (2007). The drug loading, cytotoxicty and tumor vascular targeting characteristics of magnetite in magnetic drug targeting, *Biomaterials*, **28**(31), pp. 4673–4683.

33. Zheng, W., Gao, F., and Gu, H. (2005). Magnetic polymer nanospheres with high and uniform magnetite content, *J. Magn. Magn. Mater.*, **288**, pp. 403–410.

34. Chifiriuc, M. C., Grumezescu, A. M., Saviuc, C., Croitoru, C., Mihaiescu, D. E., and Lazar, V. (2012). Improved antibacterial activity of cephalosporins loaded in magnetic chitosan microspheres, *Int. J. Pharm.*, **436**(1–2), pp. 201–205.

35. Grumezescu, A. M., Andronescu, E., Ficai, A., Bleotu, C., Mihaiescu, D. E., and Chifiriuc, M. C. (2012). Synthesis, characterization and in vitro assessment of the magnetic chitosan-carboxymethylcellulose biocomposite interactions with the prokaryotic and eukaryotic cells, *Int. J. Pharm.*, **43**, pp. 771–777.

36. Voicu, G., Andronescu, E., Grumezescu, A. M., Huang, K. S., Ficai, A., Yang, C. H., Bleotu, C., and Chifiriuc, M. C. (2013). Antitumor activity of magnetite nanoparticles: Influence of hydrocarbonated chain of saturated aliphatic monocarboxylic acids, *Curr. Org. Chem.*, **17**(8), pp. 831–840.

37. Roca, A. G., Morales, M. P., O'Grady, K., and Serna, C. J. (2006). Structural and magnetic properties of uniform magnetite nanoparticles prepared by high temperature decomposition of organic precursors, *Nanotechnology*, **17**(11), pp. 2783–2788.

38. Basak, S., Chen, D.-R., and Biswas, P. (2007). Electrospray of ionic precursor solutions to synthesize iron oxide nanoparticles: Modified scaling law, *Chem. Eng. Sci.*, **62**(4), pp. 1263–1268.

39. Kim, E. H., Lee, H. S., Kwak, B. K., and Kim, B. K. (2005). Synthesis of ferrofluid with magnetic nanoparticles by sonochemical method for MRI contrast agent, *J. Magn. Magn. Mater.*, **289**, pp. 328–330.

40. Chin, A. B. and Yaacob, I. I. (2007). Synthesis and characterization of magnetic iron oxide nanoparticles via w/o microemulsion and Massart's procedure, *J. Mater. Process. Technol.*, **191**(1), pp. 235–237.

41. Alvarez, G. S., Muhammed, M., and Zagorodni, A. A. (2006). Novel flow injection synthesis of iron oxide nanoparticles with narrow size distribution, *Chem. Eng. Sci.*, **61**(14), pp. 4625–4633.

42. Albornoz, C. and Jacobo, S. E. (2006). Preparation of a biocompatible magnetoc film from an aqueous ferrofluid, *J. Magn. Magn. Mater.*, **305**(1), pp. 12–15.

43. Kimata, M., Nakagawa, D., and Hasegawa, M. (2003). Preparation of monodisperse magnetic particles by hydrolysis of iron alkoxide, *Powder Technol.*, **132**(2), pp. 112–118.

44. Wan, J., Chen, X., Wang, Z., Yang, X., and Qian, Y. (2005). A soft-template-assisted hydrothermal approach to single-crystal Fe_3O_4 nanorods, *J. Cryst. Growth.*, **276**(3), pp. 571–576.

45. Xu, J., Yang, H., Fu, W., Du, K., Sui, Y., Chen, J., Zeng, Y., Li, M., and Zou, G. (2007). Preparation and magnetic properties of magnetite nanoparticles by sol–gel method, *J. Magn. Magn. Mater.*, **309**(2), pp. 307–311.

46. Jain, T. K., Morales, M. A., Sahoo, S. K., Leslie, D. L., and Labhasetwar, V. (2005). Iron oxide nanoparticles for sustained delivery of anticancer agents, *Mol. Pharm.*, **2**(3), pp. 194–205.

47. Tural, B., Ozkan, N., and Volkan, M. (2009). Preparation and characterization of polymer coated superparamagnetic magnetite nanoparticle agglomerates, *J. Phys. Chem. Solids.*, **70**(5), pp. 860–866.

48. Faiyas, A. P. A., Vinod, E. M., Joseph, J., Ganesan, R., and Pandey, R. K. (2010). Dependence of pH and surfactant effect in the synthesis of magnetite (Fe_3O_4) nanoparticles and its properties, *J. Magn. Magn. Mater.*, **322**(4), pp. 400–404.

49. Sun, J., Zhou, S., Hou, P., Yang, Y., Weng, J., Li, X., and Li, M. (2007). Synthesis and characterization of biocompatible Fe_3O_4 nanoparticles, *J. Biomed. Mater. Res. Part A*, **80**(2), pp. 333–341.

50. Kosa, I. N., Recnik, A., and Posfai, M. (2012). Novel methods for the synthesis of magnetite nanoparticles with special morphologies and textured assemblages, *J. Nanopart. Res.*, **14**(10), pp. 1150–1160.

51. Gupta, A. K. and Gupta, M. (2005). Synthesis and surface engineering of iron oxide nanoparticles for biomedical applications, *Biomaterials*, **26**(18), pp. 3995–4021.

52. Bergemann, C., Müller-Schulte, D., Oster, J. A., à Brassard, L., and Lübbe, A. S. (1999). Magnetic ion-exchange nano- and microparticles for medical, biochemical and molecular biological applications, *J. Magn. Magn. Mater.*, **194**(1), pp. 45–52.

53. López-Quintela, M. A. and Rivas, J. (1993). Chemical reactions in microemulsions: A powerful method to obtain ultrafine particles, *J. Colloid Interf. Sci.*, **158**(2), pp. 446–451.

54. Feltin, N. and Pileni, M. P. (1997). New technique for synthesizing iron ferrite magnetic nanosized particles, *Langmuir*, **13**(15), pp. 3927–3933.

55. Hochepied, J. F. and Pileni, M. P. (2000). Magnetic properties of mixed cobalt–zinc ferrite nanoparticles, *J. Appl. Phys.*, **87**(5), pp. 2472–2478.

56. Tourinho, F. A., Franck, R., and Massart, R. (1990). Aqueous ferrofluids based on manganese and cobalt ferrites, *J. Mater. Sci.*, **25**(7), pp. 3249–3254.

57. Ge, S., Shi, X., Sun, K., Li, C., Uher, C., Baker Jr, J. R., Banaszak, M. M., and Orr, B. G. (2009). Facile hydrothermal synthesis of iron oxide nanoparticles with tunable magnetic properties, *J. Phys. Chem. C*, **113**(31), pp. 13593–13599.

58. Niederberger, M., Krumeich, F., Hegetschweiler, K., and Nesper, R. (2002). An iron polyolate complex as a precursor for the controlled synthesis of monodispersed iron oxide colloids, *Chem. Mater.*, **14**(1), pp. 78–82.

59. Liang, M. T., Wang, S. H., Chang, Y. L., Hsiang, H. I., Huang, H. J., Tsai, M. H., Juan, W. C., and Lu, S. F. (2010). Iron oxide synthesis using a continuous hydrothermal and solvothermal system, *Ceram. Int.*, **36**(3), pp. 1131–1135.

60. Chen, F., Gao, Q., Hong, G., and Ni, J. (2008). Synthesis and characterization of magnetite dodecahedron nanostructure by hydrothermal method, *J. Magn. Mag. Mater.*, **320**(11), pp. 1775–1780.

61. Haw, C. Y., Mohamed, F., Chia, C. H., Radiman, S., Zakaria, S., Huang, N. M., and Lim, H. N. (2010). Hydrothermal synthesis of magnetite nanoparticles as MRI contrast agents, *Ceram. Int.*, **36**(4), pp. 1417–1422.

62. Zhang, Z. J., Chen, X. Y., Wang, B. N., and Shi, C. W. (2008). Hydrothermal synthesis and self-assembly of magnetite (Fe_3O_4) nanoparticles with the magnetic and electrochemical properties, *J. Crys. Growth.*, **310**(24), pp. 5453–5457.

63. Márquez, F., Campo, T., Cotto, M., Polanco, R., Roque, R., Fierro, P., Sanz, J. M., Elizalde, E., and Morant, C. (2011). Synthesis and characterization of monodisperse magnetite hollow microspheres, *Soft Nanosci. Lett.*, **1**(2), pp. 25–32.

64. Wu, M., Xiong, Y., Jia, Y., Niu, H., Qi, H., Ye, J., and Chen, Q. (2005). Magnetic field-assisted hydrothermal growth of chain-like nanostructure of magnetite, *Chem. Phy. Lett.*, **401**(4), pp. 374–379.

65. Liang, J., Li, L., Luo, M., Fang, J., and Hu, Y. (2010). Synthesis and properties of magnetite Fe_3O_4 via a simple hydrothermal route, *Solid State Sci.*, **12**(8), pp. 1422–1425.

66. Aleksenko, S. S., Shmykov, A. Y., Oszwałdowski, S., and Timerbaev, A. R. (2012). Interactions of tumour-targeting nanoparticles with proteins: Potential of using capillary electrophoresis as a direct probe, *Metallomics*, **4**(11), pp. 1141–1148.

67. Mantle, M. D. (2011). Quantitative magnetic resonance micro-imaging methods for pharmaceutical research, *Int. J. Pharm.*, **417**(1), pp. 173–195.

68. Wang, H., Wang, S., Liao, Z., Zhao, P., Su, W., Niu, R., and Chang, J. (2011). Folate-targeting magnetic core–shell nanocarriers for selective drug release and imaging, *Int. J. Pharm.*, **430**(1), pp. 342–349.

69. García-Jimeno, S., Escribano, E., Queralt, J., and Estelrich, J. (2011). Magnetoliposomes prepared by reverse-phase followed by sequential extrusion: Characterization and possibilities in the treatment of inflammation, *Int. J. Pharm.*, **405**(1–2), pp. 181–187.

70. Fan, C., Gao, W., Chen, Z., Fan, H., Li, M., Deng, F., and Chen, Z. (2011). Tumor selectivity of stealth multi-functionalized superparamagnetic iron oxide nanoparticles, *Int. J. Pharm.*, **404**(1–2), pp. 180–190.

71. Tataru, G., Popa, M., and Desbrieres, J. (2011). Magnetic microparticles based on natural polymers, *Int. J. Pharm.*, **404**(1–2), pp. 83–93.

72. Alphandéry, E., Guyot, F., and Chebbi, I. (2012). Preparation of chains of magnetosomes, isolated from *Magnetospirillum magneticum* strain AMB-1 magnetotactic bacteria, yielding efficient treatment of tumors using magnetic hyperthermia, *Int. J. Pharm.*, **434**(1–2), pp. 444–452.

73. Mihaiescu, D. E., Grumezescu, A. M., Balaure, P. C., Mogosanu, D. E., and Traistaru, V. (2011). Magnetic scaffold for drug targeting: Evaluation of cephalosporins controlled release profile, *Biointerface Res. Appl. Chem.*, **1**(5), pp. 191–195.

74. Grumezescu, A. M., Saviuc, C., Holban, A., Hristu, R., Croitoru, C., Stanciu, G., Chifiriuc, C., Mihaiescu, D., Balaure, P., and Lazar, V. (2011). Magnetic chitosan for drug targeting and in vitro drug delivery response, *Biointerface Res. Appl. Chem.*, **1**(5), pp. 160–165.

75. Liu, Y., Zhang, B., and Yan, B. (2011). Enabling anticancer therapeutics by nanoparticle carriers: The delivery of paclitaxel, *Int. J. Mol. Sci.*, **12**(7), pp. 4395–4413.

76. Mihaiescu, D. E., Grumezescu, A. M., Mogosanu, D. E., Traistaru, V., Balaure, P. C., and Buteica, A. (2011). Hybrid organic/inorganic nanomaterial for controlled cephalosporins release, *Biointerface Res. Appl. Chem.*, **1**(2), pp. 41–47.
77. Wang, M. and Thanou, M. (2010). Targeting nanoparticles to cancer, *Pharmacol. Res.*, **62**(2), pp. 90–99.
78. Phillips, M. A., Gran, M. L., and Peppas, N. A. (2010). Targeted nanodelivery of drugs and diagnostics, *Nano Today*, **5**(2), pp. 143–159.
79. Kawai, N., Ito, A., Nakahara, Y., Futakuchi, M., Shirai, T., Honda, H., Kobayashi, T., and Kohri K. (2005). Anticancer effect of hyperthermia on prostate cancer mediated by magnetite cationic liposomes and immune-response induction in transplanted syngeneic rats, *Prostate*, **64**(4), pp. 373–381.
80. Yanase, M., Shinkai, M., Honda, H., Wakabayashi, T., Yoshida, J., and Kobayashi, T. (1998). Antitumor immunity induction by intracellular hyperthermia using magnetite cationic liposomes, *Cancer Sci.*, **89**(7), pp. 775–782.
81. Ito, A., Kuga, Y., Honda, H., Kikkawa, H., Horiuchi, A., Watanabe, Y., and Kobayashi, T. (2004). Magnetite nanoparticle-loaded anti-HER2 immunoliposomes for combination of antibody therapy with hyperthermia, *Cancer Lett.*, **212**(2), pp. 167–175.
82. Masuko, Y., Tazawa, K., Sato, H., Viroonchatapan, E., Takemori, S., Shimizu, T., Ohkami, H., Nagae, H., Fujimaki, M., Horikoshi, I., and Weinstein, J. N. (1997). Antitumor activity of selective hyperthermia in tumor-bearing rats using thermosensitive magnetoliposomes as a new hyperthermic material, *Drug Deliv.*, **4**(1), pp. 37–42.
83. Hu, F. X., Neoh, K. G., and Kang, E. T. (2006). Synthesis and in vitro anti-cancer evaluation of tamoxifen-loaded magnetite/PLLA composite nanoparticles, *Biomaterials*, **27**(33), pp. 5725–5733.
84. Koppolu, B., Bhavsar, Z., Wadajkar, A. S., Nattama, S., Rahimi, M., Nwariaku, F., and Nguyen, K. T. (2012). Temperature-sensitive polymer-coated magnetic nanoparticles as a potential drug delivery system for targeted therapy of thyroid cancer, *J. Biomed. Nanotechnol.*, **8**(6), pp. 983–990.
85. Sun, X. Y. and Liang, W. Q. (2011). Comparison on antitumor activity of cisplatin-loaded liposomes and nanoparticles in vitro, *J. Zheinjang Univer. Med. Sci.*, **40**(4), pp. 408–413.
86. Gindy, M. E. and Prud'homme, R. K. (2009). Multifunctional nanoparticles for imaging, delivery and targeting in cancer therapy, *Expert Opin. Drug Deliv.*, **6**(8), pp. 865–878.

87. Legrand, P. and Rioux V. (2010). The complex and important cellular and metabolic functions of saturated fatty acids, *Lipids*, **45**(10), pp. 941–946.

88. Paneva, D., Manolova, N., Argirova, M., and Rashkov, I. (2011). Antibacterial electrospun poly(ε-caprolactone)/ascorbyl palmitate nanofibrous materials, *Int. J. Pharm.*, **416**(1), pp. 346–355.

89. Mitchell, D. A., Vasudevan, A., Linder, M. E., and Deschenes, R. J. (2006). Protein palmitoylation by a family of DHHC protein S-acyltransferases, *J. Lipid Res.*, **47**(6), pp. 1118–1127.

90. Towler, D. A., Gordon, J. I., Adams, S. P., and Glaser, L. (1988). The biology and enzymology of eukaryotic protein acylation, *Annu. Rev. Biochem.*, **57**(1), pp. 69–99.

91. Zha, J., Weiler, S., Oh, K. J., Wei, M. C., and Korsmeyer, S. J. (2000). Posttranslational N-myristoylation of BID as a molecular switch for targeting mitochondria and apoptosis, *Science*, **290**(5497), pp. 1761–1765.

92. Utsumi, T., Sakurai, N., Nakano, K., and Ishisaka, R. (2003). C-terminal 15 kDa fragment of cytoskeletal actin is posttranslationally N-myristoylated upon caspase-mediated cleavage and targeted to mitochondria, *FEBS Lett.*, **539**(1–3), pp. 37–44.

93. Sakurai, N. and Utsumi, T. (2006). Posttranslational N-myristoylation is required for the anti-apoptotic activity of human tGelsolin, the C-terminal caspase cleavage product of human gelsolin, *J. Biol. Chem.*, **281**(20), pp. 14288–14295.

94. Vilas, G. L., Corvi, M. M., Plummer, G. J., Seime, A. M., Lambkin, G. R., and Berthiaume, L. G. (2006). Posttranslational myristoylation of caspase-activated p21-activated protein kinase 2 (PAK2) potentiates late apoptotic events, *Proc. Natl. Acad. Sci. USA.*, **103**(17), pp. 6542–6547.

95. Maurer-Stroh, S., Gouda, M., Novatchkova, M., Schleiffer, A., Schneider, G., Sirota, F. L., Wildpaner, M., Hayashi, N., and Eisenhaber, F. (2004). MYRbase: Analysis of genome-wide glycine myristoylation enlarges the functional spectrum of eukaryotic myristoylated proteins, *Genome. Biol.*, **5**(3), pp. 1–16.

96. Chen, C. A. and Manning, D. R. (2001). Regulation of G proteins by covalent modification, *Oncogene*, **20**(13), pp. 1643–1652.

97. Xu, C., Chakravarty, K., Kong, X., Tuy, T. T., Arinze, I. J., Bone, F., and Massillon, D. (2007). Several transcription factors are recruited to the glucose-6-phosphatase gene promoter in response to palmitate in rat hepatocytes and H4IIE cells, *J. Nutr.*, **137**(3), pp. 554–559.

98. Budick-Harmelin, N., Anavi, S., Madar, Z., and Tirosh, O. (2012). Fatty acids-stress attenuates gluconeogenesis induction and glucose production in primary hepatocytes, *Lipids Health Dis.*, **9**(11), pp. 66.

99. Lee, J. Y., Sohn, K. H., Rhee, S. H., and Hwang, D. (2001). Saturated fatty acids, but not unsaturated fatty acids, induce the expression of cyclooxygenase-2 mediated through Toll-like receptor 4, *J. Biol. Chem.*, **276**(20), pp. 16683–16689.

100. Rada-Iglesias, A., Enroth, S., Ameur, A., Koch, K. M., Clelland, G. K., Respuela-Alonso, P., Wilcox, S., Dovey, O. M., Ellis, P. D., Langford, C. F., Dunham, I., Komorowski, J., and Wadelius, C. (2007). Butyrate mediates decrease of histone acetylation centered on transcription start sites and down-regulation of associated genes, *Genome. Res.*, **17**(6), pp. 708–719.

101. Chen, J., Ghazawi, F. M., Bakkar, W., and Li, Q. (2006). Valproic acid and butyrate induce apoptosis in human cancer cells through inhibition of gene expression of Akt/protein kinase B, *Mol. Cancer*, **5**(1), pp. 71.

102. Belakavadi, M., Prabhakar, B. T., and Salimath, B. P. (2007). Purification and characterization of butyrate-induced protein phosphatase involved in apoptosis of Ehrlich ascites tumor cells, *Biochim. Biophys. Acta*, **1770**(1), pp. 39–47.

103. Staiger, K., Staiger, H., Weigert, C., Haas, C., Haring, H. U., and Kellerer, M. (2006). Saturated, but not unsaturated, fatty acids induce apoptosis of human coronary artery endothelial cells via nuclear factor-κB activation, *Diabetes*, **55**(11), pp. 3121–3126.

104. Beauchamp, E., Tekpli, X., Marteil, G., Lagadic-Gossmann, D., Legrand, P., and Rioux, V. (2009). N-myristoylation targets dihydroceramide Δ4-desaturase 1 to mitochondria: Partial involvement in the apoptotic effect of myristic acid, *Biochimie.*, **91**(11), pp. 1411–1419.

105. Maeda, M., Scaglia, N., and Igal, R. A. (2009). Regulation of fatty acid synthesis and Δ9-desaturation in senescence of human fibroblasts, *Life Sci.*, **84**(3), pp. 119–124.

106. Ford, J. H. (2010). Saturated fatty acid metabolism is key link between cell division, cancer, and senescence in cellular and whole organism aging, *Age*, **32**(2), pp. 231–237.

107. Hunter, J. E., Zhang, J., and Kris-Etherton, P. M. (2010). Cardiovascular disease risk of dietary stearic acid compared with trans, other saturated and unsaturated fatty acids: A systematic review, *Am. J. Clin. Nutr.*, **91**(1), pp. 46–63.

108. Sampath, H., Miyazaki, M., Dobrzyn, A., and Ntambi, J. M. (2007). Stearoyl–CoA desaturase-1 mediates the pro-lipogenic effects of dietary saturated fatty acids, *J. Biol. Chem.*, **282**(4), pp. 2483–2493.

109. Legrand, P., Catheline, D., Rioux, V., and Durand, G. (2002). Lauric acid is desaturated to C12:1n-3 by rat liver homogenate and hepatocytes, *Lipids*, **37**(6), pp. 569–572.

110. Hua, M. Y., Yang, H. W., Chuang, C. K., Tsai, R. Y., Chen, W. J., Chuang, K. L., Chang, Y. H., Chuang, H. C., and Pang, S. T. (2010). Magnetic-nanoparticle-modified paclitaxel for targeted therapy for prostate cancer, *Biomaterials*, **31**(28), pp. 7355–7363.

111. Tapan, K. J., Marco, A. M., Sanjeeb, K. S., Diandra, L. L. P., and Vinod, L. (2005). Iron oxide nanoparticles for sustained delivery of anticancer agents, *Mol. Pharm.*, **2**(3), pp. 194–205.

112. Sawant, R. R., Vaze, O. S., Rockwell, K., and Torchilin, V. P. (2010). Palmitoyl ascorbate-modified liposomes as nanoparticle platform for ascorbate-mediated cytotoxicity and paclitaxel co-delivery, *Eur. J. Pharm. Biopharm.*, **75**(3), pp. 321–326.

113. Fang, J., Seki, T., and Maeda, H. (2009). Therapeutic strategies by modulating oxygen stress in cancer and inflammation, *Adv. Drug Deliv. Rev.*, **61**(4), pp. 290–302.

114. McCarty, M. F., Barroso-Aranda, J., and Contreras, F. (2010). Oxidative stress therapy for solid tumors: A proposal, *Med. Hypotheses*, **74**(6), pp. 1052–1054.

115. Foy S. P. and Labhasetwar, V. (2011). Oh the irony: Iron as a cancer cause or cure? *Biomaterials*, **32**(35), pp. 9155–9158.

116. Müller, R. H., Mäder, K., and Gohla, S. (2000). Solid lipid nanoparticles (SLN) for controlled drug delivery: A review of the state of the art, *Eur. J. Pharm. Biopharm.*, **50**(1), pp. 161–177.

117. Mehnert, W. and Mäder, K. (2001). Solid lipid nanoparticles: Production, characterization and applications, *Adv. Drug Deliv. Rev.*, **47**(2), pp. 165–196.

118. Wong, H. L., Bendayan, R., Rauth, A. M., Li, Y., and Wu, X. Y. (2007). Chemotherapy with anticancer drugs encapsulated in solid lipid nanoparticles, *Adv. Drug Deliv. Rev.*, **59**(6), pp. 491–504.

119. Puri, A., Loomis, K., Smith, B., Lee, J. H., Yavlovich, A., Heldman, E., and Blumenthal, R. (2009). Lipid-based nanoparticles as pharmaceutical drug carriers: From concepts to clinic, *Crit. Rev. Ther. Drug. Carrier. Syst.*, **26**(6), pp. 523–580.

120. Tartaj, P., del Puerto Morales, M., Veintemillas-Verdaguer, S., GonzalezCarreno, T., and Serna, C. J. (2003). The preparation of magnetic nanoparticles for applications in biomedicine, *J. Phys. D Appl. Phys.*, **36**(13), pp. R182.

121. Gupta, A. K. and Wells, S. (2004). Surface superparamagnetic nanoparticles for drug delivery: Preparation, characterization, and cytotoxicity studies, *IEEE T. Nanobiosci.*, **3**(1), pp. 66–73.

122. Denkbaş, E. B., Kiliçay, E., Birlikseven, C., and Öztürk, E. (2002). Magnetic chitosan microspheres: Preparation and characterization, *React. Funct. Polym.*, **50**(3), pp. 225–232.

123. Berry, C. C. and Curtis, A. S. G. (2003). Functionalisation of magnetic nanoparticles for applications in biomedicine, *J. Phys. D Appl. Phys.*, **36**(13), pp. R198–R206.

124. Kumar, S. S. R. and Mohammad, C. F. (2011). Magnetic nanomaterials for hyperthermia-based therapy and controlled drug delivery, *Adv. Drug Deliver. Rev.*, **63**(9), pp. 789–808.

125. Li, J., Qu, Y., Ren, J., Yuan, W., and Shi, D. (2012). Magnetocaloric effect in magnetothermally responsive nanocarriers for hyperthermia-triggered drug release, *Nanotechnology*, **23**(50), pp. 505706.

126. Yavuz, M. S., Cheng, Y., Chen, J., Cobley, C. M., Zhang, Q., Rycenga, M., Xie, J., Kim, C., Song, K. H., Schwartz, A. G., Wang, L. V., and Xia, Y. (2009). Gold nanocages covered by smart polymers for controlled release with near-infrared light, *Nat. Mater.*, 8(12), pp. 935–939.

127. Soleymani, M., Edrissi, M., and Alizadeh, M. A. (2015). Thermosensitive polymer-coated $La_{0.73}Sr_{0.27}MnO_3$ nanoparticles: Potential applications in cancer hyperthermia therapy and magnetically activated drug delivery systems, *Polym. J.*, **47**, pp. 797–801.

128. Bhayani, K. R., Kale, S. N., Arora, S., Rajagopal, R., Mamgain, H., Kaul-Ghanekar, R., Kundaliya, D. C., Kulkarni, S. D., Pasricha, R., and Dhole, S. D. (2007). Protein and polymer immobilized nanoparticles for possible biomedical applications, *Nanotechnology*, **18**(34), pp. 345108.

129. Biswas, S., Keshri, S., Goswami, S., Isaac, J., Ganguly, S., and Perov, N. (2016). Antibiotic loading and release studies of LSMO nanoparticles embedded in an acrylic polymer, *Phase Transit.*, **89**(12), pp. 1203–1212.

130. Gupta, R. and Bajpai, A. K. J. (2011). Magnetically guided release of ciprofloxacin from superparamagnetic polymer nanocomposites, *J. Biomat. Sci. Polym. E.*, **22**, pp. 893–918.

131. Weissleder, R., Bogdanov, A., Neuwelt, E. A., and Papisov, M. (1995). Long-circulating iron oxides for MR imaging, *Adv. Drug Deliver. Rev.*, **16**(2), pp. 321–334.

132. Aziz, T., Masum, S. M., Qadir, M. R., Gafur, A., and Huq, D. (2016). Physicochemical characterization of iron oxide nanoparticle coated with chitosan for biomedical application, *Int. Res. J. Pure Appl. Chem.*, **1**(1), pp. 1–9.

133. Qu, S., Yang, H., Ren, D., Kan, S., Zou, G., Li, D., and Li, M. (1999). Magnetite nanoparticles prepared by precipitation from partially reduced ferric chloride aqueous solutions, *J. Colloid Interf. Sci.*, **215**(1), pp. 190–192.

134. Mornet, S., Vasseur, S., Grasset, F., and Duguet, E. (2004). Magnetic nanoparticle design for medical diagnosis and therapy, *J. Mater. Chem.*, **14**(14), pp. 2161–2175.

135. Tiaboonchai, W. and Limpeanchob, N. (2007). Formulation and characterization of amphotericin B-chitosan-dextran sulfate nanoparticles, *Int. J. Pharm.*, **329**(1), pp. 142–149.

136. Agnihotri, S. A., Mallikarjuna, N. N., and Aminabhavi, T. M. (2004). Recent advances on chitosan-based micro and nanoparticles in drug delivery, *J. Control. Release*, **100**(1), pp. 5–28.

137. Park, J. H., Saravanakumar, G., Kim, K., and Kwon, I. C. (2010). Targeted delivery of low molecular drugs using chitosan and its derivatives, *Adv. Drug Deliver. Rev.*, **62**(1), pp. 28–41.

138. Kabiraj, M. K., Jahan, I. A., Masum, S. M., Islam, M. M., Hasan, S. M. M., Saha, B., and Nur, H. P. (2015). Effective removal of chromium (VI) ions from tannery effluent using chitosan-alumina composite, *Int. Res. J. Pure Appl. Chem.*, **10**(3), pp. 1–12.

139. Lyubutin, I. S., Starchikov, S. S., Bukreeva, T. V., Lysenko, I. A., Sulyanov, S. N., Korotkov, N. Y., Rumyantseva, S. S., Marchenko, I. V., Funtov, K. O., and Vasiliev, A. L. (2014). In situ synthesis and characterization of magnetic nanoparticles in shells of biodegradable polyelectrolyte microcapsules, *Mater. Sci. Eng. C*, **45**, pp. 225–233.

140. Rhee, S. H., Suetsugu, Y., and Tanaka, J. (2001). Biomimetic configurational arrays of hydroxyapatite nanocrystals on bio-organics, *Biomaterials*, **22**(21), pp. 2843–2847.

141. Ramesh, S. (2001). Grain size-properties correlation in polycrystalline hydroxyapatite bioceramic, *Malays. J. Chem.*, **3**(1), pp. 35–40.

142. Saraswathy, G., Pal, S., Rose, C., and Sastry, T. P. (2001). A novel bio-inorganic bone implant containing deglued bone, chitosan and gelatin, *B. Mater. Sci.*, **24**(4), pp. 415–420.

143. Wan, A. C., Khor, E., and Hastings, G. W. (1997). Hydroxyapatite modified chitin as potential hard tissue substitute material, *J. Biomed. Mater. Res.*, **38**(3), pp. 235–241.

144. Roveri, N. and Iafisco, M. (2010). Evolving application of biomimetic nanostructured hydroxyapatite, *Nanotechnol. Sci. Appl.*, **3**(1), pp. 107–125.

145. Pon-On, W., Meejoo, S., and Tang, I. M. (2008). Substitution of manganese and iron into hydroxyapatite: Core/shell nanoparticles, *Mater. Res. Bull.*, **43**(8), pp. 2137–2144.

146. Inukai, A., Sakamoto, N., Aono, H., Sakurai, O., Shinozaki, K., Suzuki, H., and Wakiya, N. (2011). Synthesis and hyperthermia property of hydroxyapatite-ferrite hybrid particles by ultrasonic spray pyrolysis, *J. Magn. Magn. Mater.*, **323**(7), pp. 965–969.

147. Pon-On, W., Meejoo, S., and Tang, I. M. (2007). Incorporation of iron into nano hydroxyapatite particles synthesized by the microwave process, *Int. J. Nanosci.*, **6**(01), pp. 9–16.

148. Tkachenko, M. V., Kamzin, A. S., Ol'khovik, L. P., Tkachenko, T. M., and Keshri, S. (2014). Synthesis and study of the new class of magnetic bioceramics for biomedical applications: Mössbauer studies. In: *Solid State Phenomena*, Vol. 215, pp. 480–488. Trans Tech Publications.

149. Markaki, A. E. and Clyne, T. W. (2004). Magneto-mechanical stimulation of bone growth in a bonded array of ferromagnetic fibres, *Biomaterials*, **25**(19), pp. 4805–4815.

150. Takegami, K., Sano, T., Wakabayashi, H., Sonoda, J., Yamazaki, T., Morita, S., Shibuya, T., and Uchida, A. (1998). New ferromagnetic bone cement for local hyperthermia, *J. Biomed. Mater. Res.*, **43**(2), pp. 210–214.

151. Baibekov, I. M. and Khanapiyaev, U. K. (2001). Healing of bone fractures of rat shin and some immunological indices during magnetic laser therapy and osteosynthesis by the Ilizarov method, *B. Exp. Biol. Med.*, **131**(4), pp. 399–402.

152. Keshri, S., Kumar, V., Wiśniewski, P., and Kamzin, A. S. (2014). Synthesis and characterization of LSMO manganite-based biocomposite, *Phase Transit.*, **87**(5), pp. 468–476.

153. Ito, M., Hidaka, Y., Nakajima, M., Yagasaki, H., and Kafrawy, A. H. (1999). Effect of hydroxyapatite content on physical properties and connective tissue reactions to a chitosan-hydroxyapatite composite membrane, *J. Biomed. Mater. Res.*, **45**(3), pp. 204–208.

154. Muzzarelli, C. and Muzzarelli, R. A. (2002). Natural and artificial chitosan–inorganic composites, *J. Inorg. Biochem.*, **92**(2), pp. 89–94.

155. Tkachenko, M. V., Ol'khovik, L. P., Kamzin, A. S., and Keshri, S. (2014). Polyfunctional bioceramics based on calcium phosphate and M-type hexagonal ferrite for medical applications, *Tech. Phys. Lett.*, **40**(1), pp. 4–6.

156. Matsumine, A., Kusuzaki, K., Matsubara, T., Shintani, K., Satonaka, H., Wakabayashi, T., Miyazaki, S., Morita, K., Takegami, K., and Uchida, A. (2007). Novel hyperthermia for metastatic bone tumors with magnetic materials by generating an alternating electromagnetic field, *Clin. Exp. Metastas.*, **24**(3), pp. 191–200.

157. Kawashita, M., Kawamura, K., and Li, Z. (2010). PMMA-based bone cements containing magnetite particles for the hyperthermia of cancer, *Acta Biomater.*, **6**(8), pp. 3187–3192.

158. Li, Z., Kawamura, K., Kawashita, M., Kudo, T., Kanetaka, H., and Hiraoka, M. (2012). In vitro heating capability, mechanical strength and biocompatibility assessment of PMMA-based bone cement containing magnetite nanoparticles for hyperthermia of cancer, *J. Biomed. Mater. Res. A*, **100**(10), pp. 2537–2545.

Chapter 5

Biocomposites Based on Natural Fibers: Concept and Biomedical Applications

Raoof Ahmad Najar, Aasim Majeed, Gagan Sharma, Villayat Ali, and Pankaj Bhardwaj

Molecular Genetics Laboratory, Centre for Plant Sciences, School of Basic and Applied Sciences, Central University of Punjab, Bathinda 151001, India
majeedaasim@gmail.com

Recent years have witnessed considerable growth in the use of biocomposites in automotive industries and for engineering applications. Biocomposites have revolutionized the different fields of human life. Different materials are being employed to generate biocomposites; however, natural fiber–based biocomposites have an advantage as they are easily available, biocompatible, renewable, cost effective, highly stiff, mechanically strong, environment friendly, and abundant. Among all the natural fibers, silk is most important as far as medical applications are concerned. The natural fiber–based composites are used in tissue engineering, drug delivery, dentistry, wound healing, and antibacterial application. This chapter focuses on natural fibers and their use in medicine.

Biocomposites: Biomedical and Environmental Applications
Edited by Shakeel Ahmed, Saiqa Ikram, Suvardhan Kanchi, and Krishna Bisetty
Copyright © 2018 Pan Stanford Publishing Pte. Ltd.
ISBN 978-981-4774-38-3 (Hardcover), 978-1-315-11080-6 (eBook)
www.panstanford.com

5.1 Introduction

A composite is made up of two or more compatible constituents with different physical and chemical properties [1]. It is a heterogeneous material with intimate contact of two or more phases, incorporated in a manner to take advantage of their positive attributes only and not of their shortcomings. Composites are more versatile as they possess high tensile strength and higher fatigue endurance limit. The properties of composites mainly depend on the interaction and composition of the constituents from which they have been made. A composite has two phases, namely continuous and discontinuous phase; the latter is comparatively harder and stronger than the former and is called reinforcement, whereas the continuous phase is also called the matrix. Reinforcement provides strength, stiffness, and ability to carry the load. Biocomposite is a composite material derived from renewable and non-renewable resources of biological origin. Natural fibers form the principal components of most of the biocomposites. They are obtained from plants such as hemp, sisal, kenaf, jute, bamboo, and banana. Silk, wool, and chicken feather fibers are fibers of animal origin [2]. The most important properties of fibers is that they can be engineered according to basic requirements.

In the recent years, composite materials have received significant interest from researchers due to their wide use in industries and in fundamental research and also due to the drive toward environmentally sustainable technologies. Natural fibers can be used to produce biofuels, textiles, and fabrics and for reinforcement of composites. Natural fiber–based biocomposites are environment friendly, used in military applications, transportation, and industrial construction, and are regaining the attention that was once shifted to synthetic products.

5.2 Types of Natural Fibers

Natural fibers are classified into two main groups: plant and animal based. Mineral-based fibers also form a substantial part of natural fibers. They are classified according to their origin (Fig. 5.1). Plants form the primary source of natural fibers. Plant-based fibers are abundantly found in nature and are easily available than animal-based ones.

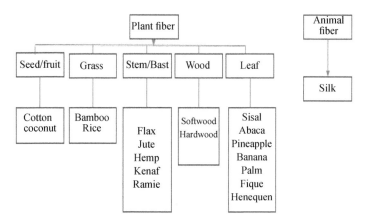

Figure 5.1 Classification of natural fibers.

Plant fibers are also called vegetable fibers and are naturally occurring composites consisting of cellulosic fibers embedded in a lignin matrix. They are non-abrasive, non-hazardous, strong, lightweight, and cost effective [3]. They can be categorized into primary and secondary fibers according to their utilities. Primary fibers include hemp, jute, kenaf, etc., while coir, pineapple, etc. belong to the secondary group. Basic types of fibers are categorized as bast fibers (ramie, jute, flax, hemp, and kenaf), leaf fibers (pineapple, sisal, and abaca), seed fiber (coir, cotton, and kapok), grass and reed fibers (wheat, corn, and rice), and other types (wood and rice) [4].

- **Sisal fiber:** Derived from agave plant, straight in shape, yellow in color, having high durability and strength. It is extracted from leaves that are sword like in shape, thick, and fleshy. It is mainly used in ropes and twines, and its reinforced composites have found place in automotive and housing sectors [5]. Its potential for being used as reinforcement in composites is reviewed by many scientific communities [3, 6].

- **Cotton fiber:** Soft white fibrous substance made into textile fiber and used for sewing. It grows around the seeds of cotton plant (*Gossypium*). It is biodegradable, water absorbent, comfortable, and has thermostatic capacity.

- **Jute fiber:** Predominately an annual rain-fed crop, obtained from the genus *Chorchorus*. It is brown in color, with soft texture and high tensile strength, environmental friendly, and biodegradable. Two species cultivated to get jute are *Chorchorus capsularis* L. and *Chorchorus olitorius* [7]. It is widely used in making carrier bags, shopping bags, home textiles, floor coverings, cushion covers, insulating materials, etc. [8]. It has been reported that more jute fiber is probably used in industrial and engineering textiles than any other fiber [9].

- **Flax fiber:** The scientific name of flax (*Linum usitatissimum* L.) is literally translated as "linen most useful" [10]. It is flexible, soft, and obtained from the stem of the flex plant. Flax bast fiber is rich in cellulose [11].

- **Coir fiber:** Coir is a natural fiber extracted from the husk surrounding the coconut seed and is divided into white and brown fiber [12]. It is mainly used for marine purposes as it shows resistance to sea water [13]. Coir is biodegradable, combustible, and compostable. It provides cooling comfort in hot climate and warmth in winter. Its natural resistance to soiling and dampness is due to high percentage of lignin. Brushes and brooms are made from coir due to their rigidity and stiffness. Nowadays coir is used as geotextiles, structural composites, sorbents, filters, molded products, and packaging materials [14].

- **Hemp fiber:** Extracted from *Cannabis sativa*, an oldest crop known to man. This plant is economically valuable, abundant, and ubiquitous. It is cultivated to obtain three products: seeds, fiber, and psychoactive substance from female inflorescence [15]. The production of insulating products and fiber-based reinforcement is the promising destination of hemp bast fibers [16]. It has been reported that after hemp cultivation, yield of wheat increases [17], which makes it a suitable crop for the modern agricultural system.

- **Abaca fiber:** Belongs to family Musaceae, produced only in two countries: Philippine and Ecuador. It has high tensile strength, which makes it favorable for producing special papers such as bank notes, tea bags, and cigarette paper [18]. Animal fibers are mostly made of proteins, for example, silk, wool, hair, etc. and is the second most important source of natural fibers after plant fibers. They have the potential to be used as reinforcement in composites [19]. Their chemical composition and physical properties render them as strong candidate for reinforcement.

- **Silk:** It consists of highly structured proteins and has high tensile strength and resistance to chemicals. It is obtained from several sources such as spiders (dragline silk, *Nephila*), which in their life time spin seven types [19]. Several insects produce silk during metamorphosis [20]. The only silk that is used as commercial application is mulberry silk obtained from *Bombyx mori*. This type of silk consists of two components: fibroin (fiber) and sericin (gum) [21]. It is used in reinforcing many blends of HDPE, LDPE, and natural rubber [22] and is also used in tissue engineering to produce scaffolds because of having biocompatibility and mechanical stability [19].

- **Wool:** It is a proteinous structure obtained from sheep skin and acts as a model for the polymer chemists searching for new fibers and protein scientists to know the secrets of nature. It is the best known representative of large class of animal hairs and is the most widely used fiber compared to shatoosh, an expensive fiber found in sheep of peaks of the Himalayan region (Tibetan antelope, *Pantholops hodgsonii*) [23]. It has been reported that wool can be used to clean the surrounding atmosphere as it has the capability to retain noxious gases because of its proteinous structure and also enhances the growth of grass [24] and nowadays is used to retain lead or iron from water supply [25].

5.3 Natural Fiber–Based Biocomposites

As environmental issues are increasing day by day, awareness of public regarding environmental protection is gaining attention. So the incorporation of natural fibers in biocomposite material is increasing rapidly in the recent years. Natural fiber–based composites have advantage over glass fiber composites in producing less pollution than synthetic polymer matrix and less weight resulting in less fuel consumption for the automotive industry [26]. A remarkable transformation of biofiber has been observed over the last few decades, gaining more and more attention in structural applications. The interest is rapidly growing, in terms of both industrial and fundamental research. They have replaced the synthetic fiber–reinforced composites in various fields such as aerospace, marine, automotive, and construction industries [4, 27]. Due to their biocompatibility, they play an important role in medical science also. They consist of biodegradable polymer and biofiber, which has low cost and high toughness [28]. Biofibers have small cross-sectional area and are embedded in a matrix (acts as a binder to bind the fibers) to form biocomposite to make them available for use in engineering applications. Due to the high performance in mechanical properties, low cost, low density, and significant processing processes, natural fiber–based composites are growing rapidly [29]. These composites have the potential to substitute wood-based materials in structural applications.

Sisal fibers are used in polymers of thermoplastics, thermosets, and rubber composites. Due to the amenability of sisal fibers to laminating and winding and their low cost of production, they have been incorporated into thermosetting plastics [30, 31]. The specific strength of sisal is comparable with glass composites, and its tensile strength is 2500–3000 MPa, half the strength of fiber glass epoxy composites [2]. Thermoplastic substances have a wide range of applications, but the filling materials, such as glass and mica, used in them are expensive. So a low cost and easily available better alternative in the form sisal fibers has reshaped the nature of thermoplastics. Further, rubber composites and plant fiber elastomer composites have sisal fibers for offering enhanced properties [32, 33]. Sisal fibers provide high modulus and tear strength to rubber [2]. Hemp fibers are considered the most ecologically friendly and are widely used, after sisal, as reinforcement in composites. The high stiffness and strength make them a strong candidate for using them as reinforcement in composite material. In 2008, a British company unveiled an ecofriendly car, Elise Eco, in which the interior trim, rooftop, and seat covers are made of hemp, wool, and sisal [34]. Also during the 2008 Beijing Olympics, window frames and floor coverings were made of hemp-reinforced composites [35]. Hemp biocomposites can be easily recycled [36] and decomposed as compared to plastics and are thus environment friendly. The mechanical properties of hemp fiber/PP composites are well preserved without any effect by reprocessing cycles [3]. They are highly used in the automotive industry. As reinforcement in composites, flax fiber has gained popularity in the recent years because of increasing requirement for developing sustainable materials. Various reasons such as oil used capacity, environmental issues, and sustainability are responsible for the increased emphasis on flax fiber to produce composites [37]. In the western hemisphere, flax was probably the first fiber used by humans to form textiles; they are natural cellulosic and multicellular fibers. Among all commercial textiles, flax has the highest heat-resistance capacity, which is why a linen sheet feels so cool and is also resistant to rotting and weathering than cotton fibers [38]. Several reports are available on the mechanical properties of flax fiber–reinforced thermoplastic composites [39], especially polylactic acid (PLA), which is a new biodegradable flax fiber–reinforced eco-biocomposite [40]. PLA is a kind of bioplastic having excellent mechanical properties [41]. It is too brittle for many commercial applications and has poor thermal properties [42], so natural fibers such as flax and hemp are used as reinforcement to improve PLA's mechanical and thermal properties [43]. PLA, which is mainly used for biodegradable products such as plastic bags and planting cups, is a thermoplastic polymer made from lactic acid, and also serves as a matrix material in composites [40]. The flax/PLA composite has a higher Young's modulus of 6.31 Gpa than cordenka/PLA composite [44]. Composites made from flax fibers with thermoplastic matrices exhibit good mechanical properties [45]. Polypropylene (PP) possesses various properties such as low density, low thermal expansion, resistance to water, and recyclability, which makes it a suitable thermoplastic matrix for flax-reinforced composites [37]. The mechanical performance of epoxy-based flax composites has been widely investigated [46, 47], and according to Oksman [47], Arctic flax/epoxy composites have excellent mechanical strength of 280 MPa and specific modulus of 29 GPa/gcm^3 than that of glass/epoxy composites. In order to reduce the environmental footprint of super electric vehicles and applications such as body panels, crash elements, side panels, and body trims, tannin resin, which is a natural phenolic resin, has been reinforced by flax fibers. Such composites offer environmental benefits also [48]. In short, flax fiber composites have a wide range of properties depending on the matrix type used, such as thermoplastic, thermosets, and biomaterials.

Due to its porous, hygroscopic, non-abrasive, viscoelastic, and biodegradable nature, jute is a versatile filler for fabrication of various biocomposites [49]. Jute fiber polyester composite has wide applications in bath units, shower, helmets, suitcases, electrical appliances, covers, pipes, roof tiles, etc. [50]. Various natural and synthetic biodegradable polymers can be combined with natural fibers such as jute and hemp to produce biocomposites. PLA is one among them as it is produced from renewable sources [51]. Jute fiber/PLA composite is gaining more interest nowadays because both resin and reinforcement material come from renewable resources. It is considered an ecofriendly alternative to wood-based panels since the resin emitting from wood-based panels is considered carcinogenic and harmful for workers [52]. Several reports state that jute fiber/PLA, when treated with NaOH and H_2O_2, enhances its tensile strength as compared to untreated one [53]. Silk fiber–based reinforced polymeric composites have emerged recently [54]. Animal fiber–based composites are the potential candidates for structural composites having various medical applications such as wound sutures and biomedical scaffolds [55]. Blending of silk sericin with other resins provides environment friendly biodegradable polymers [56]. The composites of silk and polyurethane [57] and silk fibroin/chitosan have excellent mechanical properties due to which they have potential for biomedical applications [58]. Silk fibers have high compressibility and stand bending when compared to plant fibers and even glass fibers. They provide a unique opportunity in the production of high fiber volume fraction natural fiber composites [59]. Textiles woven from silk fiber are easier to compact compared to hemp- and flax-based textiles.

5.4 Biomedical Applications of Natural Fibers

Any material used for biomedical application should possess some characteristic features such as not having any adverse effect on the host tissue during implantation and after decay. Natural fibers are biocompatible and biodegradable, so natural fiber-based biocomposites are better choice when utilized for medical applications. These biocomposites serve different medical applications, which are discussed in the following sections.

5.4.1 Tissue Engineering

Tissue engineering is a multidisciplinary field, which includes principles of engineering, life science, and molecular cell biology to develop biological substitutes that maintain, restore, and improve tissue function [60]. A basic application of tissue engineering is the use of scaffolds, which are biodegradable, biocompatible, having enough strength to stand against physical stress, not hindering cell growth, proliferation, and attachment. Tissue engineering means to restore the aim and function of a damaged tissue by developing different biological methods and can be classified as implantation of isolated cells, tissue development by providing growth substances, and placing cells on or with different matrices [61]. To create implantable pieces of organism, living cells are seeded on natural or synthetic extracellular scaffold to make them applicable for tissue engineering. Various reports are available regarding the substitution of organs by researchers, such as growing cartilage and skin [62], bone and cartilage [63], liver [64], heart valves, and arteries [65]. Scaffolds promote cell adhesion, transport of gases, regulatory factors to allow cell survival, proliferation, and differentiation and, therefore, help in tissue regeneration and repair [61]. Direct tissue regeneration can be obtained from polymer scaffold having mechanical strength, interconnected porosity, and sufficient surface area [66].

Nature is the world's best biological engineer without any doubt. The unique cells having powerful designs inspire us to produce novel technologies. For example, the characteristic features of silk such as high strength, adhesiveness, and controllable wettability suggest its potential in surgical, optical, and other biomedical applications [67]. Composite tissue engineering scaffolds loaded with BMP 2 and made from silk fibroin and hydroxyapatite nanoparticles can be generated through the electrospinning technique. Using this composite as a scaffold, bone formation is achieved in vitro by using human bone marrow derived mesenchymal cells as seeds. The mesenchymal cells successfully proliferated and differentiated in the scaffold. Both calcium deposition and bone tissue specific transcript markers show elevation for the composite scaffold than control. This is attributed to efficient and prolonged delivery of the bone morphogenetic protein by the scaffold. This composite scaffold, therefore, is capable to be used for bone tissue engineering experiments [68]. Similar composites of silk fibroin matrix and polyaspartic acid loaded with calcium and phosphorous in the form of $CaCl_2$ and Na_2HPO_4 are suitable for bone tissue engineering. Seeding of the scaffold with bone marrow stem cells in the presence of osteogenic environment provided by BMP 2 result in enhanced osteoconductivity and, therefore, bone regeneration [69]. In order to achieve enhanced repairing of inferior mandibular border defects, a composite scaffold was made from apatite-coated silk fibroin seeded with bone marrow stromal cells. The bone starts to regenerate in the scaffold in the fourth week after operation and continues till the defect is completely resolved after 12 months. Mineral deposition over the newly regenerated bone is satisfactory and close to the normal bone after 12 months [70]. In another study involving the composite scaffold having the same components, mandibular defects show enhanced recovery after eight weeks in model rats [71].

Through the electrospinning technique, a composite of poly(lactic-co-glycolic acid) and wool keratin was generated, which exhibit lesser diameter, higher thermal stability, and rough surfaces. Tensile strength and elongation break increase with the increase in wool keratin content. Bone mesenchyme stem cells show enhanced attachment and proliferation in the wool keratin/poly(lactic-co-glycolic acid) scaffold. This composite, therefore, is claimed to be suitable for bone tissue engineering applications [72]. Successful penetration and proliferation of mouse osteoblast like cells, MC3T3-E1, in the scaffold of cotton wool like poly(lactic acid) vaterite biocomposite is achieved. Further, the composite is more effective as it holds and releases calcium ions and silica up to about 56 days [73]. A novel photodynamic composite based on wool keratin was generated, which shows antimicrobial activity on exposure to light due to generation of reactive oxygen species and singlet oxygen. This composite film is doped with methylene blue and is effective against *Staphylococcus aureus*. The antibactericidal activity of the composite increases with the increase in irradiation time. This composite film is, therefore, suitable for wound healing and tissue engineering experiments to prevent sepsis at the cut tissue [74].

Mature cartilage tissue exhibits feeble vascular supply, lesser turnover of its matrix, and insufficient number of chondrocytes. These properties of cartilage render it undereffecient for regeneration [75]. Cartilage tissue reduction in osteoarthritis is one of the main reasons of associated symptoms of this disease. Current therapy involves surgically achieved allografting, autografting, or microfracturing [76]. However, these approaches are limited by their lesser success rate, so a new and robust approach is to be sought out. Cartilage tissue engineering can be a promising tool to mitigate this problem. Agarose hydrogels have been used for cartilage tissue engineering [77, 78]. However, certain properties such as poor integration of the scaffold with the tissue, lesser processing ease, and non-degradability of agarose limit its window of utility in this direction. Recently, a silk-based composite hydrogel has given promising results in cartilage engineering. Further, silk does not involve these undesirable properties, so it can form an efficient alternative system for this purpose. The composite consists of a matrix of silk hydrogel reinforced by silk microfibers. The composite shows enhanced cartilage regeneration, which leads to the formation of mechanically more robust constructs after 42 days [79]. Enhanced cartilage tissue regeneration also occurs when scaffolds of thermosensitive chitosan hydrogel matrix reinforced by silk fibers are used [80].

In order to fabricate exactly the 3D architecture of the living tissues, progenitor cells in an appropriately defined and organized biomaterial are delivered at the target site in sufficient number. This approach is commonly known as bioprinting, and the biomaterial is called bioink. Cytocompatibility and encapsulation efficiency of the bioink impart a major hurdle to this apparently looking enthusiastic technology. In order to solve this issue, researchers have tried to design new bioinks with new features. A composite of silk fibroin and gelatin laden with mesenchyme progenitor cells derived from nasal inferior turbinate tissue has been used for this purpose. The encapsulated cells undergo successful multilineage differentiation and specific tissue constructs form. Patient-specific and target-specific tissue regeneration is the future of this composite [81].

Due to its biological properties such as biocompatibility, mechanical integrity, transparency, and slow biodegradation, silk is used for eye regeneration and corneal tissue engineering [82]. Reports are available regarding preparation of SF (silk fibroin) thick transparent composite films coated with collagen IV and chondroitin sulfate-laminin. These composite films enhance successful cell proliferation and make it a potential substratum for the transplantation of tissue construction for keratoplasty [83]. With remarkable dielectric properties and mechanical flexibility, SF is a promising biofunctional material interface for nerve repair [67] and reports are available where dorsal root ganglion has been cultured in vitro on SF films, which in turn can promote repair of peripheral nervous system [84]. SF also helps in skin regeneration by stimulating the collagen synthesis of fibroblasts. For treatment of burn wounds, silk/scaffold was produced through lyophilization, which emulates the dermal extracellular matrix (ECM) [85].

5.4.2 Dental Application

The breakdown of harder elements of teeth such as enamel and dentin results into dental cavities. Restoration dentistry is a promising method to prevent tooth loss due to caries. Thus, an array of dental filling materials came into existence for this purpose. The fillers must have comparable mechanical and physical attributes like that of teeth. Further, they should function in oral environment and should possess the ability to withstand stress during chewing. In serving this purpose, resins have surpassed amalgam. However, resins have their own limitations and many times they fail mainly due to less adhesion between the matrix and the filler, thus compromising strength. This necessitated the need to reinforce the dental resins. Different reinforcing materials have been incorporated into dental resins, such as glass fibers [86], whiskers [87], and microparticles [88]. Natural fibers can also be applied for this purpose, and researchers have employed them in reinforcing dental resins. Silk, being biocompatible, mechanically tough, irritation free, and better bonding with resins, is an effective candidate for this purpose. Addition of 5% silk microfibers to bis-GMA/TEGDMA resin results in significant enhancement of its mechanical properties owing to its uniformity in distribution plus better bonding between the fiber and the resin at their interfaces [89]. Fiber-reinforced composites have now recently become center of attraction for dentists. Feather fiber, which is a protein-based fiber, can be used as reinforcement material in polymer matrix composites [90]. Polymethyl methacrylate (PMMA) is a non-biodegradable polymer and an essential material in medicine and dentistry [91], which, in combination with feather fiber, yields a biocomposite dental post because enhancement of flexural strength and modulus is observed with the addition of feather fiber [92]. Filling of dental caries, replacement of decaying tooth and Crown Bridge are the typical applications of fiber-reinforced polymer.

5.4.3 Wound Healing

Biocomposites based on natural fibers (cotton, jute, cellulose, silk, wool, hemp, and sisals) possess various biomedical properties such as antibacterial, drug delivery, and tissue engineering. Besides these biomedical activities, natural fibers have other promising applications in wound healing. Effective wound management is necessary to prevent sepsis. If left open, the ruptured tissues at the wound site get easily penetrated by the infectious bacteria, which leads to septic infections. Therefore, covering the wound effectively is the most straightforward approach in wound management. Consequently, numerous scaffolds have been prepared to cover the wound. The dressing material should be biocompatible and biodegradable. Further, it should rapidly absorb wound exudates to enhance quick drying for better healing besides possessing promising gaseous exchange properties plus barrier ability to bacterial penetration [93]. Different biomaterials have been used to prepare scaffolds and dressings for wound healing due to their excellent biodegradable, biocompatible, and bioresorbable properties such as chitosan, gelatin, collagen, and silk fibroin. They show promising advantage over synthetic polymers [94]. Among the natural fibers, silk is one of the important fibers used for wound sutures and biomedical scaffolds [95]. Silk fibroin possesses hemostatic and non-cytotoxic properties along with low antigenicity, so it can be used to produce scaffolds for biomedical use [96]. Further, it is also applicable in burn wound dressing, vascular prostheses, and structural implants [97]. Pineapple fiber has various desired characteristics for biomedical applications, such as high crosslinking, non-toxicity, durability, and biocompatibility [98], and due to these characteristic features, it is used as dressing in material for wounds.

A composite wound dressing made from silk fibroin and elastin was developed for the treatment of burn wounds. The scaffolds were prepared by lyophilization, where the solutions of both silk fibroin and elastin were blended, followed by crosslinking with genipin. The composite showed rapid healing of induced standardized burn wounds by initiating rapid re-epithelialization and wound closure. Further, the composite shows good cytocompatible property [85]. Among all the wound-dressing materials, cotton gauze has earned the fame of trust and reliability. Such dressings can be improved by conferring antibacterial and moisture-retaining property to them so as to satisfy the requirements of a modern dressing material. Impregnation of cotton gauze samples with chitosan–silver–zinc oxide nanocomposite yields an excellent modern wound-dressing composite, which shows 78% increase in drying period of the wound and 38% increase in water absorption. Further, the composite dressing shows 99% efficiency against *S. aureus* and 96% efficiency against *Escherichia coli* [99]. A spongy bilayered blend of silk fibroin/gelatin crosslinked by sericin and glutaraldehyde possesses improved homogeneous porosity and biodegradability. These blends act as important wound-dressing materials, which facilitate L929 mouse fibroblast cell proliferation and attachment. Re-epithelialization, wound closure, and collagen formation are faster in case of sericin–silk fibroin-/collagen-based dressings than clinically used ones. Moreover, these bilayered dressings are less adhesive, which facilitates easy undressing during replacement [100]. Electrospinning of nanoscale silk fibers from *B. mori* generates silk mats. Addition of epidermal growth factor (EGF) into the silk matrix forms a pharmaceutically active composite that has wound-healing properties. Here the key feature of these mats is that they release the EGF very slowly, 25% in about 172 h. This mat shows promising results in treating the human 3D skin models [101].

5.4.4 Drug Delivery

In most clinical applications, controlled and sustained release of drugs and biomaterials is highly desired for better and enhanced results. Therefore, researchers are now designing such delivery systems that facilitate controlled drug release. Moreover, the delivery system is preferred to be biocompatible and biodegradable. Silk offers these advantageous properties in addition to mechanical toughness and flexibility in processing. So it is used in producing controlled drug-delivery systems [102]. Besides, silk produces comparatively less inflammation [103]. Virgin silkworm silk elicits allergic response due to the presence of sericin [104], which thus necessitates the removal of sericin to generate a non-allergic and non-cytotoxic silk. BMP-2 is bone morphogenetic protein that induces osteogenetic differentiation of stromal cells of bone marrow. Three-dimensional scaffolds of silk after loading with BMP-2 trigger this differentiation both in vitro and in vivo [105]. A nanofilm-coated silk fibroin scaffold, on embedding adenosine, shows efficient release of adenosine up to around 1000 ng per day to suppress brain seizures during epilepsy [106]. For treating acute injuries of peripheral nerves, the standard method involves the use of nerve conduit, which is the artificial means of directing and guiding the regrowth of axons for enhanced nerve regeneration. One such nerve conduit made from nerve growth factor (NGF) loaded silk fibroin matrix shows prolonged release of the growth factor up to three weeks, which efficiently guides the sprouting axons and also protects the axonal cone for better nerve regeneration [107]. Similar scaffolds of silk matrix loaded with Insulin like growth factor 1 (IGF-1) aimed at cartilage repair show satisfying results [108]. A 3D scaffold created from blending calcium alginate beads encapsulating bovine serum albumin (BSA) and FITC-inulin with silk fibroin protein shows prolonged release of these model compounds without 35 days of initial burst. Here the silk protein provides diffusion barrier and mechanically stable shells to the encapsulated compounds [109]. After blending of silk fibroin (SF) and chitosan (CS), the resulting conjugate was loaded with the anticancer drug, curcumin, to test its efficacy in breast cancer. The results revealed the silk fiber–curcumin conjugate is more efficient than SFCS blend in terms of sustained and long-term drug release [110]. Composites made from engineered spider silk protein and polyurethanes/polyester show prolonged release of low–molecular weight drugs (methyl violet or ethacridine lactate). Further, such composite films possess tensile strength comparable to the basement membrane and are, therefore, claimed to be efficient in subcutaneous implantations [111].

Stratum corneum represents the main barrier that hinders the dermal transfer of drugs from skin to interior. High–molecular weight molecules and hydrophilic agents are especially difficult to deliver. So approaches of overcoming the dermal barrier need to be addressed. One such powerful approach is the use of microneedles. These microneedles puncture the skin to form microscale transient hydrophilic passage to efficiently enhance transdermal delivery. Vaccine-loaded microneedles made of silk/polyacrilic acid composite show enhanced release kinetics of the vaccine, resulting into increase in antigen-specific T-lymphocytes up to about tenfold, thereby conferring enhanced immunity [112]. A matrix generated by crosslinking of hyaluronic acid (HA) with polyethylene glycol (PEG), upon embedding of reinforcing material in the form of electrospun silk, resulted into the formation of a composite hydrogel, which shows sustainable delivery of antibacterial and anti-inflammatory agents [113].

Cancer is one of the most dreadful diseases in the world, consuming millions of lives. Efficient delivery systems can reduce the death toll caused by cancer. Composite microspheres made from iron oxide and silk fibroin form suitable carriers for the anticancer drug, doxorubicin hydrochloride. Both loading ability and encapsulating property of the composite are promising. The drug-loaded composite is efficiently endocytosed, resulting in comparatively less survival of cancer cells. Further, the composite is biocompatible, so it does not show any signs of cytotoxicity [114]. Using desolvation method, silk fibroin was blended with albumin to create composite nanoparticles, which act as promising drug carriers. The nanoparticles are internalized with relative ease and also show perinuclear residing ability. Upon loading with the model drug, methotrexate, they show better drug loading and encapsulating efficiency along with lesser cytotoxicity. The release of the drug prolongs up to more than 12 days [115]. Blending of poly(L-lactic acid) with keratin of wool fiber by ethanol replacement process followed by electrospinning yields composite nanofibers with superfine homogeneous organization and enhanced thermal properties. Further, the composite nanofibers show good biocompatibility and also enhances cell viability. The composite possesses promising drug-delivery profile and prolongs the release of model drug 5-flurouracil up to 120 h. Moreover, the composite, when embedded with antimicrobial peptide Attacin 2, shows antitumor ability particularly after 24 h. Thus, this composite can be used to target both tumors and bacterial infections together [116].

To the matrix of cotton fiber, researchers loaded silica particles containing the drug tetracycline by using polysiloxane as the fixing agent. The cotton fabric was then tested for the drug delivery in human skin infection. The release profile revealed sustained drug release up to 24 h [117]. In a similar study, an anti-inflammatory drug named betamethasone sodium phosphate was loaded onto silica particles, which were impregnated into a matrix of cotton fiber. Such cotton blends can be used as wound dressings to efficiently deliver the drug and to counter the bacterial infections [118]. With an intention to treat chronic venous ulcers in legs, researchers generated a blend of cotton and ascorbic acid. The cotton matrix was loaded with water-based liposomes containing ascorbic acid. The cotton matrix shows prevention of ascorbic acid degradation, thereby prolonging its life during the treatment of up to 1 month [119].

5.5 Conclusion

The recent trend to search for renewable and environment friendly biomaterials has turned the attention of researchers to delve into natural fibers as a promising biomaterial. The biocompatibility, easy availability, and abundance of natural fibers have opened the gate of medicine and pharmacology for them. Many novel medical applications are being currently served by the natural fibers, which could diversify and multiply in future.

References

1. Chandramohan, D. and Marimuthu, K. (2011). A review on natural fibers. *International Journal of Research and Reviews in Applied Sciences*, **8**(2), pp. 194–206.

2. Mukhopadhyay, S. and Fangueiro, R. (2009). Physical modification of natural fibers and thermoplastic films for composites: A review. *Journal of Thermoplastic Composite Materials,* **22**(2), pp. 135–162.

3. Joseph, K., Tolêdo Filho, R. D., James, B., Thomas, S., and Carvalho, L. H. D. (1999). A review on sisal fiber reinforced polymer composites. *Revista Brasileira de Engenharia Agrícola e Ambiental*, **3**(3), pp. 367–379.

4. Faruk, O., Bledzki, A. K., Fink, H.-P., and Sain, M. (2012). Biocomposites reinforced with natural fibers: 2000–2010. *Progress in Polymer Science*, **37**(11), pp. 1552–1596.

5. Anandjiwala, R. D. and John, M. (2010). Sisal: Cultivation, processing and products. In *Industrial Applications of Natural Fibres: Structure, Properties and Technical Applications*, pp. 181–195. John Wiley & Sons, Ltd, Chichester, UK.

6. Li, Y., Mai, Y.-W., and Ye, L. (2000). Sisal fibre and its composites: A review of recent developments. *Composites Science and Technology*, **60**(11), pp. 2037–2055.

7. Alam, M. J. and Khatun, A. (2015). Comparison between *Corchorus olitorius* and *Corchorus capsularis* at GUS histochemical assay performance for tissue culture independent transformation. *Journal of Bioscience and Biotechnology*, **4**(2), pp. 201–205.

8. Rahman, M. S. (2010). Jute: A versatile natural fibre. Cultivation, extraction and processing. In *Industrial Applications of Natural Fibres: Structure, Properties and Technical Applications*, pp. 135–161. John Wiley & Sons, Ltd, Chichester, UK.

9. Lewin, M. and Pearce, E. M. (1998). *Handbook of Fiber Chemistry, Revised and Expanded*. CRC Press.

10. Borland, V. (2002). From flower to fabric. In *Textile World*, **152**(10), pp. 52–55.

11. Akin, D. E., Gamble, G. R., Morrison III, W. H., Rigsby, L. L., and Dodd, R. B. (1996). Chemical and structural analysis of fibre and core tissues from flax. *Journal of the Science of Food and Agriculture*, **72**(2), pp. 155–165.

12. Schnegelsberg, G. (1999). *Handbuch der faser: theorie und systematik der faser*: Dt. Fachverl.

13. Jayasekara, C. and Amarasinghe, N. (2010). Coir: Coconut cultivation, extraction and processing of coir. In *Industrial Applications of Natural Fibres: Structure, Properties and Technical Applications*, pp. 197–217. John Wiley & Sons, Ltd, Chichester, UK.

14. Rowell, R. M. (1998). The state of art and future development of bio-based composite science and technology towards the 21st century. In *Proceedings: The fourth Pacific Rim Bio-Based Composite Symposium*, Y. S. Hadi (Ed.), Bogor, Indonesia.

15. Amaducci, S. and Gusovius, H.-J. (2010). Hemp: Cultivation, extraction and processing. In *Industrial Applications of Natural Fibres: Structure, Properties and Technical Applications*, pp. 109–134. John Wiley & Sons, Ltd, Chichester, UK.

16. Franck, R. R. (2005). *Bast and Other Plant Fibres*, Vol. 39. CRC Press.

17. Gorchs, G., Llovers, J., and Comas, J. (2000). Effect of hemp (*Cannabis sativa* L.) in a crop rotation hemp–wheat in the humid cool areas of north-eastern of Spain. Paper presented at the *Proceeding of the Conference: Crop Development for the Cool and Wet Regions of Europe* (COST Action 814), Pordenone, Italy.

18. Goltenboth, F. and Muhlbauer, W. (2010). Abacá: Cultivation, extraction and processing. In *Industrial Applications of Natural Fibres: Structure, Properties and Technical Applications*, pp. 163–179. John Wiley & Sons, Ltd, Chichester, UK.

19. Stevens, C. and Müssig, J. (2010). *Industrial Applications of Natural Fibres: Structure, Properties and Technical Applications*, Vol. 10. John Wiley & Sons, Ltd, Chichester, UK.

20. Kaplan, D. L., Fossey, S., Mello, C. M., Arcidiacono, S., Senecal, K., Muller, W., Stockwell, S., Beckwitt, R., Viney, C., and Kerkam, K. (1992). Biosynthesis and processing of silk proteins. *MRS Bulletin*, **17**(10), pp. 41–47.

21. Ramamoorthy, S. K., Skrifvars, M., and Persson, A. (2015). A review of natural fibers used in biocomposites: Plant, animal and regenerated cellulose fibers. *Polymer Reviews*, **55**(1), pp. 107–162.

22. Akhtar, S., De, P., and De, S. (1986). Short fiber-reinforced thermoplastic elastomers from blends of natural rubber and polyethylene. *Journal of Applied Polymer Science*, **32**(5), pp. 5123–5146.

23. Popescu, C. and Wortmann, F.-J. (2010). Wool: Structure, mechanical properties and technical products based on animal fibres. In *Industrial Applications of Natural Fibres: Structure, Properties and Technical Applications*, pp. 255–266. John Wiley & Sons, Ltd, Chichester, UK.

24. Hoecker, H. and Wortmann, G. (2003). Unconventional uses of wool. IWTO Meeting, Buenos Aires, Argentina.

25. Katoh, K., Shibayama, M., Tanabe, T., and Yamauchi, K. (2004). Preparation and properties of keratin–poly (vinyl alcohol) blend fiber. *Journal of Applied Polymer Science*, **91**(2): 756–762.

26. Zhu, J., Zhu, H., Njuguna, J., and Abhyankar, H. (2013). Recent development of flax fibres and their reinforced composites based on different polymeric matrices. *Materials*, **6**(11), pp. 5171–5198.

27. Koronis, G., Silva, A., and Fontul, M. (2013). Green composites: A review of adequate materials for automotive applications. *Composites Part B: Engineering*, **44**(1), pp. 120–127.

28. Lau, K.-T., Ho, M.-P., Au-Yeung, C.-T., and Cheung, H.-Y. (2010). Biocomposites: Their multifunctionality. *International Journal of Smart and Nano Materials*, **1**(1), pp. 13–27.

29. Satyanarayana, K., Sukumaran, K., Mukherjee, P., Pavithran, C., and Pillai, S. (1990). Natural fibre-polymer composites. *Cement and Concrete Composites*, **12**(2), pp. 117–136.

30. Pavithran, C., Mukherjee, P., Brahmakumar, M., and Damodaran, A. (1987). Impact properties of natural fibre composites. *Journal of Materials Science Letters*, **6**(8), pp. 882–884.

31. Pavithran, C., Mukherjee, P., Brahmakumar, M., and Damodaran, A. (1988). Impact performance of sisal-polyester composites. *Journal of Materials Science Letters*, **7**(8), pp. 825–826.

32. Bhagawan, S., Tripathy, D., and De, S. (1987). Stress relaxation in short jute fiber-reinforced nitrile rubber composites. *Journal of Applied Polymer Science*, **33**(5), pp. 1623–1639.

33. Geethamma, V., Joseph, R., and Thomas, S. (1995). Short coir fiber-reinforced natural rubber composites: Effects of fiber length, orientation, and alkali treatment. *Journal of Applied Polymer Science*, **55**(4), pp. 583–594.

34. Shahzad, A. (2012). Hemp fiber and its composites: A review. *Journal of Composite Materials*, **46**(8), pp. 973–986.

35. Hemp Industry on Global Course of Expansion, Online Referencing, www.jeccomposites.com (2007, accessed October 28, 2016).

36. Bourmaud, A. and Baley, C. (2009). Rigidity analysis of polypropylene/vegetal fibre composites after recycling. *Polymer Degradation and Stability*, **94**(3), pp. 297–305.

37. Xie, Y., Hill, C. A., Xiao, Z., Militz, H., and Mai, C. (2010). Silane coupling agents used for natural fiber/polymer composites: A review. *Composites Part A: Applied Science and Manufacturing*, **41**(7), pp. 806–819.

38. Raftoyiannis, I. G. (2012). Experimental testing of composite panels reinforced with cotton fibers. *Open Journal of Composite Materials*, **2**(2), pp. 31–39.

39. Bledzki, A. and Gassan, J. (1999). Composites reinforced with cellulose based fibres. *Progress in Polymer Science*, **24**(2), pp. 221–274.

40. Oksman, K., Skrifvars, M., and Selin, J.-F. (2003). Natural fibres as reinforcement in polylactic acid (PLA) composites. *Composites Science and Technology,* **63**(9), pp. 1317–1324.

41. Mohanty, A., Misra, M., and Hinrichsen, G. (2000). Biofibres, biodegradable polymers and biocomposites: An overview. *Macromolecular Materials and Engineering,* **276**(1), pp. 1–24.

42. Beckermann, G. and Pickering, K. L. (2008). Engineering and evaluation of hemp fibre reinforced polypropylene composites: Fibre treatment and matrix modification. *Composites Part A: Applied Science and Manufacturing,* **39**(6), pp. 979–988.

43. Graupner, N. (2009). Improvement of the mechanical properties of biodegradable hemp fiber reinforced poly (lactic acid)(PLA) composites by the admixture of man-made cellulose fibers. *Journal of Composite Materials,* **43**(6), pp. 689–702.

44. Bax, B. and Müssig, J. (2008). Impact and tensile properties of PLA/Cordenka and PLA/flax composites. *Composites Science and Technology,* **68**(7), pp. 1601–1607.

45. Yan, L., Chouw, N., and Jayaraman, K. (2014). Flax fibre and its composites: A review. *Composites Part B: Engineering,* **56**, pp. 296–317.

46. Liang, S., Gning, P.-B., and Guillaumat, L. (2012). A comparative study of fatigue behaviour of flax/epoxy and glass/epoxy composites. *Composites Science and Technology,* **72**(5), pp. 535–543.

47. Oksman, K. (2001). High quality flax fibre composites manufactured by the resin transfer moulding process. *Journal of Reinforced Plastics and Composites,* **20**(7), pp. 621–627.

48. Zhu, J., Abhyankar, H., Nassiopoulos, E., and Njuguna, J. (2012). Tannin-based flax fibre reinforced composites for structural applications in vehicles. *IOP Conference Series: Materials Science and Engineering,* **40**.

49. Behera, A. K., Avancha, S., Basak, R. K., Sen, R., and Adhikari, B. (2012). Fabrication and characterizations of biodegradable jute reinforced soy based green composites. *Carbohydrate Polymers,* **88**(1), pp. 329–335.

50. Gopinath, A., Kumar, M. S., and Elayaperumal, A. (2014). Experimental investigations on mechanical properties of jute fiber reinforced composites with polyester and epoxy resin matrices. *Procedia Engineering,* **97**, pp. 2052–2063.

51. Gunti, R., Ratna Prasad, A., and Gupta, A. (2016). Mechanical and degradation properties of natural fiber reinforced PLA composites:

Jute, sisal, and elephant grass. *Polymer Composites.* doi:10.1002/pc.24041

52. Nwaogu, T., Bowman, C., Marquart, H., Postle, M., and Formacare, S. (2013). Analysis of the most appropriate risk management option for formaldehyde, *TNO Triskelion and RPA: A joint report,* pp. 1–151.

53. Rajesh, G. and Prasad, A. V. R. (2014). Tensile properties of successive alkali treated short jute fiber reinforced PLA composites. *Procedia Materials Science,* **5**, pp. 2188–2196.

54. Cheung, H. Y. and Lau, A. K. T. (2007). Mechanical performance of an animal-based silk/polymer bio-composite. *Key Engineering Materials,* **334–335**, pp. 1161–1164.

55. Cheung, H.-Y., Lau, K.-T., Tao, X.-M., and Hui, D. (2008). A potential material for tissue engineering: Silkworm silk/PLA biocomposite. *Composites Part B: Engineering,* **39**(6), pp. 1026–1033.

56. Seves, A., Romanò, M., Maifreni, T., Sora, S., and Ciferri, O. (1998). The microbial degradation of silk: A laboratory investigation. *International Biodeterioration & Biodegradation,* **42**(4), pp. 203–211.

57. Nomura, M., Iwasa, Y., and Araya, H. (1995). Moisture absorbing and desorbing polyurethane foam and its production. *Japan Patent,* JP3502149.

58. Katori, S. and Kimura, T. (2002). Injection moulding of silk fiber reinforced biodegradable composites. *WIT Transactions on The Built Environment,* **59**.

59. Shah, D. U., Porter, D., and Vollrath, F. (2014). Opportunities for silk textiles in reinforced biocomposites: Studying through-thickness compaction behaviour. *Composites Part A: Applied Science and Manufacturing,* **62**, pp. 1–10.

60. De Isla, N., Huseltein, C., Jessel, N., Pinzano, A., Decot, V., Magdalou, J., Bensoussan, D, and Stoltz, J.-F. (2010). Introduction to tissue engineering and application for cartilage engineering. *Bio-medical Materials and Engineering,* **20**(3–4), pp. 127–133.

61. Dhandayuthapani, B., Yoshida, Y., Maekawa, T., and Kumar, D. S. (2011). Polymeric scaffolds in tissue engineering application: A review. *International Journal of Polymer Science,* **2011**, http://dx.doi.org/10.1155/2011/290602.

62. Eaglstein, W. H. and Falanga, V. (1997). Tissue engineering and the development of Apligraf®, a human skin equivalent. *Clinical Therapeutics,* **19**(5), pp. 894–905.

63. Boyan, B. D., Lohmann, C. H., Romero, J., and Schwartz, Z. (1999). Bone and cartilage tissue engineering. *Clinics in Plastic Surgery,* **26**(4), pp. 629–645.

64. Mayer, J., Karamuk, E., Akaike, T., and Wintermantel, E. (2000). Matrices for tissue engineering-scaffold structure for a bioartificial liver support system. *Journal of Controlled Release,* **64**(1), pp. 81–90.

65. Mayer Jr, J. E., Shin'oka, T., and Shum-Tim, D. (1997). Tissue engineering of cardiovascular structures. *Current Opinion in Cardiology,* **12**(6), pp. 528–532.

66. Hutmacher, D. W. (2001). Scaffold design and fabrication technologies for engineering tissues: State of the art and future perspectives. *Journal of Biomaterials Science, Polymer Edition,* **12**(1), pp. 107–124.

67. Jao, D., Mou, X., and Hu, X. (2016). Tissue regeneration: A silk road. *Journal of Functional Biomaterials,* **7**(3), p. 22.

68. Li, C., Vepari, C., Jin, H. J., Kim, H. J., and Kaplan, D. L. (2006). Electrospun silk-BMP-2 scaffolds for bone tissue engineering. *Biomaterials,* **27**(16), pp. 3115–3124.

69. Kim, H. J., Kim, U. J., Kim, H. S., Li, C., Wada, M., Leisk, G. G., and Kaplan, D. L. (2008). Bone tissue engineering with premineralized silk scaffolds. *Bone,* **42**(6), pp. 1226–1234.

70. Zhao, J., Zhang, Z., Wang, S., Sun, X., Zhang, X., Chen, J., and Jiang, X. (2009). Apatite-coated silk fibroin scaffolds to healing mandibular border defects in canines. *Bone,* **45**(3), pp. 517–527.

71. Jiang, X., Zhao, J., Wang, S., Sun, X., Zhang, X., Chen, J., and Zhang, Z. (2009). Mandibular repair in rats with premineralized silk scaffolds and BMP-2-modified bMSCs. *Biomaterials,* **30**(27), pp. 4522–4532.

72. Zhang, H. and Liu, J. (2013). Electrospun poly(lactic-co-glycolic acid)/wool keratin fibrous composite scaffolds potential for bone tissue engineering applications. *Journal of Bioactive and Compatible Polymers,* **28**(2), pp. 141–153.

73. Obata, A., Ozasa, H., Kasuga, T., and Jones, J. R. (2013). Cotton wool-like poly(lactic acid)/vaterite composite scaffolds releasing soluble silica for bone tissue engineering. *Journal of Materials Science: Materials in Medicine,* **24**(7), pp. 1649–1658.

74. Aluigi, A., Sotgiu, G., Torreggiani, A., Guerrini, A., Orlandi, V. T., Corticelli, F., and Varchi, G. (2015). Methylene blue doped films of wool keratin with antimicrobial photodynamic activity. *ACS Applied Materials & Interfaces,* **7**(31), pp. 17416–17424.

75. Wang, Y., Kim, U. J., Blasioli, D. J., Kim, H. J., and Kaplan, D. L. (2005). In vitro cartilage tissue engineering with 3D porous aqueous-derived silk scaffolds and mesenchymal stem cells. *Biomaterials*, **26**(34), pp. 7082–7094.

76. Detterline, A. J., Goldberg, S., Bach Jr, B. R., and Cole, B. J. (2005). Treatment options for articular cartilage defects of the knee. *Orthopaedic Nursing*, **24**(5), pp. 361–366.

77. Mouw, J. K., Case, N. D., Guldberg, R. E., Plaas, A. H. K., and Levenston, M. E. (2005). Variations in matrix composition and GAG fine structure among scaffolds for cartilage tissue engineering. *Osteoarthritis and Cartilage*, **13**(9), pp. 828–836.

78. Hunter, C. J. and Levenston, M. E. (2004). Maturation and integration of tissue-engineered cartilages within an in vitro defect repair model. *Tissue Engineering*, **10**(5–6), pp. 736–746.

79. Yodmuang, S., McNamara, S. L., Nover, A. B., Mandal, B. B., Agarwal, M., Kelly, T. A. N., Chao, P. H., Hung, C., Kaplan, D. L., and Vunjak-Novakovic, G. (2015). Silk microfiber-reinforced silk hydrogel composites for functional cartilage tissue repair. *Acta Biomaterialia*, **11**, pp. 27–36.

80. Mirahmadi, F., Tafazzoli-Shadpour, M., Shokrgozar, M. A., and Bonakdar, S. (2013). Enhanced mechanical properties of thermosensitive chitosan hydrogel by silk fibers for cartilage tissue engineering. *Materials Science and Engineering: C*, **33**(8), pp. 4786–4794.

81. Das, S., Pati, F., Choi, Y. J., Rijal, G., Shim, J. H., Kim, S. W., and Ghosh, S. (2015). Bioprintable, cell-laden silk fibroin–gelatin hydrogel supporting multilineage differentiation of stem cells for fabrication of three-dimensional tissue constructs. *Acta Biomaterialia*, **11**, pp. 233–246.

82. Lawrence, B. D., Marchant, J. K., Pindrus, M. A., Omenetto, F. G., and Kaplan, D. L. (2009). Silk film biomaterials for cornea tissue engineering. *Biomaterials*, **30**(7), pp. 1299–1308.

83. Suzuki, S., Dawson, R. A., Chirila, T. V., Shadforth, A., Hogerheyde, T. A., Edwards, G. A., and Harkin, D. G. (2015). Treatment of silk fibroin with poly(ethylene glycol) for the enhancement of corneal epithelial cell growth. *Journal of Functional Biomaterials*, **6**(2), pp. 345–366.

84. Benfenati, V., Stahl, K., Gomis-Perez, C., Toffanin, S., Sagnella, A., Torp, R., Kaplan, D. L., Ruani, G., Omenetto, F. G., Zamboni, R., and Zamboni, R. (2012). Biofunctional silk/neuron interfaces. *Advanced Functional Materials*, **22**(9), pp. 1871–1884.

85. Vasconcelos, A., Gomes, A. C., and Cavaco-Paulo, A. (2012). Novel silk fibroin/elastin wound dressings. *Acta Biomaterialia*, **8**(8), pp. 3049–3060.
86. Abdulmajeed, A. A., Närhi, T. O., Vallittu, P. K., and Lassila, L. V. (2011). The effect of high fiber fraction on some mechanical properties of unidirectional glass fiber-reinforced composite. *Dental Materials*, **27**(4), pp. 313–321.
87. Profeta, A. C., Mannocci, F., Foxton, R., Watson, T. F., Feitosa, V. P., De Carlo, B., Mongiorgi, R., Valdré, G., and Sauro, S. (2013). Experimental etch-and-rinse adhesives doped with bioactive calcium silicate-based micro-fillers to generate therapeutic resin–dentin interfaces. *Dental Materials*, **29**(7), pp. 729–741.
88. Xu, H. H., Eichmiller, F. C., Antonucci, J. M., Schumacher, G. E., and Ives, L. K. (2000). Dental resin composites containing ceramic whiskers and precured glass ionomer particles. *Dental Materials*, **16**(5), pp. 356–363.
89. Rameshbabu, A. P., Mohanty, S., Bankoti, K., Ghosh, P., and Dhara, S. (2015). Effect of alumina, silk and ceria short fibers in reinforcement of Bis-GMA/TEGDMA dental resin. *Composites Part B: Engineering*, **70**, pp. 238–246.
90. Kock, J. W. (2006). Physical and mechanical properties of chicken feather materials. Masters Theses, Georgia Institute of Technology, May 2006.
91. Unemori, M., Matsuya, Y., Matsuya, S., Akashi, A., and Akamine, A. (2003). Water absorption of poly(methyl methacrylate) containing 4-methacryloxyethyl trimellitic anhydride. *Biomaterials*, **24**(8), pp. 1381–1387.
92. Salehuddin, S. M. F., Wahit, M. U., Kadir, M. R. A., Sulaiman, E., and Kasim, N. H. A. (2014). Mechanical and morphology properties of feather fiber, composite for dental post application. *Malaysian Journal of Analytical Sciences*, **18**(2), pp. 368–375.
93. Turner, T. (1979). Hospital usage of absorbent dressings. *The Pharmaceutical Journal*, **222**, pp. 421–426.
94. Kearns, V., MacIntosh, A., Crawford, A., and Hatton, P. (2008). Silk-based biomaterials for tissue engineering. In *Topics in Tissue Engineering*, N. Ashammakhi, R. Reis, and F. Chiellini (Eds.), Vol 4.
95. Couet, F., Rajan, N., Vesentini, S., and Mantovani, D. (2007). Design of a collagen/silk mechano-compatible composite scaffold for the vascular

tissue engineering: Focus on compliance. *Key Engineering Materials,* **334–335**, pp. 1169–1172.

96. Ha, T. L. B., Quan, T. M., Vu, D. N., Si, D. M., and Andrades, J. A. (2013). Naturally derived biomaterials: Preparation and application. In *Regenerative Medicine and Tissue Engineering,* J. A. Andrades (Ed.), pp. 247–274. InTech.

97. Acharya, C., Kumar, V., Sen, R., and Kundu, S. C. (2008). Performance evaluation of a silk protein-based matrix for the enzymatic conversion of tyrosine to L-DOPA. *Biotechnology Journal,* **3**(2), pp. 226–233.

98. Cherian, B. M., Leão, A. L., de Souza, S. F., Thomas, S., Pothan, L. A., and Kottaisamy, M. (2010). Isolation of nanocellulose from pineapple leaf fibres by steam explosion. *Carbohydrate Polymers,* **81**(3), pp. 720–725.

99. Abbasipour, M., Mirjalili, M., Khajavi, R., and Majidi, M. M. (2014). Coated cotton gauze with Ag/ZnO/chitosan nanocomposite as a modern wound dressing. *Journal of Engineered Fabrics & Fibers,* **9**(1), pp. 124–130.

100. Kanokpanont, S., Damrongsakkul, S., Ratanavaraporn, J., and Aramwit, P. (2012). An innovative bi-layered wound dressing made of silk and gelatin for accelerated wound healing. *International Journal of Pharmaceutics,* **436**(1), pp. 141–153.

101. Schneider, A., Wang, X. Y., Kaplan, D. L., Garlick, J. A., and Egles, C. (2009). Biofunctionalized electrospun silk mats as a topical bioactive dressing for accelerated wound healing. *Acta Biomaterialia,* **5**(7), pp. 2570–2578.

102. Numata, K. and Kaplan, D. L. (2010). Silk-based delivery systems of bioactive molecules. *Advanced Drug Delivery Reviews,* **62**(15), pp. 1497–1508.

103. Meinel, L., Hofmann, S., Karageorgiou, V., Zichner, L., Langer, R., Kaplan, D., and Vunjak-Novakovic, G. (2004). Engineering cartilage-like tissue using human mesenchymal stem cells and silk protein scaffolds. *Biotechnology and Bioengineering,* **88**(3), pp. 379–391.

104. Zaoming, W., Codina, R., Fernandez-Caldas, E., and Lockey, R. F. (1995). Partial characterization of the silk allergens in mulberry silk extract. *Journal of Investigational Allergology & Clinical Immunology,* **6**(4), pp. 237–241.

105. Karageorgiou, V., Tomkins, M., Fajardo, R., Meinel, L., Snyder, B., Wade, K., and Kaplan, D. L. (2006). Porous silk fibroin 3-D scaffolds for delivery of bone morphogenetic protein-2 in vitro and in vivo. *Journal of Biomedical Materials Research Part A,* **78**(2), pp. 324–334.

106. Wilz, A., Pritchard, E. M., Li, T., Lan, J. Q., Kaplan, D. L., and Boison, D. (2008). Silk polymer-based adenosine release: Therapeutic potential for epilepsy. *Biomaterials*, **29**(26), pp. 3609–3616.

107. Uebersax, L., Mattotti, M., Papaloïzos, M., Merkle, H. P., Gander, B., and Meinel, L. (2007). Silk fibroin matrices for the controlled release of nerve growth factor (NGF). *Biomaterials*, **28**(30), pp. 4449–4460.

108. Uebersax, L., Merkle, H. P., and Meinel, L. (2008). Insulin-like growth factor I releasing silk fibroin scaffolds induce chondrogenic differentiation of human mesenchymal stem cells. *Journal of Controlled Release*, **127**(1), pp. 12–21.

109. Mandal, B. B. and Kundu, S. C. (2009). Calcium alginate beads embedded in silk fibroin as 3D dual drug releasing scaffolds. *Biomaterials*, **30**(28), pp. 5170–5177.

110. Gupta, V., Aseh, A., Rios, C. N., Aggarwal, B. B., and Mathur, A. B. (2009). Fabrication and characterization of silk fibroin-derived curcumin nanoparticles for cancer therapy. *International Journal of Nanomedicine*, **4**, pp. 115–122.

111. Hardy, J. G., Leal-Egaña, A., and Scheibel, T. R. (2013). Engineered spider silk protein-based composites for drug delivery. *Macromolecular Bioscience*, **13**(10), pp. 1431–1437.

112. DeMuth, P. C., Min, Y., Irvine, D. J., and Hammond, P. T. (2014). Implantable silk composite microneedles for programmable vaccine release kinetics and enhanced immunogenicity in transcutaneous immunization. *Advanced Healthcare Materials*, **3**(1), pp. 47–58.

113. Elia, R., Newhide, D. R., Pedevillano, P. D., Reiss, G. R., Firpo, M. A., Hsu, E. W., Kaplan, D. L., Prestwich, G. D., and Peattie, R. A. (2013). Silk-hyaluronan-based composite hydrogels: A novel, securable vehicle for drug delivery. *Journal of Biomaterials Applications*, **27**(6), pp. 749–762.

114. Zhang, H., Ma, X., Cao, C., Wang, M., and Zhu, Y. (2014). Multifunctional iron oxide/silk-fibroin (Fe_3O_4–SF) composite microspheres for the delivery of cancer therapeutics. *RSC Advances*, **4**(78), pp. 41572–41577.

115. Subia, B. and Kundu, S. C. (2012). Drug loading and release on tumor cells using silk fibroin–albumin nanoparticles as carriers. *Nanotechnology*, **24**(3), pp. 035103.

116. Zhang, J. (2014). *Keratin Composite Nanofibrous Anti-Tumor Drug Delivery System*, Doctoral dissertation, The Hong Kong Polytechnic University.

117. Hashemikia, S., Hemmatinejad, N., Ahmadi, E., and Montazer, M. (2016). A novel cotton fabric with anti-bacterial and drug delivery properties using SBA-15-NH 2/polysiloxane hybrid containing tetracycline. *Materials Science and Engineering: C*, **59**, pp. 429–437.

118. Hashemikia, S., Hemmatinejad, N., Ahmadi, E., and Montazer, M. (2016). Antibacterial and anti-inflammatory drug delivery properties on cotton fabric using betamethasone-loaded mesoporous silica particles stabilized with chitosan and silicone softener. *Drug Delivery*, **23**(8), pp. 2946–2955.

119. Bennett, I. M. (2013). *Textile Dressing for Drug Delivery: Ascorbic Acid on Cotton Fabric*, Doctoral dissertation, University of Otago.

Chapter 6

Algae-Based Composites and Their Applications

Richa Mehra,[a] Satej Bhushan,[a] Balraj Singh Gill,[a]
Wahid Ul Rehman,[a] and Felix Bast[b]
[a]*Centre for Biosciences, School of Basic and Applied Sciences, Central University of Punjab, Bathinda 151001, India*
[b]*Centre for Plant Sciences, School of Basic and Applied Sciences, Central University of Punjab, Bathinda 151001, India*
r.richamehra@gmail.com

Demand for bio-based products is increasing rapidly because of environmental awareness and dwindling resources. Biocomposites have found their place in market and research owing to their processing advantages, biodegradability, low relative density, high strength, low cost, non-toxicity, and renewability. Algae have an edge, as compared to other natural resources, to be used as composites as they are abundant globally and can be procured as by-products of the biofuel industry. Research is in progress to explore more applications and to address the issues related to biomass and processing techniques. Algae-based composites are seen as the future of the industry with more reduction in costs and better quality in the

---

Biocomposites: Biomedical and Environmental Applications
Edited by Shakeel Ahmed, Saiqa Ikram, Suvardhan Kanchi, and Krishna Bisetty
Copyright © 2018 Pan Stanford Publishing Pte. Ltd.
ISBN 978-981-4774-38-3 (Hardcover), 978-1-315-11080-6 (eBook)
www.panstanford.com

coming years. This chapter highlights the importance of algal fibers over synthetic and natural fibers, processing technique, commercial applications, and future scope of algal biocomposites.

6.1 Introduction

Environmental awareness and stricter laws related to biodegradation of industrial wastes and by-products have resulted in lots of "green" initiatives, which is why synthetic composites are losing credibility globally. Consequentially, biocomposites, defined as composite materials containing at least one natural constituent, have grabbed lots of attention recently due to their renewability, biodegradability, lesser toxicity, and low cost [1]. A plethora of natural resources can be utilized for the synthesis of biocomposites. However, algae stand aside in the competition. Algae represent a major proportion of earth's biodiversity and exhibit considerable variability in terms of structure and composition. In some countries, a few algal species are edible, while in rest of the world, these are still being ignored as "waste" [2, 3]. Besides, several invasive algal species along the coasts are posing threat to marine flora and fauna but can otherwise be exploited for good. Algal biomass can be utilized as either filler or reinforcement fibers. When used as filler, it is not treated, rather milled and pulverized, in order to reduce the overall cost, while as reinforcement fiber, algae are first bleached to get rid of all soluble components and keep cellulosic fibers. For example, bleached red algae fibers (BRAF) admixed with polypropylene (PP), poly(L-lactic acid) (PLLA), and poly(butylene succinate) (PBS) have shown improved thermal and mechanical properties along with better environmental impact [4].

Many industries are exploring alternative means of revenue in addition to those obtained from mainstream products such as biofuels, agar production, paper, and food industry. Various techniques for cultivation, extraction of commercially viable components from algae and synthesis of biocomposites are being explored. Fundamentally, these processes involve two stages: first, wherein algal growth is initiated and second, where the biocomposite-compound accumulation is promoted. Although a number of studies related to the scope of algae as biocomposites are being carried out, most of them are in infancy, hitherto, and have not penetrated the industry yet. However, it is expected that after reaching the industrial scale, it is most likely that they would replace their synthetic counterparts. Possible routes to employ algae-derived monomers for PLLA synthesis are being investigated, while composites containing algae-derived fibers have found their place in the commercial market [5]. Several initiatives such as BRIGIT, INNOBITE, and Coir Kerala Fair for promoting the biocomposites at the global level are being taken with positive impacts at the socio-economic and environment levels.

6.2 Bio-based/Natural Fibers

Fibers originating from natural sources such as plants, animals, or algae are considered natural fibers. These are cheap, renewable, partially or completely recyclable, and biodegradable. The history of utilization of natural fibers dates back to around 8000 BC. For example, hemp and linen textiles are reported to exist in Europe around 4000 BC. Likewise, ramie has been reportedly used in Egypt for mummy cloths during 5000–3300 BC. Cotton fibers were discovered in Mexico caves dating back over 7000 years [6]. However, plants have always remained as the source of natural fibers apart from exhibiting medicinal properties [7]. In 21st century, with the advancement in science and technology and environment awareness, it is known to all that non-renewable resources are getting scarce and the burden on frequently used renewable resources is also increasing. Thus, overall interest is shifting toward alternative sources of natural fibers such as algae.

Natural fibers are classified mostly on the basis of their source of origin. They can be obtained from plant, animal, and marine sources [8]. Plant fibers can be obtained from either wood or non-wood sources and can be further separated into stem/bast, leaf, seed, core, grass/reed, and other types, including wood and root. Animal fibers, more appropriately called protein-based fibers, are obtained from wool or hairs, feathers, and cocoons. Marine fibers are obtained from marine organisms such as algae, sponges, and jellyfish. The schematic classification of natural fibers is shown in Fig. 6.1.

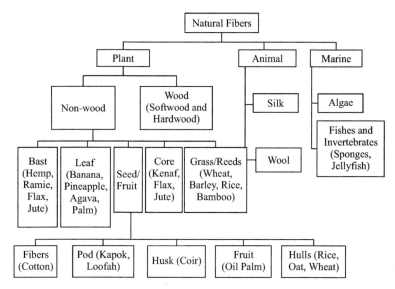

Figure 6.1 Schematic diagram for classification of natural fibers.

Natural/bio-based fibers are preferred choice over synthetic fibers for commercial applications. Biocomposites represent a potentially more reliable, environment friendly, and value-added source of income in the agriculture sector. India accounts for more than 20% of the world's total coir production; jute is also produced majorly by India and Bangladesh; sisal is extensively grown in tropical countries with Tanzania and Brazil being the main producers; kenaf originated from the United States and ramie fibers from China, Malaysia, and Japan. Most of the synthetic plastics cannot withstand load-bearing applications by themselves due to their insufficient strength, dimensional stability, and stiffness. On the contrary, natural fibers are known for high strength and stiffness but cannot be directly used in load-bearing functions. Thus, the concept of hybrid composites originated where fiber-reinforced composites are produced with plastic serving as the matrix and fibers serving as reinforcement material, proving overall strength and stiffness for load-bearing applications.

6.2.1 Algal versus Other Natural and Synthetic Fibers

Biocomposites use natural fibers as the major constituent, and the source of these natural fibers ranges from cereals to fruits such as banana and perennial grasses such as sugarcane. Nowadays, marine algae have gained much attention as the source of natural fibers in biocomposites. In some comparative studies, algae have even been observed to be more promising than cotton linters, plant wood fibers, and other natural fibers. Algal fibers have shown to possess more rigidity, higher thermal degradation temperatures [9] as compared to other natural fibers. Various algal taxa, such as *Gelidium*, *Cladophora*, *Gracilaria*, *Zostera*, and *Lyngbya*, have been reported to have the potential to be used as biocomposite constituent fibers. Some of the distinct algal taxa and their potential applications are summarized in Table 6.1.

Table 6.1 Algal species and their proven applications as biocomposites

Algal Species	Applications
Gelidium sesquipedale	Fillers in soy protein isolate (SPI) biocomposites
Cladophora	Drug carriers, reinforcement material in polyurethane foams
Ulva armoricana	Thermoplastic composites
Jania rubens	Biosorption of heavy metals
Sargassum swartzii	Removal of crystal violet from aqueous solutions
Nannochloropsis salina	PVA fabrication
Gelidium amansii and *Gelidium corneum*	Paper making
Gelidium elegance	Reinforcement material in PBS composites

6.2.2 Algal Constituents as Biocomposite Candidate

6.2.2.1 Alginate

Alginate is a linear anionic polysaccharide found in the cell walls of brown algae and *Pseudomonas aeruginosa* (pathogenic) biofilms. It consists of β-D-mannuronic acid (M blocks) and α-L-guluronic acid (G blocks), which can be joined either as (1→4)-linked homopolymers of G blocks or (1→4)-linked homopolymers of M blocks or (1→4)-linked alternating M and G blocks. Alginates with high G content are industrially more important. The most common form of alginate in industries is sodium alginate as it is the first by-product obtained during algal purification. Alginates have various industrial applications ranging from manufacturing of ceramics, textile printing, stabilization, gel formation to viscosification. Recent researches have shown that alginates can be effective against obesity, and currently many functional alginates are in human clinical trials.

6.2.2.2 Cellulose

Cellulose, the most abundant polymer on earth, is a polysaccharide found in the cell walls of many plant and algal species. It is a linear polymer of $\beta(1{\rightarrow}4)$-linked D-glucose units. The most common raw materials for the synthesis of cellulosic bio-plastic are cotton fibers and wood. Algae such as *Cladophora* and many red algae are the recent choice of raw material owing to their better physical and mechanical parameters. Cellulosic polymers are produced by chemical modifications of cellulose and are further employed for various applications. Three main classes of cellulosic polymers are cellulose esters such as cellulose acetate and cellulose nitrate (film and fiber applications); cellulose ethers such as hydroxyethyl cellulose and carboxymethyl cellulose (food, construction, personal care, pharmaceuticals, and paint); and regenerated cellulose (textiles, home furnishing, and hygienic disposables).

6.2.2.3 Agar

Agar is a jelly like substance composed of a mixture of agarose (linear polysaccharide) and agropectin (heterogenous mixture of smaller molecules). Chemically, agar is made up of β-D-galactopyranosyl-linked (1→4) 3,6-anhydro-α-L-galatopyranosyl. It is found abundantly in the cell walls of many red algae such as *Gracilaria* spp. and *Gelidium* spp. These algae are commonly known as agarophytes. Traditionally, agar has been used as a gelling agent in the food industry and as a solid substrate in culture media. More recently, agar has been approved to be used in packaging materials such as films, foams, and coatings; as additives in biopolymers for better mechanical and water barrier properties and in nanocomposite films with promising results [10].

6.2.2.4 Carrageenan

Carrageenans include a family of water-soluble, linear sulfated polysaccharides extracted from red algae. Carrageenan is a copolymer of alternating units of α-(1→3)-D-galactose and β-(1→4)-3,6-anhydro-D- or L-galactose. It has three isomers: κ, λ, and ι-carrageenans; differing in the degree of sulfation of the galactose units with κ having one, ι having two, and λ having three sulfate groups per disaccharide. κ and ι-carrageenans, because of their lower level of sulfation, exhibit excellent film-forming properties. Also, κ-carrageenan has been tested in combination with chitosan and turned out to be having good tensile strength, elongation property, and water vapor permeability, making them suitable for the biocomposite industry [11].

6.3 Synthesis of Biocomposites

6.3.1 Algae Culture

Algae are simple photosynthetic organisms ranging from microscopic species (microalgae) to large seaweeds (macroalgae). They can be cultured on land, in ponds, in specialized bioreactors, or in near-shore open systems. They are fast growing and reproduce very fast in comparison to plants. The concentration of cells in culture systems is usually high as compared to natural conditions. Thus, cultures are enriched with nutrients to fulfil their nutritional requirements. Media formulations such as Walne medium, Guillard's Fl_2 medium can be used for laboratory or commercial culturing [12, 13]. Other important parameters for the growth of algae include light (1000–10,000 lux depending on the depth and density of culture), pH (7–9), temperature (20–24°C), salinity (20–24 g/L), sufficient aeration and mixing to prevent sedimentation of algae and for proper supply of nutrients and light exposure.

6.3.2 Extraction of Algal Fiber

The extraction of algae generally recommended for the paper and pulp industry involves sequential steps of chemical treatments to obtain high yields of cellulose fibers. The procedure is divided into two major steps: (a) Kraft cooking and (b) multistage bleaching. The commonly used reagents for bleaching are chlorine dioxide (ClO_2), sodium hydroxide (NaOH), and hydrogen peroxide (H_2O_2) diluted at varying concentrations with distilled water [2]. The multistage process of bleaching includes immersion of algae in bleaching agent and distilled water mixture with intermittent stirring at the designated temperatures followed by straining of algae fibers and thorough washing of algae fibers with distilled water. The outline of the extraction process is depicted in Fig. 6.2.

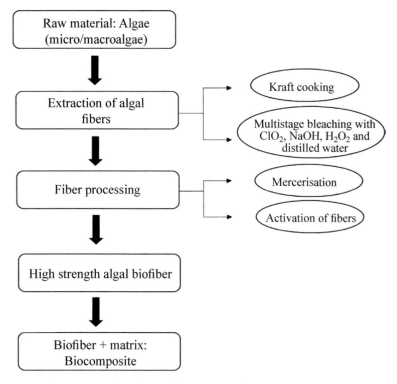

Figure 6.2 Layout of synthesis of biocomposite from algal biomass.

6.3.3 Natural Fiber Processing

Natural fibers are processed to enhance the fiber strength, facilitate handling, and endure the downstream processing equipment such as looms. When used as reinforcement fiber, two types of treatments are given, first to improve the wet-out using resins and the second to improve the fiber-matrix interfacial bond. In the wet-out treatment, atmospheric moisture is reduced through an alkaline treatment, called mercerization, which modifies the cellulose chain and thus reduces its ability to entice moisture that can otherwise create voids in the final product. Mercerization results in the swelling of fibers and increases the amount of type II cellulose fibers. The second treatment partially coincides with the first one since alkaline treatment, besides making the fibers more hydrophobic, strengthens their bond with thermosetting resins. After mercerization, fibers are commonly treated with silane and maleated polyolefins for activation of fibers [14]. However, many of these treatments reduce the fiber strength to some extent but result in an overall net increase in biocomposite strength, highlighting the significance of analyzing the biocomposite as a whole entity.

For processing, algal fibers are thoroughly dried and crushed, dissociating the fibers at 5000–10,000 rpm for around 100 s at 70–100°C. The crushed material is then sieved to collect fine fibers. These fibers are mixed with molten polymeric agents such as PBS, poly(lactic acid) (PLA), or polycarprolactone (PCL) and the temperature is elevated at the rate of 5°C/min up to 200°C for 25–20 min. After this retention period, compression molding is done at 1000 psi for 3–15 min followed by cooling at room temperature. The molded biocomposite is later separated from the mold [15].

6.4 Applications of Algae-Based Composites

The global market of algae-based products is expected to grow in the next decade. In the United States alone, growing demand for clean fuels and biodiesels bears immense opportunities for algae. Likewise, the global trend is shifting toward the utilization of biofuel obtained from algae. At present, there is negligible viable application of algal residues generated from the biofuel industry. However, biocomposite synthesis can exploit this waste for good (Fig. 6.3).

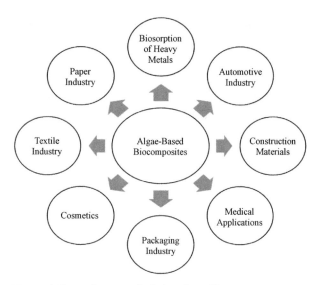

Figure 6.3 Multifaceted potential of algae-based biocomposites.

6.4.1 Biosorption of Heavy Metals

Algae–silica-based biocomposites, biocers, prepared using the sol–gel technique are reported to exhibit ability for biosorption of heavy metals. These biocers retained mechanical stability up to 30–50% algal content and 40–60% porosity [16]. Different micro- and macroalgae can be immobilized within the silica nanosols keeping in mind the stability of the granules in water. Using relatively inexpensive commercially available nanosols such as Nyacol can result in the cost-effective production of biocers, which is a promising technique to integrate biocers with the conventional water treatment plants.

6.4.2 Automotive Industry

Algae have proven potential to be used as biocomposites in the automotive industry, with comparable density and tensile strength with the routinely used fibers in the industry, such as sisal, jute, and flax. Besides additional advantages of lower cost and density, *Lyngbya* fibers have shown to exhibit 10% lower specific tensile strength than jute fibers and 40% higher specific modulus than sisal fibers [2]. Biocomposites are already being used by the automotive industry in European countries for their environmental impacts. Biocomposites in the automotive industry have twofold advantage of reduction in waste disposal and better fuel efficiency. Germany is leading the use of biocomposites where auto manufacturers—BMW, Mercedes, Volkswagen, and Audi—have introduced natural fiber-based composites for interior and exterior applications. Ecobasic, a small prototype car by Fiat, had been developed, which consumes 3 liters fuel per 100 km [17].

6.4.3 Construction Materials

Algae fibrils from *Cladophora*, *Lyngbya*, and *Gelidium* are suggested to be used as structural components in construction materials such as hurricane-resistant houses, door panels, and armrests. Cellulose fibers are inexpensive, abundant, and compatible with composite materials such as polyurethanes. The surface hydroxyl groups of cellulose fibers covalently bond with polyurethane matrix and thus improve the elastic modulus, increase thermal resistance, and impact strength resulting in better biodegradability and lowered cost [18]. These natural fibers generally reduce the stress load and increase the toughness of composites by absorbing energy at the time of debonding and cracks. Johnson and Shiv Kumar have also suggested the use of *Cladophora* fibrils as reinforcement material in polyurethane foams [19].

6.4.4 Medical Applications

Natural products are highly endorsed with myriad therapeutics effect modulating cancer signaling, having an edge of specificity, without detrimental effects [20]. Algae themselves possess various bioactivities such as immuno-modulatory, antiherpetic, antibacterial, antidiabetic, antioxidant, and anticancer. Besides these bioactivities, algae have other promising applications in biomedical industry, such as drug carriers, bone tissue engineering, and wound dressing. Alginate-based microspheres, in combination with suitable compounds to improve stability, have been tested as drug carriers for oral controlled-release system and are considered a better alternative to MCC (microcrystalline cellulose)-based drug carriers

[21]. *Cladophora* cellulose has been proved as a promising candidate for even liquid drugs, for example, nicotine. The stability tests for nicotine with drug carriers revealed that it remained almost intact with 0.9% degradation inside *Cladophora* cellulose in comparison to 23.6% degradation in MCC blends [22]. Chitosan–alginate–fucoidan (Chi-Alg-fucoidan) has been suggested as a biomaterial for artificial bone scaffolds with 56–437 μm, respectively. In vitro studies with MG-63 (human osteosarcoma) cell line have revealed their cytocompatibility, enhanced cell proliferation, and increased alkaline phosphatase secretion capabilities, thus presenting Chi-Alg-fucoidan as a promising candidate for bone tissue regeneration [23]. Also, sodium alginate, extracted from brown algae, has been studied for its potential as wound dressings owing to its biocompatibility and non-toxic nature [24].

6.4.5 Packaging Industry

Recent trends in this era of bioplastics have shifted toward the use of algae for the production of plastic formulations and polymer production. For example, polyhydroxyalkanoate (PHA) polymers and some grades of poly-3-hydroxybutyrate (PHB) have comparable properties to polypropylene (PP) and exhibit moisture resistance and aroma barrier characteristics. Besides these, PHA has the following features: insolubility in water and relatively resistant to hydrolytic degradation than PHB, solubility in chlorinated hydrocarbons such as chloroform, UV resistance, poorly resistant to acids and bases, sinks in water and thus anaerobically biodegradable, non-toxicity and biocompatibility, less sticky on melting as compared to other traditional polymers, making it a better alternative [5].

6.4.6 Cosmetics

Chitin extracted from calcified algal species serves as an active ingredient in cosmetic products. It has been proved that chitin-nanofibrils (CNs) embedded with antioxidant agents (melatonin, ectoin, or lutein) improved their penetration through skin layers, thus can be used in antiaging and antiwrinkle products. Test analyses have revealed tolerance for CN, absence of erythema, and improved skin-barrier system. These biocomposites are used in a range of skin care (lotions, creams, make-up, and nail lacquers), hair care (hair sprays, shampoos, and hair colors), and oral care (toothpaste, chewing gums, and mouthwashes) products. CNs are also used in cosmetic dermatology because of their backbone similarity with hyaluronic acids that can be metabolized by endogenous enzymes [25]. Besides, alginates and agar from red and brown seaweeds are used as thickener and stabilizers in cosmetics by industries such as American Agar Company and FMC BioPolymer.

6.4.7 Textiles

Textile manufacturers are now fond of "smart textiles" exhibiting properties such as heating fabrics, shielding of electromagnetic radiations, transfer of signals, and piezoelectric fibers. Research is in progress for application of nanocomposites in textiles to impart them antibacterial, self-cleaning, and UV-blocking properties [26]. Besides, algae such as *Caulerpa lentillifera* have been exploited to develop eco-friendly textile dyes in conjunction with mordants. These dyes fall in good to excellent ratings as per MS ISO standard for fastness and color strength properties except for light fastness, which still needs to be improved [27].

6.4.8 Paper Industry

Global warming and restrictions on tree cutting, globally, have resulted in difficulties for the paper industry at the global level because wood serves as the primary raw material. Consequently, interests are shifting toward alternative fiber-based products such as algae. Countries such as China, Japan, Philippines, and Korea are following aquaculture at the commercial scale. *Gracilariopsis lemaneiformis*, for example, is used in farming, producing million tonnes of algae annually, which is primarily used for agar extraction, while the residues are indiscriminately discharged into the sea or other waterbodies. Interestingly, these agar residues have fiber-like constituents that have been explored for their use in paper making as a fiber source or functional filler. The evaluation of the hand-sheet samples when the algal material was used as a partial substitute for wood pulp revealed that the paper exhibits waterproof, greaseproof, and antimicrobial properties in addition to improved paper density [28].

6.5 Challenges and Future Prospects

Biocomposites are not a novel concept anymore and are being used at the industrial scale for over a decade now. From offering a huge market of non-food products from crop-derived components to contributing in cosmetics, paper, healthcare products, biocomposites have proven significantly important to mankind. The current industries are looking for bio-based alternatives to the already existing synthetic monomers and polymers, for instance, new grades of PLA introduced by Nature Works, having higher mechanical and thermal properties. However, major challenges faced by biocomposite industries include raw material management, performance, efficiency, and cost of production [29]. Keeping in mind the lack of experience of the relatively newer techniques and uncertainty of demand/supply balance, it would not be feasible to build large-scale plants at this point of time. For the economic viability of this industry, it would be just to develop (a) biomass logistics, (b) cheaper alternative techniques for extraction of bio-components, and (c) efficient recovery methods and downstream processing [30].

There are no doubts that the global demand for food and energy is going to increase with the ever-increasing rates of growing population and biocomposites would be serving as safer and efficient alternatives to their synthetic counterparts. Algae-based biocomposites are definitely going to reduce the burden from plants as sources of biocomposite fibers. There are several technologies in the pipeline, exploring alternative synthesis pathways and exploring many more applications of biocomposites. In addition, tailoring their properties by suitable physical and chemical changes and alternating processing parameters can also improve their efficiency. Thus, identifying the major areas of applications, synthesizing prototypes, and fabricating beneficial products need to be investigated further in order to overcome the global demands and environmental issues.

Acknowledgments

All the Authors thank Vice Chancellor, Central University of Punjab, Bathinda (India) for providing infrastructural support. RM acknowledges ICMR for providing financial support as JRF. SB thanks MoES for financial assistance as JRF.

References

1. Fowler, P. A., J. M. Hughes, and R. M. Elias. (2006). Biocomposites: Technology, environmental credentials and market forces. *J. Sci. Food Agr.*, **86**(12): 1781–1789.
2. Constante, A., S. Pillay, H. Ning, and U. K. Vaidya. (2015). Utilization of algae blooms as a source of natural fibers for biocomposite materials: Study of morphology and mechanical performance of Lyngbya fibers. *Algal Res.*, **12**: 412–420.
3. Toro, C., M. M. Reddy, R. Navia, M. Rivas, M. Misra, and A. K. Mohanty. (2013). Characterization and application in biocomposites of residual microalgal biomass generated in third generation biodiesel. *J. Polym. Environ.*, **21**(4): 944–951.
4. Sim, K. J., S. O. Han, and Y. B. Seo. (2010). Dynamic mechanical and thermal properties of red algae fiber reinforced poly(lactic acid) biocomposites. *Macromol. Res.*, **18**(5): 489–495.
5. Bugnicourt, E., P. Cinelli, A. Lazzeri, and V. A. Alvarez. (2014). Polyhydroxyalkanoate (PHA): Review of synthesis, characteristics, processing and potential applications in packaging. *Express Polym. Lett.*, **8**(11): 791–808.
6. Pickering, K. (2008). *Properties and Performance of Natural-Fibre Composites*. Woodhead Publishing, Cambridge.
7. Gill, B. S. and S. Kumar. (2016). Triterpenes in cancer: Significance and their influence. *Mol. Biol. Rep.*, **43**(9): 881–896.
8. Biagiotti, J., D. Puglia, and J. M. Kenny. (2004). A review on natural fibre-based composites-part I: Structure, processing and properties of vegetable fibres. *J. Nat. Fibers*, **1**(2): 37–68.
9. Hai, L. V., Son, H. N., and Seo, Y. B. (2015). Physical and bio-composite properties of nanocrystalline cellulose from wood, cotton linters, cattail, and red algae. *Cellulose*, **22**(3): 1789–1798.
10. Rhim, J.-W. (2011). Effect of clay contents on mechanical and water vapor barrier properties of agar-based nanocomposite films. *Carbohyd. Polym.*, **86**(2): 691–699.
11. Park, S. Y., B. I. Lee, S. T. Jung, and H. J. Park. (2001). Biopolymer composite films based on κ-carrageenan and chitosan. *Mater. Res. Bull.*, **36**(3): 511–519.
12. Azma, M., M. S. Mohamed, R. Mohamad, R. A. Rahim, and A. B. Ariff. (2011). Improvement of medium composition for heterotrophic cultivation of green microalgae, *Tetraselmis suecica*, using response surface methodology. *Biochem. Eng. J.*, **53**(2): 187–195.

13. Roleda, M. Y., S. P. Slocombe, R. J. Leakey, J. G. Day, E. M. Bell, and M. S. Stanley. (2013). Effects of temperature and nutrient regimes on biomass and lipid production by six oleaginous microalgae in batch culture employing a two-phase cultivation strategy. *Bioresource Technol.*, **129**: 439–449.

14. Sobczak, L., O. Brüggemann, and R. Putz. (2013). Polyolefin composites with natural fibers and wood-modification of the fiber/filler–matrix interaction. *J. Appl. Polym. Sci.*, **127**(1): 1–17.

15. Han, S.-O., H.-S. Kim, Y. J. Yoo, Y. B. Seo, and M. W. Lee. (2007). Algae fiber-reinforced bicomposite and method for preparing the same. Google Patents, US 20090197994 A1.

16. Ulrich, S., M. Sabine, K. Gunter, P. Wolfgang, and B. Horst. (2010). Algae-silica hybrid materials for biosorption of heavy metals. *J. Water Resource Prot.*, **2**(2): 115–122.

17. Puglia, D., J. Biagiotti, and J. Kenny. (2005). A review on natural fibre-based composites—Part II: Application of natural reinforcements in composite materials for automotive industry. *J. Nat. Fibers*, **1**(3): 23–65.

18. Pavlik, R. (2011). *From the Protean to the Systematized: The Development of Novel Construction Methods Utilizing Bio-based Polymer Composite Materials*, Master's Thesis, Harvard University Graduate School of Design.

19. Johnson, M. and S. Shivkumar. (2004). Filamentous green algae additions to isocyanate based foams. *J. Appl. Polym. Sci.*, **93**(5): 2469–2477.

20. Gill, B. S. and S. Kumar. (2016). Ganoderic acid targeting multiple receptors in cancer: In silico and in vitro study. *Tumor Biol.*, **37**(10): 14271–14290.

21. Remminghorst, U. (2007). Polymerisation and export of alginate in *Pseudomanas aeruginosa*: Functional assignment and catalytic mechanism of Alg8/44: A thesis presented to Massey University in partial fulfilment of the requirement for the degree of Doctor of Philosophy in Microbiology, Department of Microbiology, Massey University, New Zealand.

22. Mihranyan, A. (2011). Cellulose from Cladophorales green algae: From environmental problem to high-tech composite materials. *J. Appl. Polym. Sci.*, **119**(4): 2449–2460.

23. Venkatesan, J., I. Bhatnagar, and S.-K. Kim. (2014). Chitosan-alginate biocomposite containing fucoidan for bone tissue engineering. *Mar. Drugs*, **12**(1): 300–316.
24. De Moraes, M. A. and M. M. Beppu. (2013). Biocomposite membranes of sodium alginate and silk fibroin fibers for biomedical applications. *J. Appl. Polym. Sci.*, **130**(5): 3451–3457.
25. Hamed, I., F. Özogul, and J. M. Regenstein. (2016). Industrial applications of crustacean by-products (chitin, chitosan, and chitooligosaccharides): A review. *Trends Food Sci. Tech.*, **48**: 40–50.
26. El-Rafie, H., M. El-Rafie, and M. Zahran. (2013). Green synthesis of silver nanoparticles using polysaccharides extracted from marine macro algae. *Carbohyd. Pol.*, **96**(2): 403–410.
27. Ab Kadir, M., W. W. Ahmad, M. Ahmad, M. Misnon, W. Ruznan, H. Abdul Jabbar, K. Ngalib, and A. Ismail. (2014). Utilization of eco-colourant from green seaweed on textile dyeing. In: Ahmad M., Yahya M. (Eds.), *Proceedings of the International Colloquium in Textile Engineering, Fashion, Apparel and Design 2014 (ICTEFAD 2014)*. Springer, Singapore.
28. Pei, J., A. Lin, F. Zhang, D. Zhu, J. Li, and G. Wang. (2013). Using agar extraction waste of *Gracilaria lemaneiformis* in the papermaking industry. *J. Appl. Phycol.*, **25**(4): 1135–1141.
29. Sahari, J. and S. Sapuan. (2011). Natural fibre reinforced biodegradable polymer composites. *Rev. Adv. Mater. Sci.*, **30**(2): 166–174.
30. Babu, R. P., K. O'Connor, and R. Seeram. (2013). Current progress on bio-based polymers and their future trends. *Prog. Biomater.*, **2**(1): 1–16.

Chapter 7

Going Green Using *Colocasia esculenta* Starch and Starch Nanocrystals in Food Packaging

Bruce Saunders Chakara and Shalini Singh
*Department of Operations and Quality Management, Durban University of Technology,
P.O. Box 1334, Durban 4001, South Africa*
shalinis@dut.ac.za

Pollution from food packaging has become a major problem in the well-being of fauna and flora, resulting in initiatives to replace conventional raw materials with natural options. Selected synthetic and natural raw materials have been presented in this review of food-packaging materials. Of particular focus is starch derived from *Colocasia esculenta*, an underutilized root crop of the *Araceae acroideae* family. It is grown in the tropical regions, and the corms are believed to contain a substantial quantity of starch (70–80% dry *C. esculenta*), but it also varies depending on the location where it was cultivated. Biodegradable *C. esculenta* starch nanocrystals are presented and characterized using SEM and TEM. *C. esculenta* starch-based film, reinforced with starch nanocrystals for improved

---

Biocomposites: Biomedical and Environmental Applications
Edited by Shakeel Ahmed, Saiqa Ikram, Suvardhan Kanchi, and Krishna Bisetty
Copyright © 2018 Pan Stanford Publishing Pte. Ltd.
ISBN 978-981-4774-38-3 (Hardcover), 978-1-315-11080-6 (eBook)
www.panstanford.com

tensile strength, water and oxygen barrier properties and sorbitol as a plasticizer was demonstrated. Economic value can be added to *C. esculenta* by the mass production of environmentally friendly biodegradable starch based biofilm reinforced with sorbitol and starch nanocrystals. By doing so, the environmental impact from food-packaging waste is reduced.

7.1 Introduction

Polymeric materials developed in the past century have proved to be robust and inert in the nature. Despite the presence of varying environmental factors, these materials have been consistent and durable, thus resulting in their long-term performance. Nevertheless, in light of the existing importance on environmental contamination challenges combined with the scarcity of land to dump rubbish, there is now a major rise in the need for eco-friendly biodegradable polymers [1–3]. In spite of the numerous advances in these packaging materials to promote their reuse and recycling, the entire processes give off toxic residues or gases, which further pollute the environment [2]. This, however, poses a contradiction and a major setback to the concept of going green and preserving the environment. As such industries have evolved food packaging to an extent that it fully serves the function of preserving food and also can be recycled at the end of its life cycle without an adverse effect on the environment. This chapter will review current food-packaging materials and outline their strengths and weaknesses with a view to draw on possible opportunities of fully biodegradable material sources.

7.2 Food Packaging

The packaging sector represents about 2% of the gross national product (GNP) in developed countries, and about half of all packaging produced is used to package food [4]. Food packaging is mainly used to cover the food and predominantly acts as a barrier that protects food products from external influences. It also serves as a platform where consumers can get the nutritional composition and ingredients information of the product. Coles et al. [5] and Marsh and

Bugusu [6] add that food packaging has multifaceted duties, some of which are to provide food containment, protection, preservation, convenience, presentation, brand communication, promotion (from a marketing perspective), economy and environmental responsibility. Significantly, at the end of packaging life, the industry typically focuses on reuse and recycling, while very little focus is regarded to the end of life and to the final disposal of packaging material and its effects on the landfill site and the environment.

Notwithstanding the safeguards offered by food packaging, it in itself can as well be a source of chemical food contagion. The coating surface that touches the food product is termed "food contact material." Numerous forms of food contact materials are generally used, each with unrelated properties. Generally, any food contact material ought not to emit chemicals into the food at magnitudes that can cause any impairment to human health [7, 8]. Food-packaging materials are typically made from glass, metal, paper, and a large range of polymeric (plastic) materials or combinations of these as laminates or coated products [5, 9].

7.2.1 Conventional Synthetic Packaging

Glass packaging has been used for a variety of food products because it is chemically inert and odorless, rendering an advantage as it does not react with food. Glass maintains the food products' original state as it is impermeable to vapor or gases, thus preserving the product for an extended period without any alterations in the flavor or taste. Once set and tempered correctly, glass can withstand processing temperatures and this makes it ideal for heat sterilized products of any pH range in foods. Glass is used to offer insulation and can be molded into any shape due its rigid nature. Its transparency allows consumers to inspect the product and can be colored in order to protect products that are sensitive to light. Although it is recyclable and reusable, it is not biodegradable. It is brittle and prone to breakages from either strong impact or thermal shock, thus hindering the efforts to make it thinner and lighter [5, 6].

Metal packaging is one of the most adaptable materials of all. It has impeccable tensile strength and provides exceptional barrier properties when it comes to light, foods, and liquids. The two leading sources used in food packaging are aluminum (Al) and steel. Aluminum is low in density, while steel is high in density. They are both rigid, and Al has an added advantage over steel of being malleable depending on the intended use and focus. Al is silvery white and, due to its reactive nature, exists as aluminum oxide (Al_2O_3) and is used in the forging of Al cans, Al foil, and laminated plastic and paper packaging. Its main disadvantage is that it is very expensive when compared to other metals and it cannot be welded, thus rendering it useful only when creating seamless containers [5, 10]. **Steel**, on the other hand, is used on the making of tinplate and tin-free steel. **Tinplate** is made by dipping low carbon steel sheets into liquefied tin and thus providing an inert barrier between the metal the product. It can withstand high temperatures, making it ideal for pasteurization, retorting, and hermetically sealing. The tinplate is mainly used in the making of beverage cans, processed foodstuffs, and packaging for powdered foods. **Tin-free steel** is made by coating steel with chrome or chrome oxide, and despite making it incompatible to weld, it provides a surface that is excellent for adhesion of dyes, varnishes, and inks. It is slightly less costly than tinplate. Tin-free steel is used to make big vessels for bulk storage [11] and cans for food, bottle caps, trays, and can ends [5, 6]. The nature of the metal packaging is ideal because of its durability and resistance to degradation, but this, in the long term, is detrimental to the environment as it causes pollution, considering that metal is not biodegradable.

Paper and paperboard have been used as packaging since the 17th century. Paper originates from cellulose fibers derived from wood, which is chemically treated to give the ideal final product. The materials are low in density, thus being favored, but they provide poor barrier properties to light, liquids, gases, and vapors. This is counteracted by coating, lamination, or wrapping the paper by sulfate, sulfite, plastic, or acid depending on the use. Examples of treated paper are kraft, sulfite, greaseproof, glassine, and parchment paper. The main difference between paper and paperboard is that paperboard is heavier since it is made of several layers, which provides better stiffness properties. Examples are whiteboard, solid board used for cartons, chipboard used to make cereal boxes, and fiberboard used for transporting bulk food and case packing. Paper and paperboard can both be resilient to grease and penetrable to liquids and vapors. They can be creased, folded, glued, and can also tear easily. It might not be brittle and does not provide as much tensile strength as metal. Looking at the properties of paper and paperboard packaging, it still lacks the features of plastic, the most popular packaging material. This gives rise to **paper laminates** with improved properties such as being able to be heat sealed with better gas and liquid barrier properties.

Plastic packaging possesses an eclectic collection of properties, some of which are permeability to gases and vapors at variable temperatures. The density of the material is very low, and it provides a vast range of optical and physical properties. The tensile and tear strengths are flexible, and the rigidity is usually low. Despite being transparent, they can be colored just like glass. Depending on the treatment, plastic can be used over a wide range of temperatures; it is flexible when need be and can be creased. Conventional synthetic packaging has always been petrochemical based, for example, polyethylene terephthalate (PET), polyvinylchloride (PVC), polyethylene (PE), polypropylene (PP), polystyrene (PS), and polyamide (PA), to mention a few [7]. These have always been used due to their exceptional properties such as tensile and tear strengths, O_2 barrier, CO_2, anhydride and odor compound, and ability to be heat sealed [2, 12]. The downfall of all these plastics is their inability to easily degrade, arousing poignancy due to a lack of control and its high volumes of pollution.

7.2.2 Biofilms, Edible Films, and Coatings

The word "biodegradable" is used to define constituents that can be broken down completely with the aid of enzymatic action, for instance bacteria, yeasts, and fungi, resulting eventually at the end with CO_2, H_2O, and biomass under aerobic conditions and hydrocarbons, methane and biomass under anaerobic conditions [1, 13]. Biodegradable, however, does not mean compostable since compostable materials belong to a subgroup of biodegradable products that are biologically decomposed under composting conditions within a short period of a composting cycle [14, 15].

Composting is defined as the conversion of organic constituents into soil-like steady produce by thermophilic microorganisms naturally through an aerobic biochemical process [16, 17]. Plastic packaging materials are at the forefront of packaging materials, typically because of their toughness and flexibility, but this also makes them hard to deteriorate. As a result when consumers discard the packaging from their products, some materials break down into miniscule particles, while the rest remains intact, thus causing pollution. This pollution affects a continuum of areas from land and sea. As a result of swift industrial development and automation of the packaging sector, the mortality of animals has also increased. A survey carried out at an abattoir in Sudan showed that 77% of sheep and 20.7% of goats had indigestible debris from waste materials in their digestive system [18]. Furthermore, marine pollution kills marine life directly through ingestion, which leads to blockages of their digestive system, poisoning due to the toxins in the waste and false stomach filling, which leads to death from starvation and, in the long run, affects the food chain in the marine world (ecosystem and biodiversity) [19]. Due to the upsurge of pollution from packaging wastes, the hazards involved, and the shortage of space in dumping sites, composting is a well-researched and documented procedure in several literature [17, 20–23].

The ability of a material to be compostable is a crucial characteristics [2] because recycling consumes energy, while with the aid of biological degradation, composting breaks down the materials into H_2O, CO_2, and inorganic compounds without the toxic residue that comes from recycling, which affects the environment. Another benefit of compostable materials is that when they break down, they become fertilizers and soil conditioners from which the environment can benefit [3]. Figure 7.1 depicts a model of a life cycle on the reuse and breakdown of bioplastics, which can be used as biomass to facilitate plant growth.

There are several sources of materials that can be used to make biodegradable packaging. The main focus of this chapter is on the alternative source of plastic raw materials. Against this backdrop, starch is a natural polymer that can be manipulated to produce desired properties similar to traditional non-biodegradable plastic. Starch films are stronger than other biopolymer films, and the mechanical properties of starch films are better than polysaccharides and protein films [24].

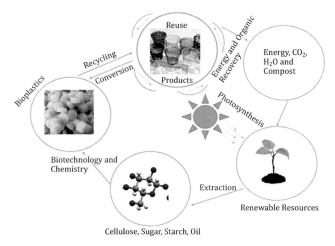

Figure 7.1 Life cycle of biomass.

7.3 Starch

Starch is a polysaccharide carbohydrate encompassing a colossal number of glucose units linked together by glycosidic bonds. It is produced by mainly green plants as an energy store. It is the most vital carbohydrate in the human diet and is encompassed in staple foods such as rice, potatoes, maize, cassava, and wheat. Pure starch is a white, flavorless, and odorless powder, which does not dissolve in unheated water or alcohol. It consists of two kinds of polymers: the linear and helical amylose and the branched amylopectin (Fig. 7.2) [25].

Starch is present in higher plants as semi-crystalline granules of polymers of glucose molecules, which are linked genetically to straight-chain (amylose) and branched-chain (amylopectin) structures. Starches having great economic value are mainly obtained from root crops and seeds of cereals [27]. The crystalline structure of starch is centered on the micellar nature of the starch chains in the starch granules. The granules display a variety of shapes, and the sizes are often distinctively characteristic of the cultivar or variety from which the starch is sequestered [28]. When starch is hydrolyzed at a specified temperature, it prevents starch gelatinization and allows the acid to attack the amorphous region. The regions of starch granules that are crystalline in nature are rapidly isolated by either HCl or H_2SO_4 acid. Sulfuric acid is preferred to HCl since the sulfate group is more stable and hydrolysis is complete in 5 days instead of 15 days [29]. Figure 7.3 is a diagrammatic illustration of the crystalline and amorphous rings in a starch granule.

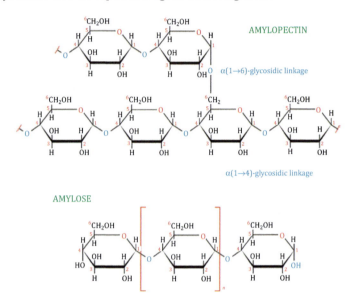

Figure 7.2   Starch structure. Reprinted with permission from Ref. [26].

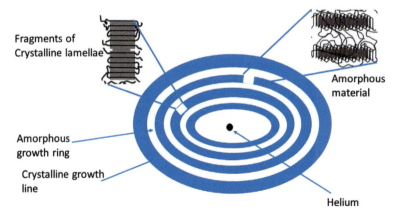

Figure 7.3   Schematic illustration of starch granule structure.

7.3.1 Potato

Potato, scientifically known as *Solanum tuberosum* L. [30], is rich in starch ranking as the world's fourth most important food crop, after maize, wheat, and rice [31, 32]. It is believed that potatoes were initially cultivated eight centuries ago in Peru's Central Andes, but their value was only realized in the 19th century when the continent of Europe was enduring starvation [33], because it was cheap and required less growth time.

The amylose content in potato starch is close to 20%, and granules are big with a smooth plump oval nature with a size range between 15 and 75 µm, as shown in Fig. 7.4 [34, 35]. Potato starch has several admirable properties, which improve the solidity and firmness of the gel in some food products as compared to other starches. The phosphorus content in the amylopectin has a negative charge and repulsive at a greater speed due to the swelling of the potato starch granules in heated H_2O and elevated thickness, elevated clearness, and it is involved in low retro-gradation quickness of their pastes [25, 36, 37].

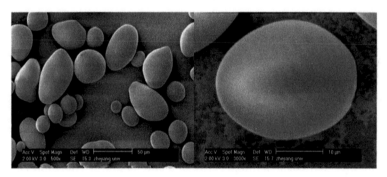

Figure 7.4 SEM micrographs of potato starch granules. Reprinted from Ref. [34], with permission from Elsevier.

7.3.2 Cassava

Cassava, scientifically known as *Manihot esculenta* [38], is the source of tapioca starch, which is used in various industrialized and food applications, such as water binding and texturizing agent. It contains high viscosity, water-holding capacity, and binding abilities, thus also performing as a bonding agent for paper [35]. The amylose portion in the starch constituent of the fusions is reported by Oladunmoye, Aworh [39] and Kim and Wiesenborn [40] to vary between 15% and 19.49%. The tapioca granules are smooth, irregular spheres, and their dimensions range between 5 and 25 μm, as shown in Fig. 7.5.

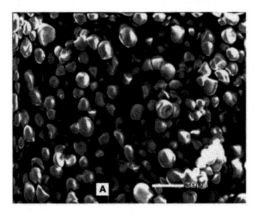

Figure 7.5 SEM micrograph of cassava granules. Reprinted from Ref. [45], with permission from Elsevier.

7.3.3 Maize

Maize or corn, scientifically called *Zea mays*, is the most popular and traditional source of starch. Based on the amylose and amylopectin ratio, maize is classified into normal, waxy, and high amylose [41]. Waxy maize is the most common type used for the formation of biofilms and nanocrystals due to its high concentration in amylopectin [42]. The granules are irregular polyhedron shaped, and their dimensions range between 5 and 20 μm, as shown in Fig. 7.6 [41, 43, 44].

7.3.4 Amadumbe

Amadumbe, taro, or cocoyam has three varieties, namely, *Colocasia esculenta*, *Xanthosoma sagittifolium* (red flesh), and *Xanthosoma sagittifolium* (white flesh). Among the three, *C. esculenta* has the smallest granules size of about 0.25 μm, and they are polygonal in shape (Fig. 7.7) [28, 45, 46]. *C. esculenta* has a low pasting temperature when compared to the other two varieties, and this allows it to be easy to cook and manipulate into biofilms [28]. *C. Esculenta* is rich in starch and has a composition of 72% amylopectin and 28% amylose, which is a favorable trait in the making of starch nanocrystals [47].

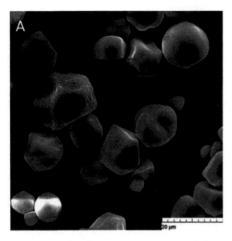

Figure 7.6 SEM micrograph of *Zea mays*. Reprinted from Ref. [43], with permission from Elsevier.

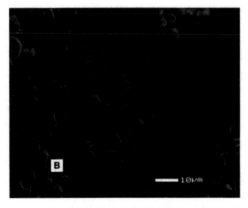

Figure 7.7 SEM micrograph of *C. esculenta* (cocoyam). Reprinted from Ref. [45], with permission from Elsevier.

7.4 Methods

The process of starch extraction is general, regardless of the source. The following methods show how starch is extracted, modified, and molded into biodegradable films and then analyzed under several specialized microscopes.

7.4.1 Starch Extraction

Two common starch extraction methods are water extraction and alkaline extraction. The two only differ on the use of a base (NaOH) or water. The yields of both methods are similar.

7.4.1.1 Water extraction method

One part of *C. esculenta* powder is to be dispersed in five parts of distilled water and let to stand for 2 h. The suspension is later screened through 200-mesh and 300-mesh sifters, respectively. The suspension is centrifuged at 3000× g and 4°C for 10 min, after which the supernatant is decanted. The sediment is re-suspended in five parts of distilled water. The centrifugation step is repeated four times. The sediment is finally dried in a hot-air oven at 40°C for 16 h, ground, and sieved through a 100-mesh sifter. The flour is sealed in a plastic bag and kept in a desiccator for further analyses [48].

7.4.1.2 Alkaline extraction method

In this extraction method, 0.05% (w/v) NaOH solution is used in place of distilled water in the first extraction. After the suspension has been centrifuged at 3000× g and 4°C for 10 min, the sediment is re-suspended in five parts of distilled water and the centrifugation is carried out. The washing step using distilled water is repeated four times. The drying procedure is carried out in the same manner as in the water extraction method [48].

7.4.2 Preparation of Starch Nanocrystals

The starch obtained is then modified into starch nanocrystals using acid hydrolysis. The details for the preparation of nanocrystals by H_2SO_4 hydrolysis of native starch granules have been previously described [49]. The conditions of hydrolysis differed from those of the so-called "lintnerization" procedure and were defined as the result of the optimization of the treatment of nanocrystals using a response surface methodology. Native waxy maize starch granules (37 g) is mixed with 250 mL of 3.16 M H_2SO_4 over 5 days at 40°C, with continuous stirring at 100 rpm. The suspension is then washed by successive centrifugations in distilled water until neutral and finally freeze-dried [49, 50]. The starch nanocrystals obtained are then used in the fortification of the biofilm matrix to be made in the next step.

7.4.3 Film Preparation

A starch solution with a concentration of 3% (w/v) is prepared by dispersing starch in distilled water and heating the mixtures and stirring until it gelatinized (85°C for 5 min). It is then cooled to 45±2°C. Sorbitol is added as 40% of the starch. Subsequently, the starch nanocrystals dispersion is added at 5, 10, 15, 20, 25, and 30% of starch and stirred for 2 min. The mixtures are cast onto flat, leveled, non-stick trays to set. Once set, the trays are held overnight undisturbed at 55°C for 10 h and then cooled to ambient temperature before peeling the films off the plates. The film samples are stored in plastic bags and held in desiccators at 60% RH for further testing. All treatments should be made in triplicate [50]. A scanning electron microscope and a transmission electron microscope are used for the characterization of the starch, starch nanocrystals, and biofilms and the methods are as follows.

7.4.3.1 Scanning electron microscopy

The starch samples are sprinkled onto the aluminum specimen stubs with double-sided adhesive tape, while the non-sticking portion is blown off. The samples are coated with a 30 nm layer of gold using a sputter coater [Polaron (Fisons) SC 515 VG Microtech, Sussex, UK]. The coated starch samples are observed using a scanning electron microscope (FESEM Leo Supra 50VP, Carl-Zeiss SMT, Oberkochen, Germany). Images are captured at different magnifications of 1000 K ×, 2000 K ×, and 5000 K × for morphological studies [51]. SEM is typically performed to illustrate the morphology of the particle sizes. This instrument is operated at controlled atmospheric conditions at 20 kV to characterize the surface morphology and the elemental composition of the selected samples. Samples are prepared prior to SEM observations, where the surface of the sample is coated with a thin, electric conductive gold film to prevent the accumulation of electrostatic charge [52].

7.4.3.2 Transmission electron microscopy

A drop of dilute nanocrystal suspension is spread on a glow-discharged carbon-coated TEM grid. The preparation is negatively stained with 2% (w/v) uranyl acetate and is observed using a Philips CM200 microscope (FEI Company, Eindhoven, The Netherlands) operating at 80 kV. Images are recorded on Kodak S0163 film [49]. The transmission electron microscope is primarily used for understanding the internal microstructure of materials at the nanometer level. This instrument uses electrons as a "light source" as their much lower wavelength allows for a resolution a thousand times better than a light microscope [53].

7.5 Conclusion

With the current impacts of food-packaging waste materials on the environment and all the focus toward trying to reduce or totally eradicate pollution and its harm to the environment and its ecosystems, focusing on green initiatives is the preferred solution. The use of natural raw materials that can be recycled allows humanity to secure the future against consequences such as food shortages, global warming, and climate changes. An excellent example of such raw materials is shown by starch, which considerably is of low costs and is plentiful in nature. Starch can be easily modified to give the desired functional properties; it is ideal in the formation of starch nanocrystals, which are used in the making of biocomposite films. The main researched sources of starch are maize, rice, potato, and cassava, which may, however, bring the controversy of food security. Amadumbe, on the other hand, is a documented underutilized tuber crop similar to potato and cassava and is an abundant source of starch, which is also ideal in the making of starch nanocrystals. These nanocrystals are used in the making of biocomposite films. This, in summary, provides potential large-scale farming and increased utilization of this abundant and cheaper starch source, which in turn provides employment to nation without job insecurity.

References

1. Arvanitoyannis, I., et al., Biodegradable films made from low-density polyethylene (LDPE), rice starch and potato starch for food packaging applications: Part 1. *Carbohydrate Polymers*, 1998, **36**(2): 89–104.
2. Siracusa, V., et al., Biodegradable polymers for food packaging: A review. *Trends in Food Science & Technology*, 2008, **19**(12): 634–643.
3. www.european-bioplastics.org. European Bioplastics. 2016 [cited 2016; Available from: http://www.european-bioplastics.org/].
4. Robertson, G. L., *Food Packaging: Principles and Practice*. 2016: CRC Press.
5. Coles, R., D. McDowell, and M. J. Kirwan, *Food Packaging Technology*, Vol. 5. 2003: CRC Press.
6. Marsh, K. and B. Bugusu, Food packaging: Roles, materials, and environmental issues. *Journal of Food Science*, 2007, **72**(3): R39–R55.
7. Restuccia, D., et al., New EU regulation aspects and global market of active and intelligent packaging for food industry applications. *Food Control*, 2010, **21**(11): 1425–1435.
8. 21CFR174, U.S., Food and Drugs, D.o.H.a.H. Services, Editor. 2015.
9. Shah, A. A., et al., Biological degradation of plastics: A comprehensive review. *Biotechnology Advances*, 2008, **26**(3): 246–265.
10. The Aluminum Association. The strength of aluminum, 2016 [cited 2016; Available from: http://www.aluminum.org/strength-aluminum].
11. Fellows, P. and B. L. Axtell, *Appropriate Food Packaging: Materials and Methods for Small Businesses*. 1993: Practical Action Publishing.
12. Sorrentino, A., G. Gorrasi, and V. Vittoria, Potential perspectives of bio-nanocomposites for food packaging applications. *Trends in Food Science & Technology*, 2007, **18**(2): 84–95.
13. Petersen, K., et al., Potential of biobased materials for food packaging. *Trends in Food Science & Technology*, 1999, **10**(2): 52–68.
14. Avella, M., et al., Biodegradable starch/clay nanocomposite films for food packaging applications. *Food Chemistry*, 2005, **93**(3): 467–474.
15. Yoshiharu, D., Biodegradable plastics and polymers. *Journal of Pesticide Science*, 1994, **19**(1): S11–S14.
16. Schaub, S. M. and J. J. Leonard, Composting: An alternative waste management option for food processing industries. *Trends in Food Science & Technology*, 1996, **7**(8): 263–268.

17. Westlake, K., *Landfill Waste Pollution and Control.* 2014: Woodhead Publishing.
18. Reddy, M. V. B. and P. Sasikala, A review on foreign bodies with special reference to plastic pollution threat to livestock and environment in Tirupati rural areas. *International Journal of Scientific and Research Publications,* 2012, **2**(12): 1–8.
19. Todd, P. A., X. Ong, and L. M. Chou, Impacts of pollution on marine life in Southeast Asia. *Biodiversity and Conservation,* 2010, **19**(4): 1063–1082.
20. Ivar do Sul, J. A. and M. F. Costa, The present and future of microplastic pollution in the marine environment. *Environmental Pollution,* 2014, **185**: 352–364.
21. Finstein, M. and J. Hogan, Integration of composting process microbiology, facility structure and decision-making. *Science and Engineering of Composting,* 1993: 1–23.
22. Haug, R. T., *The Practical Handbook of Compost Engineering.* 1993: CRC Press.
23. Leonard, J. and S. Ramer. Physical properties of compost: What do we know and why should we care? In *Proceedings of the 4th Annual Meeting of the Composting Council of Canada,* 1994: Environment Canada Toronto, Ontario, Canada.
24. Masmoudi, F., et al., Biodegradable packaging materials conception based on starch and polylactic acid (PLA) reinforced with cellulose. *Environmental Science and Pollution Research,* 2016: 1–11.
25. BeMiller, J. N. and R. L. Whistler, Starch: Chemistry and technology. 2009: Academic Press.
26. E. Generalic, https://glossary.periodni.com/glossary.php?en=starch.
27. Carr, J., K. Sufferling, and J. Poppe, Hydrocolloids and their use in the confectionery industry. *Food Technology,* 1995.
28. Sefa-Dedeh, S. and E. Kofi-Agyir Sackey, Starch structure and some properties of cocoyam (*Xanthosoma sagittifolium* and *Colocasia esculenta*) starch and raphides. *Food Chemistry,* 2002, **79**(4): 435–444.
29. Lin, N., et al., Preparation, modification, and application of starch nanocrystals in nanomaterials: A review. *Journal of Nanomaterials,* 2011, **2011**: 13.
30. Consortium, P. G. S., Genome sequence and analysis of the tuber crop potato. *Nature,* 2011, **475**(7355): 189–195.

31. Hawkes, J. G., *The Potato: Evolution, Biodiversity and Genetic Resources*. 1990: Belhaven Press.
32. Burton, W. G., *The Potato*. 1948: London, Chapman & Hall.
33. Lutaladio, N. and L. Castaldi, Potato: The hidden treasure. *Journal of Food Composition and Analysis*, 2009, **22**(6): 491–493.
34. Hui, R., et al., Preparation and properties of octenyl succinic anhydride modified potato starch. *Food Chemistry*, 2009, **114**(1): 81–86.
35. Chaisawang, M. and M. Suphantharika, Pasting and rheological properties of native and anionic tapioca starches as modified by guar gum and xanthan gum. *Food Hydrocolloids*, 2006, **20**(5): 641–649.
36. Rajisha, K. R., et al., Preparation and characterization of potato starch nanocrystal reinforced natural rubber nanocomposites. *International Journal of Biological Macromolecules*, 2014, **67**: 147–153.
37. Morrison, I. M., et al., Potato starches: Variation in composition and properties between three genotypes grown at two different sites and in two different years. *Journal of the Science of Food and Agriculture*, 2001, **81**(3): 319–328.
38. Cock, J. H., *Cassava. New Potential for a Neglected Crop*. 1985: Westview Press.
39. Oladunmoye, O. O., et al., Chemical and functional properties of cassava starch, durum wheat semolina flour, and their blends. *Food Science & Nutrition*, 2014, **2**(2): 132–138.
40. KIM, Y. S. and D. P. Wiesenborn, Starch noodle quality as related to potato genotypes. *Journal of Food Science*, 1996, **61**(1): 248–252.
41. Singh, N., K. S. Sandhu, and M. Kaur, Physicochemical properties including granular morphology, amylose content, swelling and solubility, thermal and pasting properties of starches from normal, waxy, high amylose and sugary corn. *Progress in Food Biopolymer Research*, 2005, **1**(2): 43–55.
42. Peat, S., W. Whelan, and G. J. Thomas, Evidence of multiple branching in waxy maize starch. *Journal of the Chemical Society* (*Resumed*), 1952: 4536–4538.
43. Sujka, M. and J. Jamroz, Ultrasound-treated starch: SEM and TEM imaging, and functional behaviour. *Food Hydrocolloids*, 2013, **31**(2): 413–419.
44. Network, G. H. N. Understanding starch functionality, 1996 [cited 2016; Available from: http://www.naturalproductsinsider.com/articles/1996/01/understanding-starch-functionality.aspx].

45. Nwokocha, L. M., et al., A comparative study of some properties of cassava (*Manihot esculenta*, Crantz) and cocoyam (*Colocasia esculenta*, Linn) starches. *Carbohydrate Polymers*, 2009, **76**(3): 362–367.

46. Purseglove, J. W., *Monocotyledons* (*Tropical Crops S*). 1972: Longman.

47. Cambie, R. C. and L. R. Ferguson, Potential functional foods in the traditional Maori diet. *Mutation Research/Fundamental and Molecular Mechanisms of Mutagenesis*, 2003, **523–524**(0): 109–117.

48. Tattiyakul, J., S. Asavasaksakul, and P. Pradipasena, Chemical and physical properties of flour extracted from taro *Colocasia esculenta* (L.) Schott grown in different regions of Thailand. *Science Asia*, 2006, **32**(3): 279–284.

49. Angellier-Coussy, H., et al., The molecular structure of waxy maize starch nanocrystals. *Carbohydrate Research*, 2009, **344**(12): 1558–1566.

50. Piyada, K., S. Waranyou, and W. Thawien, Mechanical, thermal and structural properties of rice starch films reinforced with rice starch nanocrystals. *International Food Research Journal*, 2013, **20**(1): 439–449.

51. Oladebeye, A. O., et al., Morphology, X-ray diffraction and solubility of underutilized legume starch nanocrystals. *International Journal of Science and Research*, 2013, **3**(9): 497–503.

52. Zhang, L., et al., Investigating into the antibacterial behavior of suspensions of ZnO nanoparticles (ZnO nanofluids). *Journal of Nanoparticle Research*, 2007, **9**(3): 479–489.

53. Howe, J. M., B. Fultz, and S. Miao, *Transmission Electron Microscopy*, 2nd ed., 2012: Wiley and Sons, Inc., New York.

Chapter 8

Bionanocomposite Materials: Concept, Applications, and Recent Advancements

Nafees Ahmad,[a] Saima Sultana,[a] Suhail Sabir,[a] Ameer Azam,[b] and Mohammad Zain Khan[a]

[a]*Environmental Research Laboratory, Department of Chemistry, Aligarh Muslim University, Aligarh 202 002, India*
[b]*Centre of Excellence in Nanomaterials, Department of Applied Physics, Aligarh Muslim University, Aligarh 202 002, India*
zn.khan1@gmail.com

Bionanocomposites are an important class of nanosized materials in which both the filler and the matrix are obtained from biological resources. It is a hybrid material formed by the combination of natural polymers and inorganic solids that have at least one nanometer dimension. They are similar to nanocomposites, but the basic differences are in the methods of preparation, properties, biocompatibility, biodegradability, functionalities, and their application. Researchers all over the world, with their tremendous efforts, made extraordinary progress to create a new product of bionanocomposites. Research on bionanocomposites sets a new interdisciplinary field similar to biomineralization

---

Biocomposites: Biomedical and Environmental Applications
Edited by Shakeel Ahmed, Saiqa Ikram, Suvardhan Kanchi, and Krishna Bisetty
Copyright © 2018 Pan Stanford Publishing Pte. Ltd.
ISBN 978-981-4774-38-3 (Hardcover), 978-1-315-11080-6 (eBook)
www.panstanford.com

process, biomimetic system, and bioinspired materials. Nowadays, researchers are interested in bio-based polymers that can reduce the dependence on fossil fuel and can utilize a sustainable material basis. Bionanocomposites create an opportunity for the utilization of new, high-performance, lightweight green nanocomposite materials to replace conventional non-biodegradable petroleum-based products. Biopolymers are also used for biomedical purposes such as drug delivery, tissue engineering, and bone replacement and also have some application in electronics, sensors, and energy regeneration. Starch, cellulose derivative polylactic acid (PLA) and polycaprolactone (PCL) are most widely used matrices suitable for the packaging application.

8.1 Introduction

Biodegradable polymers are the material produced by plant microorganisms or bioprocess, while bionanocomposites are the combination of natural polymers and inorganic solids. In the recent years, "bionanocomposite" has attracted wide attention and has become a common term for the formation of those nanocomposite that involved a naturally occurring polymer (biopolymer) in combination with an inorganic moiety, and showing at least one dimension on the nanometer scale [1]. The non-degradability and non-renewability of some polymers such as polyethene, plastics, have created a new interest in many industries especially for the packaging material to use bio-based polymer derived from renewable sources. Polymers that are completely degradable at the end of their use are suitable materials for the development of bionanocomposites, because these materials do not put an extra burden on the environment and will be beneficial from the perspective of sustainability and environmental problems [2]. The polymer matrices that are generally used to synthesize the polymer nanocomposite are non-biodegradable, which create environmental hazard. So in order to make it environmentally friendly and to improve its performance and activity, a number of biopolymers have been developed and used. Nanocomposites from biopolymers exhibit several useful properties such as enhanced mechanical strength and improved heat resistance as compared to other conventional composites [3].

Polymers that replace non-biodegradable polymers include starch, chitosan, chitin, lignin, cellulose, pectin, and poly(lactic acid) (PLA). They are also referred to as green polymers as they are sustainable and mostly derived from natural sources.

The biodegradation of such polymers can also be enhanced by incorporation of clays. Properties of these biopolymers are quite good, but the incorporation of different nanofillers such as organically modified layered silicates, cellulose nanofibers, carbon nanotubes, and halloysites nanotubes enhances their material properties [4]. Although bionanocomposites offers many applications in various fields such as electronics, medicine, packaging industry, some of their inherent properties such as brittleness, low melt viscosity, high gas and vapor permeability restrict their use in various area [2]. Bionanocomposites create an interdisciplinary area involving biology, chemistry, material science, engineering, and nanotechnology. Sometimes, bionanocomposites are called biocomposites, nanocomposites, nanobiocomposites, green composites as well as bioplastics. Biopolymers containing composite materials are a topic of recent interest.

8.2 Types of Bionanocomposites

8.2.1 Polysaccharide-Based Bionanocomposites

8.2.1.1 Chitosan-based bionanocomposites

Chitosan is a linear copolymer of β-(1–4)-linked 2-acetamido-2-deoxy-β-D-glucopyranose, and 2-amino-2-deoxy-β-D-glycopyranose [5] is N-deacetylated product of chitin. It is a cationic biopolymer [6] soluble in aqueous and acidic media [7] and has been utilized as a matrix for bionanocomposites with a range of nano-reinforcements such as clays, chitin, and cellulose nanofibers [8, 9]. It may be categorized as a semi-crystalline polymer because its degree of crystallinity depends on the amount of deacetylation. Bionanocomposites of chitosan can also be used as adsorbent for immobilization [2]. By preparing a compound of chitosan with montmorillonite, it can be effectively employed for the removal of acidic pesticides and water from the acidic environment [10] and made water free from pollution.

8.2.1.2 Cellulose-based bionanocomposites

Cellulose, the most abundant renewable resource on earth, is a polysaccharide linear polymer consisting of long chains of sugar molecules [11]. Cellulose is also known as the most abundant agropolymer with the primary components in the structure of plant cells [4]. The properties of cellulose depend on its chain length and degree of polymerization. A variety of agro-based biopolymers such as wood cellulose and cotton can be used as a raw material for the production of cellulose esters polymers in the powder form when using appropriate plasticizers and additives. In cellulose-based bionanocomposites, the polar surface can hinder its dispersion in non-polar polymer [12]. The tensile strength and rigidity of cellulose-based material can be enhanced by the addition of nanocomposites such as organoclay and nanofibers [13].

8.2.1.3 Starch-based bionanocomposites

Starch is mainly composed of two major carbohydrate units: amylase and amylopectin [14]. It is an abundant, non-toxic, inexpensive biopolymer by which a number of products can be recovered by the processing of starch source and can be utilized in a number of ways [15, 16]. The main source of starch is cereals (wheat, maize, etc.), tubers (potato), and peas. The basic form of starch is quiet useful for the storage of energy in plants and microorganisms in the form of isolate granules with different size range depending on starch source [17]. The melting point of dry starch is in the range 220–240°C, which is almost equal to the initial decomposition temperature of starch. Starch montmorillonite matrix incorporated with silver nanoparticles enhances its activity. The same can be used in various other fields, that is, catalysis, dentistry, clothing, electronic, and food industries [18].

8.2.1.4 Chitin-based bionanocomposites

Chitin, poly[β-(1-4)-N-acetyl-D-glucosamine], is a natural polysaccharide and acetylated form of chitosan. It is modified cellulose that has a high–molecular weight, highly insoluble material resembling cellulose in its solubility with low chemical reactivity [2, 19]. It is found in exoskeletons as well as internal structure of invertebrates. Due to its excellent biodegradability, biocompatibility, absorptivity, and non-toxic nature, chitin can be utilized in many applications. Chitin can also be employed as an effective binder for dye and fabric in industries and also to improve crop yields [17]. The chief sources of chitin are crustaceans, shrimps, and crab shells. Chitin-based polyurethane bionanocomposites have been used by Zia et al. [20] with some clay content to give better performance and thermal stability of the matrix. Its remarkable properties and high strength per unit mass with excellent reinforcing performance provide polyethylene oxide with chitin nanofibers an efficient stress transfer from matrix to fiber [21].

8.2.2 Nanoclay-Based Nanocomposites

Nanoclays are the nanoparticle of tetrahedral sheet of silicates. Nanoclay, due to its excellent nanometric structure and thermally stability, is a perfect matrix for nanocomposites [22]. There are many types of nanoclays (e.g., montmorillonite, bentonite, kaolinite) due to their different chemical composition and sizes. The unique properties of nanoclay, that is, low weight, low moisture absorption, low cost, and low density, make it an excellent tool for petrochemical applications [23]. Nanoclay-based nanocomposites have become an interesting topic for researchers due to their structural behavior as well as electrical and electrochemical properties. The nanoclay–biopolymer (e.g., montmorillonite–chitosan) matrix can be used to enhance its thermal properties. Various analytical techniques (e.g., XRD, SEM, TGA) show high affinity between the clay substrate and biopolymer [6].

8.2.3 Hallyosite-Based Nanocomposites

Halloysites mainly formed naturally on the earth over millions of years by the surface weathering of aluminosilicates that composed of aluminum, hydrogen, silicon, and oxygen, with a chemical composition of $Al_2(OH)_4Si_2O_5(2H_2O)$. Hallyosite is mainly composed of aluminosilicates with hollow tubular structure. Hallyosite-based nanocomposites are used as additives to improve the mechanical, thermal, and fire-retardant properties of polymers [24]. It is formed in the form of nanotubes that are ultra-tiny hollow tubes and then coated with metallic substances to enhance mechanical and thermal properties [25]. It is a potential option to expensive CNTs for nanocomposites where advanced mechanical properties are concerned.

8.3 Preparation and Modifications

Bionanocomposites can be prepared usually by four methods: in situ polymerization, solution casting, melt processing, and in situ template synthesis [26]. Nanoclay-, cellulose-, and halloysites-based nanocomposites can be processed by these methods. By the incorporation of different nanoparticles and nanofillers (e.g., ZnO and Ag nanoparticles) to the biopolymer such as starch, cellulose, PLA, etc., composite polymers with enhanced properties and good performance are produced. In the process of in situ polymerization, nanoparticles are pre-mixed with the liquid monomer and the polymerization is then initiated by a suitable indicator. In the solution-casting method, both the polymers and nanoparticles are dissolved in suitable solvents, while in melt processing, nanoparticles are mixed with the polymer in the molten state [27]. Melt processing is a green technique because in this technique, no solvents are required for synthesis.

Nanoparticles have the tendency to enhance mechanical and thermal properties and show some barrier characteristics. Use of a biopolymer source such as polysaccharides and PLA has given a large contribution in the processing of bionanocomposites. The sensitivity of biopolymers toward water and barrier films and their mechanical weakness require careful attention for their modification [28]. One of the modification methods is the combination of polysaccharides with protein molecules [29, 30]. Another effective method for the preparation of bionanocomposites is emulsion polymerization by incorporating any biopolymer within the matrix as done by Zuber et al. [31], who prepared chitin-based polyurethane bionanocomposites. By the addition of nanofillers or nanocomposites to the biopolymer, the properties of that matrix can be enhanced. However, sometimes it has been reported that after the incorporation of the bionanocomposite polymer, the properties are somewhat less than those of the pure biopolymer; thus, there is a need to modify the structure altogether. Wang et al. [32] studied about the chitosan clay nanocomposites and found slightly improved tensile property while inferior thermal property than that of pure chitosan. Zia et al. [20] improved the properties of chitin-based polyurethane composites by incorporating bentonite clay into the polymer matrix.

8.4 Special Properties of Bionanocomposites

8.4.1 Mechanical and Barrier Properties

Some special properties of bionanocomposites are shown in Fig. 8.1. Mechanical properties can be attributed to high rigidity and aspect ratios of nanoparticles together with good affinity. Polymer bionanocomposites have good barrier properties against gases and water vapor. Best gas barrier properties can be obtained in polymer nanocomposites with fully exfoliated nanoclay mineral with large aspect ratio [33]. Many polysaccharides and polymer films of bionanocomposites can be used as barrier film with its effective characteristics to enhance the barrier film activity. Nanoclay plays a very important role in barrier enhancement. Mechanical properties can be defined mainly by the following:

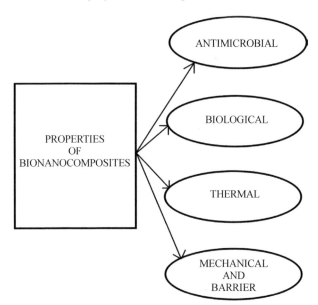

Figure 8.1 Some special properties of bionanocomposites.

8.4.1.1 Young's modulus and tensile strength

Young's modulus and tensile strength mainly explain the reinforcement effect of fillers in bionanocomposites. It enables the filler to carry a disproportionality high fraction of an applied load provided that the interfacial bonding between polymer matrices and fillers is quiet sufficient [11], and by using a filler with a large surface area, greater reinforcement effect can be attained. Young's modulus of nanocomposites is a function of clay content [34]. It can also be observed that there is a change not only in Young's modulus of the bionanocomposites upon the incorporation of organic clay but also on the tensile strength of the bionanocomposites [35].

8.4.1.2 Toughness and strain

Toughness and strain are quiet useful for the nanocomposites when used in industries because in working conditions, hardness and toughness are important parameters. Low toughness or brittleness is a drawback of bionanocomposites, which must be removed to enhance their usage. By the inclusion of poly(lactic acid) to nanocomposites, their elongation is increased by 40% as compared to neat PLA [36], thereby decreasing brittleness.

8.4.2 Biological Properties

Biological properties are mainly defined through the biodegradation of bionanocomposites. Biodegradation can be defined as the decomposition of materials when they are exposed to bacteria or any other biological condition. It can be enhanced in bionanocomposites by the addition of certain additives. Tetto and co-workers (1999) reported enhanced biodegradation rates of polycaprolactone (PCL) upon the addition of montmorillonite [37].

8.4.3 Thermal Properties

The thermal properties of polymer bionanocomposites can be explained by many techniques. Glass transition temperature (T_g), melting temperature (T_m), and differential scanning calorimetry can be used to see the weight loss with temperature as well as the degree of crystallinity [38]. Upon heating the sample under vacuum or in inert atmosphere, non-oxidative degradation is achieved, and in the presence of air, oxidative degradation is achieved. The thermal stability of bionanocomposites can be improved by the incorporation of layered silicates and various other nanoparticles [39–41]. As in the case of polymer clay nanocomposites, inclusion of layered silicates can improve thermal stability by acting as insulator and mass transport barrier [39, 42].

8.4.4 Antimicrobial Properties

The antimicrobial properties of bionanocomposites are an important factor in various industries. Antimicrobial agents inhibit the growth of microorganisms (above a particular level of concentration) and prevent the material from decay. Bionanocomposites are used as antimicrobial agents and antimicrobial carrier in paints, coatings, and packing materials [43]. The nanoparticles are quite effective in their activity due to their high surface-to-volume ratio and improved surface activity of the nanosized antimicrobial agents [44]. There are many agents that can be effectively used as antimicrobial agents, including natural antimicrobial agents (nisin, thymol, and isothocyanate), synthetic antimicrobial agents (EDTA, propono-ic acid, and benzoic acid), and some metal oxide (ZnO, TiO_2). Some metal ions (Au, Ag, Pt) also show effective antimicrobial properties.

8.5 Recent Advances in the Field of Bionanocomposites

During the past few years, a lot of work has been done in the field of bionanocomposites. The work mainly focused on how to improve the mechanical, thermal, and biological properties of bionanocomposites. Mousa et al. [11] improved the mechanical properties of bionanocomposites in solid and melt state along with enhanced thermal stability and biodegradability with the addition of nanofillers, which work as heat barriers. Hosseini [45] reported that the incorporation of chitosan nanoparticles to fish gelatin results in an increased water vapor barrier, and upon the incorporation of layered silicates to the polymer clay nanocomposites, thermal stability of the matrix can be improved. The materials also show better elastic properties, which help in film applicability. The biocompatibility and biodegradability of bionanocomposites along with other properties (especially mechanical and thermal properties) filled the gap between functional and structural materials. The increasing demand of bionanocomposites and biopolymers is mainly attributed to the environmental concern and also to the limitation of petroleum products [28].

A wide and considerable application and research have been developed in the field of bionanocomposites by using renewable resources based biopolymers [46], which exhibit improvement in thermal, mechanical, and other functional properties. So in order to improve the properties of bionanocomposites, adding nanostructured filler to the biopolymer is an excellent and viable option. As in the case of starch-based biopolymers, poor moisture barrier and high humidity sensitivity restrict their application, and addition of a few nanofillers such as nanofibers, CNTs, and nanoclays has shown to improve these properties [47].

8.6 Applications of Bionanocomposites

Being environment friendly, biodegradable, and biocompatible, bionanocomposites offer numerous applications in different fields such as biomedicine, electronics, environment, membrane separation, sensors, and packaging (Fig. 8.2).

8.6.1 Electronic, Sensor, and Energy Generation

Bionanocomposites can be used as membrane in different instruments as well as in fuel cells where the reaction takes place by the transfer of electrons. Bionanocomposite membranes are also employed in the process of water purification by reverse osmosis. Bionanocomposites can be used effectively for protein separation, and pervaporation is another useful application of bionanocomposites [48]. They can also be used for energy generation in solar cells (due to high solar absorptivity). Polymer nanocomposites assisted with carbon nanotubes are quite flexible materials and can be used in photovoltaic cells as well [49].

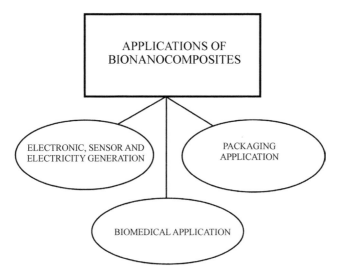

Figure 8.2 Some important applications of bionanocomposites.

8.6.2 Biomedical Applications

Bionanocomposites can be used in biomedical sciences due to their important properties such as biocompatibility, environmental friendliness, and natural abundance. They are used for tissue engineering, kidney dialysis, bone replacement, skin graft, and also used in heart surgery [11]. They are chosen for biomedical applications as the material used for medical purposes is derived from bio-derived polymer and possesses tunable mechanical properties. For example, plastics and films of bio-based polymers made from corn-derived PDO (1,3-propanediol) clearly show non-cytotoxic and non-inflammatory properties [50].

8.6.3 Packaging Applications

The main purpose of packaging food or any product is to protect and preserve it from any kind of damage and to increase its shelf life. While packaging any product, many factors should be kept in mind. Permeability is one of the most important factors for the packaging industry [2]. Due to some unique properties of bionanocomposites, for example, excellent barrier properties (gas and water vapor), high mechanical strength, high thermal stability, chemical inertness, improved recyclability, dimensional stability, and heat resistance, packaging application has been regarded as one of the advanced nanocomposite technologies [51].

8.7 Challenges

The main challenge related with the application of bionanocomposite is their complicated synthesis and processing. Uniform dispersion of nanoparticles in the polymer matrix is also necessary during the synthesis of bionanocomposites. A better dispersion can be achieved by using the solvent-casting method and melt compounding. However, during in situ polymerization, different additives and catalysts are added in order to enhance mechanical, thermal, and biological properties [26]. Different fillers and films (montmorillonite/chitosan, PLA, etc.) are incorporated in the bionanocomposites to make them more useful in different applications. The properties and production rate of the material must be maintained. One of the applications of bionanocomposites is energy generation, but there is a challenging issue with this application to enhance the conductivity of polymer, which is directly controlled by the conduction of photogenerated carrier to the electrode.

The exact stiffness and strength of the composite materials must also be known. The proportion of the additives to the polymer matrix should be such that the coupling of the filler to the matrix gives quality products [46]. The most important parameter related to the formation of bionanocomposites is its design so that maximum advantages can be taken from the products.

8.8 Conclusion and Future Trends

The chapter showed the current status of bionanocomposites, various methods of their synthesis, modification, and applications. The rate of production should be enhanced in order to cope with the growing demands of biopolymer. Some of the biopolymers do not have good properties (film barrier, mechanical, thermal properties); therefore, it has been realized that incorporating nanoparticles or nanofillers such as nanoclays, nanocellulose, and carbon nanotubes to biopolymer will improve its properties and make the processing trouble-free. There are many areas in which bionanocomposites can be utilized. Due to the biodegradable and biocompatible nature of bionanocomposites, they can be used for biomedical applications such as tissue engineering, bone replacement, and drug delivery. They also possess good thermal and mechanical properties. The film formed by bionanocomposites can be used for packaging food with high barrier properties and long shelf life. They are also environment friendly and low cost. It has been found that the antimicrobial properties of bionanocomposites are improved by adding clay, montmorillonite, some metal oxides (TiO_2, ZnO, MgO) as well as some metal ions (Ag, Pt, Cu, Au) in the nanorange. Significant research in the field of bionanocomposites has been in progress to extend the application in electronics and medicines.

Acknowledgment

The authors are thankful to all those who have done valuable work in the field of bionanocomposites and to those who are consistently working in this area to develop novel bionanocomposites for the benefit of humans. The authors acknowledge the Department of Chemistry, Aligarh Muslim University, for providing necessary research facilities.

References

1. Ruiz-Hitzky, E., Darder, M., and Aranda, P. (2005). Functional biopolymer nanocomposites based on layered solids. *J. Mater. Chem.*, **15**(35–36), pp. 3650–3662.

2. Ray, S. S. and Bousmina, M. (2005). Biodegradable polymers and their layered silicate nanocomposites: In greening the 21st century materials world. *Prog. Mater. Sci.*, **50**(8), pp. 962–1079.

3. Sorrentino, A., Gorrasi, G., and Vittoria, V. (2007). Potential perspectives of bionanocomposites for food packaging applications. *Trends Food Sci. Technol.*, **18**, pp. 84–95.

4. Averous, L. and Boquillon, N. (2004). Biocomposites based on plasticized starch: Thermal and mechanical behaviours. *Carbohydr. Polym.*, **56**(2), pp. 111–122.

5. Dash, M., et al. (2011). Chitosan: A versatile semi-synthetic polymer in biomedical applications. *Prog. Polym. Sci.*, **36**(8), pp. 981–1014.
6. Darder, M., Montserrat, C., and Ruiz-Hitzky, E. (2003). Biopolymer-clay nanocomposites based on chitosan intercalated in montmorillonite. *Chem. Mater.*, **15**(20), pp. 3774–3780.
7. Marguerite, R. (2006). Chitin and chitosan: Properties and applications. *Prog. Polym. Sci.*, **31**(7), pp. 603–632.
8. Sriupayo, J., et al. (2005). Preparation and characterization of a chitin whisker reinforced chitosn nanocomposites films with or without heat treatment. *Carbohydr. Polym.*, **62**, pp. 130–136.
9. Mathew, A. P., Laborie, G., and Oksman, K. (2009). Cross-linked chitosan/chitin crystal nanocomposites with improved permeation selectivity and pH stability. *Biomacromolecules*, **10**(6), pp. 1627–1632.
10. Celis, R., et al. (2012). Montmorillonite–chitosan bionanocomposites as adsorbents of the herbicide clopyralid in aqueous solution and soil/water suspensions. *J. Hazard Mater.*, **209**, pp. 67–76.
11. Mousa, M. H., Dong, Y., and Davies, I. J. (2016). Recent advances in bionanocomposites: Preparation, properties, and applications. *Int. J. Polym. Mater.*, **65**(5), pp. 225–254, DOI:10.1080/00914037.2015.1103240.
12. Oksman, K., et al. (2006). Manufacturing process of cellulose whiskers/polylactic acid nanocomposites. *Compos. Sci. Technol.*, **66**(15), pp. 2776–2784.
13. Sultana, S., et al. (2016). Natural polymer based composite materials: Recent advances, perspectives, modifications and approaches. In *Natural Polymers: Derivatives, Blends and Composites*, S. Ikram and S. Ahmed (Eds.), Vol. I., Nova Science Publisher, pp. 171–196.
14. Brown, P. W. H. (2005). *Introduction to Organic Chemistry*, 3rd edition, Wiley.
15. Dufresne, T. S. and Pothan, L. A. (2013). *Biopolymer Nanocomposites: Processing, Properties, and Applications*, John Wiley & Sons.
16. Ahmad, N. (2016). *Natural Polymers Based Hydrogels: Preparation, Classification, Properties and Applications*, Nova Science Publishers. *In press*.
17. Reddy, M. M., Mishra, M., and Mohanty, A. (2012). Bio-based materials in the new bio-economy. *Chem. Eng. Prog.*, **108**(5), pp. 37–42.
18. Mahendra, R., Yadav, A., and Gade, A. (2009). Silver nanoparticles as a new generation of antimicrobials. *Biotechnol. Adv.*, **27**(1), pp. 76–83.

19. Ravi Kumar, M. N. V. (2000). A review of chitin and chitosan applications. *React. Funct. Polym.*, **46**, pp. 1–27.
20. Zia, K. M., et al. (2010). XRD pattern of chitin based polyurethane bionanocomposites. *Carbohydr. Polym.*, **80**(2), pp. 539–543.
21. Jie, W., Lin, H., and Meredith, J. C. (2016). Poly(ethylene oxide) bionanocomposites reinforced with chitin nanofiber networks. *Polymer*, **84**, pp. 267–274.
22. Jawaid, M., Qaiss, A. K., and Bouhfid, R. (2016). *Nanoclay Reinforced Polymer Composites: Nanocomposites and Bionanocomposites*, Springer.
23. Hossen, M. F., et al. (2016). Effect of clay content on the morphological, thermo-mechanical and chemical resistance properties of propionic anhydride treated jute fiber/polyethylene/nanoclay nanocomposites. *Measurement*, **90**, pp. 404–411.
24. Guo, B., et al. (2008). Styrene–butadiene rubber/halloysite nanotubes nano-composites modified by methacrylic acid. *Appl. Surf. Sci.*, **255**, pp. 2715–2722. DOI: 10.1016/j.apsusc.2008.07.188.
25. Tate, J. S., Akinola, A. T, and Kabakov, D. (2009). Bio-based nanocomposites: An alternative to traditional composites. *J. Tech. Studies*, pp. 25–32.
26. Ojijo, V. and Ray, S. S. (2013). Processing strategies in bionanocomposites. *Prog. Polym. Sci.*, **38**(10), pp. 1543–1589.
27. Vaia, R. A., et al. (1996). Microstructural evolution of melt intercalated polymer organically modified layered silicates nanocomposites. *Chem. Mater.*, **8**, pp. 2628–2635.
28. Hassannia, K. M., et al. (2016). Development of ecofriendly bionanocomposite: Whey protein isolate/pullulan films with nano-SiO_2. *Int. J. Biol. Macromol.*, **86**, pp. 139–144.
29. Zolfi, M., et al. (2014). Development and characterization of the kefiran-whey protein isolate-TiO_2 nanocomposite films. *Int. J. Biol. Macromol.*, **65**, pp. 340–345.
30. Gounga, M. E., Xu, S., and Wang, Z. (2007). Whey protein isolate-based edible films as affected by protein concentration, glycerol ratio and pullulan addition in film formation. *J. Food Eng.*, **83**, pp. 521–530.
31. Zuber, M., et al. (2010). Synthesis of chitin–bentonite clay based polyurethane bionanocomposites. *Int. J. Biol. Macromol.*, **47**(2), pp. 196–200.
32. Wang, S., Chen, L., and Ton, Y. (2006). Structure–property relationship in chitosan-based biopolymer/montmorillonite nanocomposites. *J. Polym. Sci. Part A. Polym. Chem.*, **44**, pp. 686–696.

33. Choudalakis, G. and Gotsis, A. D. (2009). Permeability of polymer/clay nanocomposites: A review. *Eur. Polym. J.*, **45**, pp. 967–984.
34. Pavlidou, S. and Papaspyrides, C. D. (2008). A review on polymer-layered silicate nanocomposites. *Prog. Polym. Sci.*, **33**(12), pp. 1119–1198.
35. Chang, J. H., Yeong, U. A., and Gil, S. S. (2003). Poly(lactic acid) nanocomposites with various organoclays. I. Thermomechanical properties, morphology, and gas permeability. *J. Polym. Sci. Part B Polym. Phys.*, **41**(1), pp. 94–103.
36. Christopher, T., et al. (2005). Influence of montmorillonite layered silicate on plasticized poly(L-lactide) blown films. *Polymer*, **46**(25), pp. 11716–11727.
37. Tetto, J. A., et al. (1999). Biodegradable poly(caprolactone)/clay nanocomposites. *ANTEC Proc.*, **99**, pp. 1628–1632.
38. Siqueira, G., et al. (2013). Thermal and mechanical properties of bionanocomposites reinforced by Luffacylindrica cellulose nanocrystals. *Carbohydr. Chem.*, **91**(2), pp. 711–717.
39. Becker, O., Varley, R. J., and Simon, G. P. (2004). Thermal stability and water uptake of high performance epoxy layered silicate nanocomposites. *Eur. Polym. J.*, **40**(1), pp. 187–195.
40. Sultana, S., Khan, M. Z., and Umar, K. (2012). Synthesis and characterization of copper ferrite nanoparticles doped polyaniline. *J. Alloy Compd.*, **535**, pp. 44–49.
41. Sultana, S., et al. (2013). Electrical, thermal, photocatalytic and antibacterial studies of metallic oxide nanocomposite doped polyaniline. *J. Mater. Sci. Technol.*, **29**(9), pp. 795–800.
42. Zhu, J., et al. (2001). Studies on the mechanism by which the formation of nanocomposites enhances thermal stability. *Chem. Mater.*, **13**(12), pp. 4649–4654.
43. Bi, L., et al. (2011). Designing carbohydrate nanoparticles for prolonged efficacy of antimicrobial peptide. *J. Control. Release*, **150**, pp. 150–156.
44. Damm, C., Münsted, H., and Rösch, A. (2008). The antimicrobial efficacy of polyamide 6/silver nano- and microcomposites. *Mater. Chem. Phys.*, **108**, pp. 61–66.
45. Hosseini, S. F., et al. (2015). Fabrication of bionanocomposite films based on fish gelatin reinforced with chitosan nanoparticles. *Food Hydrocoll.*, **44**, pp. 172–182.

46. Reddy, M. M., et al. (2013). Biobased plastics and bionanocomposites: Current status and future opportunities. *Prog. Polym. Sci.*, **38**(10), pp. 1653–1689.
47. Gao, W., Dong, H., Hou, H., and Zhang, H. (2012). Effects of clays with various hydrophilicities on properties of starch-clay nanocomposites by film blowing. *Carbohydr. Polym.*, **88**, pp. 321–328.
48. Nogi, M. and Yano, H. (2008). Transparent nanocomposites based on cellulose produced by bacteria offer potential innovation in the electronics device industry. *Adv. Mater.*, **20**(10), pp. 1849–1852.
49. Kymakis, E., Alexandrou, I., and Amaratunga, G. (2003). High open-circuit voltage photovoltaic devices from carbon-nanotube-polymer composites. *J. Appl. Phys.*, **93**, pp. 1764–1768.
50. Bhatia, S. K. and Kurian, J. V. (2008). Biological characterization of Sorona polymer from corn-derived 1,3-propanediol. *Biotechnol. Lett.*, **30**, pp. 619–623.
51. Rhim, J.-W., Park, H. M., and Ha, C. K. (2013). Bionanocomposites for food packaging applications. *Prog. Polym. Sci.*, **38**(10), pp. 1629–1652.

Chapter 9

Plant Fiber–Reinforced Thermoset and Thermoplastic-Based Biocomposites

T. P. Mohan and Krishnan Kanny
*Composites Research Group, Department of Mechanical Engineering,
Durban University of Technology, PO Box 1334, Durban 4000, South Africa*
mohanp@dut.ac.za, kannyk@dut.ac.za

This chapter reviews the recent progress in plant fiber–reinforced composites and their applications. Composites with thermoplastic, thermoset, and rubber matrices were reviewed. Different types of commonly used natural fibers as reinforcement, their chemical treatments, thermal and mechanical properties were reviewed. The processing of natural fiber–reinforced composites and their structure–property relations were discussed. The physical, thermal, and mechanical properties of thermoplastic, thermoset, and rubber-based composites with respect to processing, fiber content, and matrix type were evaluated. The current application of the natural fiber–reinforced composites and their futuristic scope were also discussed.

Biocomposites: Biomedical and Environmental Applications
Edited by Shakeel Ahmed, Saiqa Ikram, Suvardhan Kanchi, and Krishna Bisetty
Copyright © 2018 Pan Stanford Publishing Pte. Ltd.
ISBN 978-981-4774-38-3 (Hardcover), 978-1-315-11080-6 (eBook)
www.panstanford.com

9.1 Introduction

Natural fibers are obtained from plant, animal, and mineral sources. The fibers from plant sources include cotton, flax, hemp, sisal, jute, kenaf, and coconut. Fibers from animal sources include silk, wool, and mohair [1]. Natural fibers can be classified according to their origin, as shown in Fig. 9.1. The figure shows the various types of natural and human-made fibers that can be used in the engineering world for different purposes. Later on in this chapter, we will be expanding mostly on cellulose-based fibers that you see in Fig. 9.1, as well as the different types of uses as natural fiber composites.

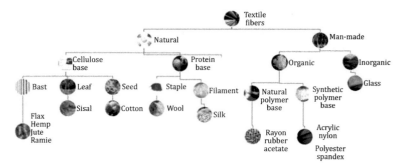

Figure 9.1 Family tree of natural fibers.

9.2 Natural Fibers as Reinforcement

We use natural fibers as reinforcement because they contain properties similar to those of synthetic fibers as they contain cellulose. The growing interest in natural fibers as reinforcement material in the polymer composite world is mainly due to their ease of access, low cost, relatively high specific strength, low density, and minimal hazards [1]. Besides cellulose, these fibers are a compound of hemicellulose and lignin. These components are responsible for different mechanical properties; for instance, hemicellulose is responsible for moisture absorption, whereas lignin is responsible for thermal stability [2]. The presence of surface impurities and the large amount of hydroxyl groups make plant fibers less attractive for reinforcement; however, by the use of additives such as sodium hydroxide and silane, the fibers can be strengthened.

Ecological problems in the recent decades have created the necessity to look for new alternatives that could replace the traditional fiber-reinforced composites with materials having lower environmental impact. This created a renewed interest in natural materials, which could be used as reinforcements or fillers in composites and are thus referred to as "natural fiber–reinforced composites" [3]. Fiber-reinforced composites with thermoplastic matrices have successfully proven their high qualities in many applications. Besides materials such as Kevlar, plant fibers are now replacing synthetic fibers in the industry. In comparison to glass and carbon fibers, natural fibers are better because of the cost of production as well as being greener and biodegradable. The advantages of natural fibers as reinforcement for polymers include low density, wide availability, and higher specific strength than that of glass. With these properties and cheaper ways of attaining these fibers, natural fibers have become theoretically desirable at a cheaper cost. Another important aspect regarding the replacement of glass fiber by natural fibers as the reinforcing component in thermoplastic composites is the distinctive improvement in crash behavior (transport industry). It can be assume that automotive interiors with a reinforcement of natural fibers are safer than glass fiber parts, as no sharp edges occur in the case of a crash [4].

Many different parameters effect the performance of natural fiber reinforcements, one being fiber length. Fiber orientation is an important characteristic in getting optimum results as reinforcement. Fibers tend to orientate along the flow direction, causing the mechanical properties of the material to differ. Tensile strength and Young's modulus increase along fiber direction as length increases. However, fiber strands that are too long decrease the mechanical properties of the material due to fiber entanglement [5]. Natural fibers with small diameter generally possess high mechanical properties, while their permeability is relatively low compared to those with large diameters. By hybridizing these two kinds of natural fibers, a composite with both high permeability and good mechanical properties can be achieved.

Table 9.1 gives a technical understanding with regards to the strength of some of the main natural fibers that are commonly used today.

Table 9.1 Properties of natural fibers

Fiber	Density (g/cm³)	Tensile strength (MPa)	Young's modulus (GPa)	Elongation at break (%)	Specific tensile strength (MPa)	Specific Young's modulus (MPa)
Banana	1.35	222.3–780.3	25.6	1–3.5	392–677	19
Kenaf	1.3	393–773	13–26.5	3	286–562	9–19
Sisal	1.5	468–640	12	3–7	323–441	6–15
Glass	2.55–2.58	500	10–12	3.1–5.3	364–784	15
Carbon	1.79	350–600	14–16	1.5–2.0	195–355	12.8
Coir	2.57	210	1.46–1.96	23.9–51.4	81.7	8
Ramie	1.89	250–400	1.56–1.92	4.2–4.8	456–522	7
Cotton	1.2	150–180	1.11–1.35	0.89–1.2	222–251	4.8
Pineapple	1.48	166–175	60–82	2.78–3.34	112–118	40.54–55.41
Sugarcane bagasse	0.9–1.0	257.3–290.5	15–18	6.2–8.2	285.89–322.78	16.67–20.00
Jute	1.46	300–700	26.5	1.0–1.8	205.48–479.45	18.15
Flax	1.5	500–900	27.6	1.3–3.3	333.33–600.00	18.4
Rice	0.86	435–450	24.67–26.63	2.1–2.25	505.81–523.26	28.69–30.97
Abaca	1.4	879–980	38.45	9–11	627.86–700	27.46
Bamboo	0.6–1.1	140–230	11–17	—	312	13.75–21.25
Hemp	1.15	441.2	26.5	1.6	3.65	23.04

Source: Reprinted from Ref. [6], with permission from Elsevier.

We notice that these different types of fibers possess varied strengths, as well as different densities. Densities are very important and come into play when we discuss specific tensile strengths. We can see, for instance, that fibers from banana and kenaf have low densities with excellent strength values. This is why they are very commonly used in the engineering field as reinforcements.

Table 9.2 shows various natural fibers as well as important quantities such as lignin content. This information is important as we can see which fibers are best to fit certain situations. For instance, in situations where thermal stability is important, lignin content will have to be taken into consideration.

Table 9.2 Properties of natural fibers

Fiber	Aspect ratio (length/diameter) of fiber microfibrils	Lignin (%)
Sugarcane bagasse	1–10	20–25
Banana	10–20	5–15
Jute	5–30	10–15
Ramie	10–100	0–5
Flax	10–20	0–5
Sisal	10–50	5–15
Cotton	3–45	0–3
Coir	20–50	30–50
Pineapple	3–80	0–15
Bamboo	1–10	10–15
hemp	1–10	0–15
Flax	10–25	0–5
Rice husk	1–5	5–15
Abaca	1–10	5–15

Table 9.3 shows the approximate world population of various natural fibers. This gives us a better understanding of which

fibers are widely available and which are scarce. These factors will definitely affect the cost of the material. The mechanical properties of different plant fibers vary due to their different structures as they grow naturally. For instance, ramie and flax fibers possess better mechanical properties owing to their smaller diameters and lumen sizes. However, the permeability of these fabrics is relatively low due to their smaller flow channels. Some other kinds of plant fibers possess larger fiber diameters and lumen sizes, such as jute and sisal fibers, which may lead to a high permeability of their fabrics. However, the mechanical properties of these fibers are not high enough due to the more existing defects caused by the larger fiber diameters. Therefore, combining these two kinds of plant fiber fabrics may lead to a reinforcing material for composites, which possesses both high permeability and good mechanical properties [8].

Table 9.3 Production of natural fibers

Fiber source	World production (1000 ton)
Bamboo	30,000
Jute	2300
Kenaf	970
Flax	830
Sisal	378
Hemp	214
Coir	100
Ramie	100
Abaca	70
Sugarcane bagasse	75,000
Grass	700
Banana	52,000
Pineapple	45,000
Rice husk	60,000

Source: Reprinted from Ref. [9], with permission from Elsevier.

In Table 9.4, we see that if cellulose is high, hemicellulose is low. As illustrated above, the cellulose content determines the properties of the plant cell wall, which gives its key characteristics of, for example, strength, which make flax, kenaf, pineapple, and jute suitable candidates for applications where a high strength-to-weight ratio is required.

Table 9.4 Chemical composition of some common natural fibers

Fiber	Cellulose (wt%)	Hemicellulose (wt%)	Waxes (wt%)
Bamboo	26–45	20–30	0–2
Flax	65–75	15–25	0–5
Kenaf	70–75	15–25	0–2
Banana	60–65	10–20	0–2
Jute	60–75	10–20	0–5
Hemp	65–70	10–20	0–5
Ramie	65–80	10–20	0–5
Sisal	55–65	10–20	0–5
Coir	30–45	0–5	0–2
Pineapple	75–85	0–5	0–2
Rice husk	30–45	15–25	0–2
Bagasse	50–60	15–20	0–2

9.3 Woven and Non-woven Fabric

9.3.1 Woven Fabric

Woven fabrics are principally produced by multiple fill and warp weaving method and usually consist of two sets of interlacing yarn or roving to form three-dimensional fabric structure. Warp runs parallel to the machine direction, while fill runs in the horizontal or perpendicular direction. Mats fiber is consider a blanket of continuous strands laid down as a continuous flat thin sheet. This structure is held together by an adhesive resinous binder or by mechanical bound normally compression stress. Figure 9.2 shows an example of a woven banana mat [11].

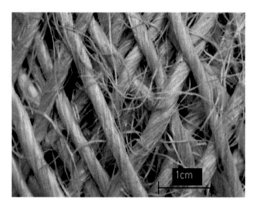

Figure 9.2 Banana fiber woven mat. Reprinted from Ref. [12], with permission from Taylor & Francis.

9.3.2 Non-woven Fabric

Non-woven fabric is a fabric-like material made from long fibers, bonded together by chemical, mechanical, heat, or solvent treatment. The term is used in the textile manufacturing industry to denote fabrics such as felt, which are neither woven nor knitted. Some non-woven materials lack sufficient strength unless made dense or reinforced by a backing. In the recent years, non-wovens have become an alternative to polyurethane foam.

There is a debate in the materials world over the use of woven and non-woven fibers. The trade-off between directional fibers weaved together and put into a lay-up is at odds with the random dispersion of fibers in some kind of thermoset or even thermoplastic resin. The uniform dispersion of shorter fibers in a resin system is seemingly random, yet produces close to isotropic properties in the final cured material. Non-woven fibers and resin systems are much easier to apply to an automated process and are, in general, less costly to produce than weaved, aligned fibers [13].

9.4 Comparison of Non-woven and Woven Fabrics

The effects of woven and non-woven kenaf fibers on the mechanical properties of polyester composites were studied at different types of perform structures. Composite polyester–reinforced kenaf fiber has been prepared via hand lay-up process by varying fiber forms into plain weave, twill, and mat structure. The reinforcing efficiency of different fiber structure was compared with the control of unreinforced polyester sample. It was found that the strength and stiffness of the composites are largely affected by the fiber structure. A maximum value for tensile strength of composite was obtained for weave pattern of fiber structure, while no significant difference for plain weave and mat structure. The elastic modulus of composite has shown some improvement on plain and will weave pattern [14]. Meanwhile, lower value of modulus elasticity was achieved by mats structure composite as well as control sample. The modulus of rupture and impact resistance were also analyzed. An improvement in the modulus of rupture can be seen on plain and twill weave pattern. However, impact resistance does not show significant improvement in all types of structures, except for mat fiber. The mechanical properties of kenaf fiber–reinforced polyester composite were found to be increased with woven and non-woven fiber structures in the composite [15].

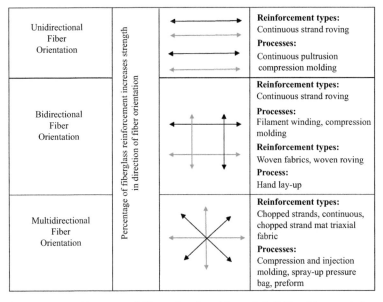

Figure 9.3 Architecture of fibers. Reprinted from Ref. [15], with permission from Elsevier.

Figure 9.3 shows the different types of mats that can be made. Each type of fiber orientation affects the composite as a whole. The different orientation of fibers determines the mechanical characteristics of the material. In unidirectional fiber orientation, fibers are parallel to one another and go in a uniform direction. In bidirectional fiber orientation, the fibers are interlaced between one another; this orientation is used in the textile industry. Multidirectional orientation is a random distribution of fibers as shown in Fig. 9.4. As depicted above, the multidirectional fiber orientation illustrates a higher strength-to-weight ratio in comparison to unidirectional and bidirectional fiber orientations.

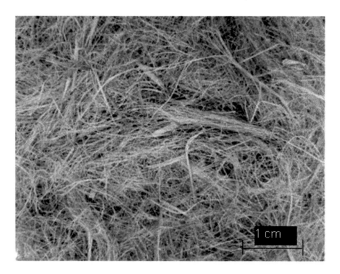

Figure 9.4 Kenaf fiber non-woven mat. Reprinted from Ref. [16], with permission from Elsevier.

9.5 Mechanical Properties: Woven versus Non-woven Kenaf Fibers

As illustrated in Fig. 9.5, plain and twill weave possess the same tensile strength in comparison to mat. This is due to the fiber orientation in plain and twill weave at a higher fiber loading.

Mechanical Properties | 227

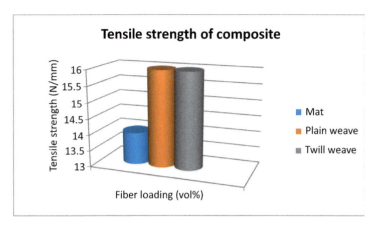

Figure 9.5 Tensile strength of composite. Reprinted from Ref. [17], with permission from Elsevier.

As shown in Fig. 9.6, twill weave possesses a slightly higher Young's modulus than plain weave due to fiber loading, whereas mat has a significantly lower Young's modulus in comparison to plain and twill weave.

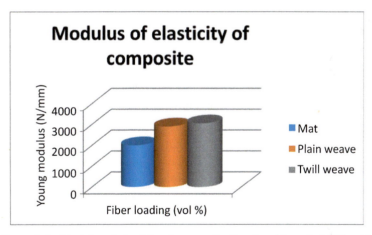

Figure 9.6 Modulus of elasticity of composite. Reprinted from Ref. [17], with permission from Elsevier.

As shown in Fig. 9.7, twill weave possesses a slightly higher elongation at break than plain weave due to the performance type, whereas mat has a significantly lower elongation at break in comparison to plain and twill weave.

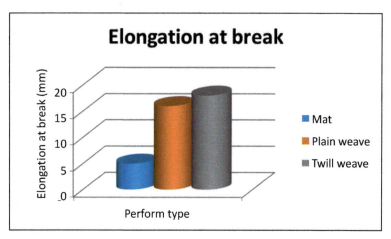

Figure 9.7 Elongation at break. Reprinted from Ref. [17], with permission from Elsevier.

9.6 Types of Plant Fibers and Chemical Treatments

9.6.1 Types of Plant Fiber

Cellulose is the main component of **vegetable fibers**. Examples include cotton, jute, flax, ramie, sisal, and hemp. Vegetable fibers can be further categorized into the following types:

- **Seed fibers** are collected from seeds or seed cases. An example is cotton, a soft fluffy fiber that grows in a ball or protective case, around the seeds of the cotton plants. The fiber is almost pure cellulose. Another example is kapok, a given name for a tree and may also refer to the cotton-like fluff obtained from its seed pods.
- **Leaf fibers** are collected from leaves. Examples are sisal and agave.
- **Fruit fibers** are collected from the fruit of certain plants, such as coconut (coir fiber).
- **Stalk fibers** are actually stalks of plants, such as straws of wheat, rice, barley, and other crops, including bamboo and grass. Tree wood is also such a fiber.

- **Bast fiber and skin fiber** are collected from the skin of bast surrounding the stem of their respective plant. These fibers have higher tensile strength than other fibers. Therefore, these fibers are used for durable yarn, fabric, packaging, and paper. Some examples are flax, jute, kenaf, and industrial hemp.

Table 9.5 represents the different types of fibers used. Each fiber possesses a unique property and origin in relevance to its desired environment. Some of these natural fibers are scarce, while others are abundant, increasing the demand and supply of these fibers. Natural fibers are extracted without damaging the integrity of an ecosystem, thus making them a valuable entity. The huge variety of natural fibers justifies the need to incorporate this natural resource in more of our lives.

Table 9.5 Types of natural fibers

Category	Description
Seed fiber	Fibers collected from seeds or seed cases, e.g., cotton and kapok
Leaf fiber	Fibers collected from leaves, e.g., sansevieria, sisal, banana, and agave
Bast fiber Skin fiber	Fibers collected from the skin or bast surrounding the stem of their respective plant. These fibers have higher tensile strength than other fibers. Therefore, these fibers are used for durable yarn, fabric, packaging, and paper. Some examples are flax, jute, kenaf, industrial hemp, ramie, rattan, and vine fibers.
Fruit fiber	Fibers are collected from the fruit of the plant, e.g., coconut (coir) fiber.
Stalk fiber	Fibers are actually the stalks of the plant, e.g., straws of wheat, rice, barley, and other crops including bamboo and grass. Tree wood is also such a fiber.

Source: Reprinted from Ref. [18], with permission from Taylor & Francis.

9.6.2 Chemical and Thermal Treatment of Fibers

To improve the behavior under aging of natural fibers–reinforced composites, there are two techniques: modification of the matrix [19] and fiber treatment [20]. The second section can represent the advantage of improving the fiber/matrix interface. Many treatments have been applied to natural fibers in the effort to prepare them for practical applications [21]. The chemical treatments most widely used on fibers are acid hydrolysis and alkaline treatment [22]. These treatments include delignification processes. Natural fibers have also been subjected to modifications that accelerate their degradation into monosaccharides. Pulping of natural fibers is also used in the paper industry to eliminate the amounts of lignin and hemicellulose [23].

9.6.2.1 Alkali treatments

All ester-linked molecules of the hemicellulose and other cell-wall components can be cleaved by alkali. This tends to increase the hydrophilicity and hence the solubility of the material [23].

Alkali treatment of lignocellulosic substances disrupts the cell wall, dissolves hemicellulose and lignin by hydrolyzing acetic acid esters and by swelling cellulose, and decreases the crystallinity of cellulose. The biodegradability of the cell wall increases due to the cleavage of the bonds between lignin and hemicellulose or between lignin and cellulose [24].

Fiber cell-OH + NaOH ⟶ Fiber cell-O-Na+ H_2O+ impurities
Chemical reaction

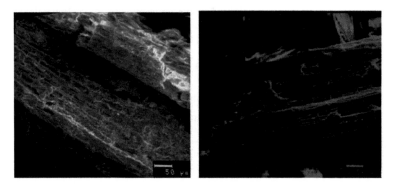

Figure 9.8 SEM image of alkali treatment banana fiber before and after. Reprinted from Ref. [24], with permission from Elsevier.

Figure 9.8 shows banana fiber undergoing alkali treatment. Results show that treated fiber surface is more ridged than that of untreated fibers. Mechanical characteristics indicated that Young's modulus, among other properties, increased. When banana fibers undergo alkali treatment, the strength of the fiber becomes higher than that of the untreated versions due to the intrinsically increased strength of the fibers.

9.6.2.2 Acid treatments

The effects of acid treatments on vegetable fibers [25] differ with the nature and concentration of the acid and with the temperature of the experiment. Hemicelluloses are very sensitive to acid hydrolysis and are easily hydrolyzed by acids [26]. By hydrolysis, they form their corresponding monomer elements.

The actuation of the acid on the cellulose chain can entail the attack of glucosidic bonds by hydronium ions. It also induces the failure of the microfibrils and the separation of the constituents of the fiber.

The lignin in hardwood species is partly dissolved by sulfuric acid during acid hydrolysis [27]. The acid treatment decreases the aliphatic hydroxyl content and consequently decreases the polarity of the lignin molecules without derivatization, but enhances the antioxidant properties [28].

$$\text{Fiber-OH} + CH_3(CH_2)16COOH \longrightarrow CH_3(CH_2)16COO\text{-O-Fiber} + H_2O$$

Figure 9.9 shows that the surface roughness decreases in the sample. It is also found that treating the fiber decreases the magnitude of loss modulus. The flexural strength of composites made from this fiber increased.

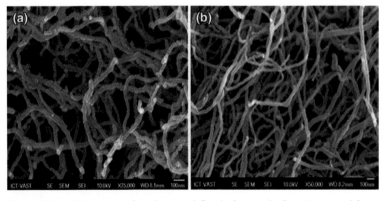

Figure 9.9 SEM image of acid-treated flax before and after. Reprinted from Ref. [29], with permission from Elsevier.

9.6.2.3 Pyrolysis treatments

The first process in the thermal decomposition of vegetable materials corresponds to hemicellulose decomposition [30]. In the thermal decomposition of natural fibers, it was found that below 300°C, this reaction results in the formation of char, water, carbon monoxide, and carbon dioxide. However, between 300 and 500°C, pyrolysis results in the formation of tars, which consist largely of anhydrous sugars, oligosaccharides, and dehydration of pyrans and furans. Above 500°C, flash pyrolysis produces volatiles or gaseous molecules of low molecular weight from secondary reactions of tars and the interaction between char, water, and CO_2 at high temperature. Cellulose degradation is the second process in the decomposition of lignocellulosic materials [31].

The pyrolysis of lignin occurs in inert atmospheres at high temperatures over a wide temperature domain [32, 33]. The thermal decomposition of lignin is also affected by the acid pretreatment used for cellulose extraction [34]. This is responsible for the breakdown of the three-dimensional structure of lignin. A combination of chemical or thermal treatment can also be carried out [35, 36]. For sugarcane delignification, hydrothermal and alkali pulp treatment [37, 38] and acid and thermal treatment [39] can be used.

Figure 9.10 indicates that as the diameter of the fiber decreases, the surface roughness also decreases. The strength of the fiber increases. The tensile strength values of coir fiber increased with the increase in concentration of treatment up to a certain level and then remains constant. This treatment was more effective than silane treatment in enhancing the mechanical properties of cellulose fiber.

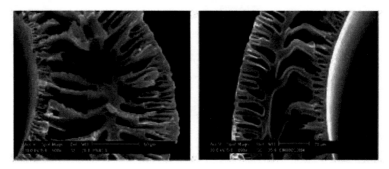

Figure 9.10 SEM image of pyrolysis-treated coir before and after. Reprinted from Ref. [39], with permission from Elsevier.

9.6.2.4 Coating with silane treatment

Alkyltrialkoxysilanes, R'Si(OR)$_3$, are used in many industrial applications as coupling agents to improve the adhesion between polymeric matrices and inorganic materials. They have also been used in vegetable fiber polymer composites [41, 41] to modify fiber surface. The mechanism of these coupling reactions is related to the effect of two reactive surface groups, and these reactions are different according to the substrate in contact. Alkoxy groups (OR) allow silane to bind to surface OH groups after hydrolysis. Additionally, the alkyl groups R' increase the compatibility with the organic compounds and the hydrophobic character of the surface, leading to an enhancement in the strength of the interface in the polymer matrix. Usually, silane treatment is carried out with a diluted silane solution at 0.2% to 20% by weight [42, 43]. These conditions have the following advantages:

- Increase in silane solubility
- Improvement in the thickness of the surface film
- Development of a uniform cover on the surface

Water produces moderate hydrolysis of silane and leads to silanol. This behavior allows the adhesion of silanes onto the OH groups of the fiber substrate.

After solvent evaporation, the residual silanol groups can condense with the hydroxyl groups of the substrate or can lead, by self-condensation reactions, to a polysiloxane network on the surface. In aqueous media, partially or totally hydrolyzed silanes are reactive molecules that change with time by self-condensation of silanol groups or condensation of silanol with alkoxy groups to form dimers or oligomers. They are commonly used as commercial water repellents [44].

Figure 9.11 shows that silane-treated fibers have less impurities and lignin and hemicelluloses removed than those by other treatments. After treatment, there is a significant increase in the interfacial strength of the fibers. The fibers also possess a higher tensile strength from silane-treated than alkali-treated fibers.

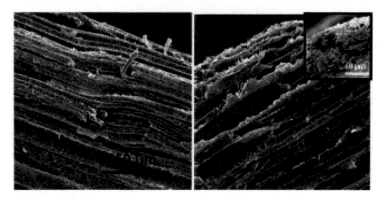

Figure 9.11 SEM images of surface before and after silane treatment of kenaf fibers. Reprinted from Ref. [45], with permission from Elsevier.

9.6.2.5 Benzoylation treatment

Benzoylation is an important transformation in organic synthesis [46]. It involves reaction of the cellulosic hydroxyl group of the fiber and benzoyl chloride, which is most commonly used in fiber treatment [47]. The benzoyl group ($C_6H_5C=O$) of benzoyl chloride is responsible for the decreased hydrophilic nature of the treated fiber and improved interaction with the hydrophobic polymer matrix. Benzoylation of fiber improves fiber matrix adhesion, thereby considerably increasing the strength of the composite, decreasing its water absorption, and improving its thermal stability.

Figure 9.12 shows that the surface of the treated fiber is significantly smoother than the untreated fiber. This treatment improves fiber matrix adhesion, thereby considerably increasing the strength of the fiber, decreasing its water absorption rate, and improving its thermal stability.

9.7 Plant Fiber–Reinforced Thermoplastic Composites

In technical application, fiber-reinforced composites have been proven to be successful in various fields. Natural fibers such as hemp and flax are being used for reinforcement, apart from the usual materials such as Kevlar or glass fiber.

Acetylation with acid catalyst

$$\text{Fiber–OH} + \text{CH}_3\text{COOH} \xrightarrow[\text{Conc. H}_2\text{SO}_4]{(\text{CH}_3\text{CO})2\text{O}} \text{Fiber} - \text{O} - \overset{\overset{\displaystyle O}{\|}}{\text{C}} - \text{CH}_3 + \text{H}_2\text{O}$$

Acetylation without acid catalyst

$$\text{Fiber–OH} + \text{CH}_3 - \overset{\overset{\displaystyle O}{\|}}{\text{C}} - \text{O} - \overset{\overset{\displaystyle O}{\|}}{\text{C}} - \text{CH}_3 \longrightarrow \text{Fiber} - \text{O} - \overset{\overset{\displaystyle O}{\|}}{\text{C}} - \text{CH}_3 + \text{CH}_3\text{C} - \text{OH}$$

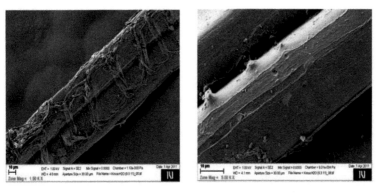

Figure 9.12 SEM image of benzoylation-treated banana before and after. Reprinted from Ref. [47], with permission from Springer Nature.

In the field of thermoplastics and thermosets, many different natural fibers are now being used, including kenaf and sisal. Most cellulose-based fibers are being used, even the likes of agricultural materials such as rice straw, corn cobs, and corn stalks, even though they have lower cellulose content compared to wood and other plant fibers. However, these materials are being used more due to their lower cost and wide availability, which makes the mass production of these natural fiber composites less expensive [48].

9.7.1 Processing and Characterization for the Processing of Natural Fiber–Reinforced Thermoplastics

For the use of lightweight structures, natural fibers offer superior results with regards to reinforcement. As discussed before, due to the improvement in crash behavior from natural fibers, they are quickly replacing glass fibers in the industry. Alternatively, natural fibers have an advantage that they offer great acoustics due to their high absorptivity. Unlike glass fibers, natural fibers hardly cause irritation to skin, so they are industrially better to work with. Alternatively, an important advantage in the processing of natural fibers is that they are a source of renewable material; thus, they are a positive influence in the promotion of "green" composites [49].

There are many different methods in the manufacturing of thermoplastic natural fibers. In this section, we are mainly going to discuss solution casting, compression molding, and injection molding. Mostly in these processes, fibers are chopped during process; therefore, composites have short fibers. The composites' orientation depends on the method used to create the composite; for instance, in injection molding, it will depend on the mold. For a more continuous process, thermoplastic pultrusion can be used. For a more plain orientation in a composite, longer fibers are used, as in pultrusion. Elementary fiber rather than technical fiber should be used in the manufacturing of natural fiber composites. However, if the aim is to create longer fiber composites, technical fiber should be used to get optimum results [50].

9.7.1.1 Polymer solution casting

This technique can deliver high-quality films with excellent mechanical and physical properties. In the process of polymer solution casting, a solution dissolves the polymer, coated onto a carrier substrate, and then the water or solvent is removed by drying to create a solid layer on the carrier. To produce a standalone film, it is possible for the resulting cast layer to be stripped from the carrier. It is common to create multilayer products by laminating the cast film with other materials [51].

The manufacturing advantages of polymer solution casting over traditional film extrusion methods include the following:

- It can be processed at low temperatures, which can be of great help when dealing with temperature-sensitive materials.
- Using non-thermoplastics to produce high-temperature resistant films.

- Simplified incorporation of additives and fillers.
- Quicker changeovers for platforms with many part numbers that are differentiated based on formula.
- Single-pass manufacturing of multilayer films (e.g., the ability to cast a free film, then coat an adhesive and laminate release liner on one side, and coat a top coat on the other side).
- Wider range of material choices with casting from either aqueous or solvent-based solutions.

Advantages of the resulting film include the following:

- Greater film thickness uniformity, as tight as +/−2%.
- Wider range of film thickness, from 150 microns down to less than 12 microns.
- Films that are gel and pinhole free.
- Excellent flatness and dimensional stability.
- Isotropic orientation (mechanical and optical) as film is not stretched during manufacture.
- Absence of typical extrusion process lubricants.

The suitability of polymer solution casting is evaluated on a case-by-case basis according to the product application, base material, intended use, and numerous other considerations. Specific benefits are realized for the following applications, among others [52].

- **Acrylic and other polymer films**: deliver superior optical properties and thickness uniformity.
- **Polyurethane (PU) films**: improve mechanical properties such as elimination of pinholes or voids; also ensures film uniformity, high optical clarity and production of thin films, which can be easily customized with added functional layers and properties. Thermoset adhesive films where melt extrusion is not feasible.
- **Thermal interface materials**: enable the addition of more concentrated thermally conductive fillers than are feasible with the melt extrusion process.
- **Electro-active polymer films**: deliver superior optical properties, uniformity, and gel and pinhole-free materials that do not provide a path for high-voltage breakdown failure.

Due to the environmental concern of petroleum-based materials, natural fibers are becoming the obvious choice forward in many molding methods, especially solvent casting. The advantages of using the solvent-casting method, as shown in Fig. 9.13, are its ease of fabrication and no need of advanced equipment. Natural fibers are also low-cost fibers, have low densities and high specific properties. This then makes the polymer cheaper and stronger for the mold. They are also biodegradable and non-abrasive.

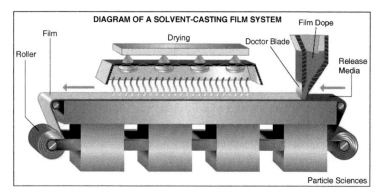

Figure 9.13 Diagram of a solvent-casting film system. Reprinted from Ref. [52], with permission from John Wiley and Sons.

9.7.1.2 Compression molding

This process uses a heated mold cavity, into which a polymer is poured. Pressure is put on the material to ensure that all areas of the mold are covered. Until the polymer has cured fully, the heat and pressure remain constant.

Natural fiber moldings are now being manufactured using this compression molding method in the engineering industry. This is where a combination of natural fiber and polypropylene non-woven mats is needle punched into a sandwich-like structure. The sandwich is then heated until soft and then transferred to a cold press, where it can be compression molded. Most applications use thermosets; however, compression molding can use both thermoplastics and thermosets. Natural fibers can be used as a mat or chopped and can be compression molded to create a composite thermoplastic [53]. High-strength objects are suitable to be made by compression molding as it is a high-volume, high-pressure plastic molding method. It is being used more in the automotive industry as it has a short cycle time and a high production rate; therefore, producing parts are easier and quicker.

Figure 9.14 gives us a brief idea of how compression molding system works.

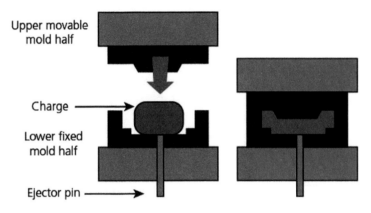

Figure 9.14 Compression molding.

9.7.1.3 Injection molding

For the fabrication of plastic parts, injection molding is the most common and best manufacturing process. Many different products are being manufactured by the injection mold; all vary due to their size and complexity. The injection molding process needs the use of an injection molding machine, raw plastic material, and a mold. The injection process is rather simple. The plastic is melted in the injection molding machine and then injected into the mold, where it cools and solidifies into the final part [54].

A common product that injection moldings are used for is plastic housings and other thin-walled plastic parts. Many electronic components and household appliances make use of these plastic housings. Other common items that use injection moldings are buckets and toothbrushes. Also products such as syringes, which are used in the medical field, make use of injection molding [55].

Due to the always increasing price level of conventional plastics, natural fibers are quickly gaining importance in today's world.

Natural fiber–reinforced plastics are filled or reinforced with natural fibers; therefore, it can be easily used for injection molding as a replacement for the normal expensive and less "green" plastics.

Figure 9.15 shows how an injection mold works. The feeder hopper is where the raw material is added to be heated. Once heating has been completed, the screw pushes the polymer (raw material) into the mold.

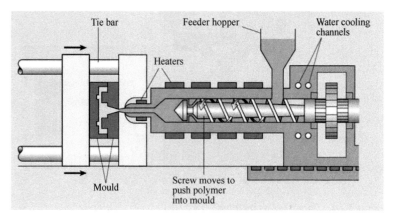

Figure 9.15 Injection molding. Reprinted from Ref. [55], with permission from John Wiley and Sons.

Figure 9.16 shows an example of a natural fiber–reinforced plastic. It is a cork using elastic-reinforced natural fiber.

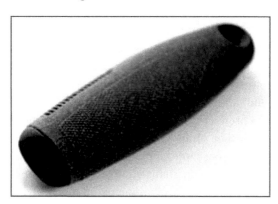

Figure 9.16 Cork produced using injection molding. Reprinted from Ref. [56], with permission from Elsevier.

9.7.2 Mechanical, Thermal, and Physical Properties

Natural fibers are characterized by the same parameters and properties as all other fibers. However, they show much higher variability of the various parameters than their synthetic counterparts, due to natural origin. Chemical composition, crystallinity, surface properties, diameter, cross-sectional shape, length, strength, and stiffness vary from fiber to fiber. Moreover, their properties depend on harvesting conditions and processing. This poses two problems: quality characterization of fibers and difficulties in application of traditional composite theories. Natural plant fiber materials to be used include cellulose, hemicellulose, and lignin components. In order to separate cellulose, hemicellulose, and lignin fractions, such that the cellulose fraction can be chemically treated and removed from the hemicellulose and lignin fractions, the fibers have to be treated prior to the formation of composite materials. The fibers of the cellulose component of the plant materials can be substituted for the synthetic fibers used to achieve similar mechanical characteristics for the composite material as when synthetic fibers are used, particularly tensile and flexural strength as well as impact toughness. In addition, the cellulose fraction of the natural plant materials does not absorb and retain water, thus does not detrimentally affect the waterproof properties of the composite material. Furthermore, the cellulose fraction enables the composite material to be readily disposed of.

Natural plant fibers are mechanically treated prior to chemical treatment in order to obtain relatively pure plant material for use in the chemical extraction process. The particular mechanical treatment is accomplished in a manner that reduces the breakage of the core fibers, resulting in longer cellulose fibers from the chemical extraction process, which in turn provide a stronger composite composition with enhanced strength and lighter weight than glass fiber-filled composite materials [57, 58].

In Table 9.6, it can be seen that NFC composites with aligned fibers are produced by hand if the fiber is in a reasonably raw form. Although yarn gives good performance, processing is particularly intensive with many stages, including carding and spinning for which each stage requires specialist equipment.

Table 9.6 Mechanical, thermal, and physical properties of natural fibers

Fiber	Matrix	Fiber content (m%)	Tensile strength (MPa)	Stiffness/ Young's modulus (GPa)	Flexural strength (MPa)	Flexural modulus (GPa)	Notes: Processing/length/ treatment
Flax yarn (aligned)	PP	72	321	29	—	—	Filament wound
Flax (aligned)	PP	50	40	7	—	—	Needle punched flax/PP mats CM
Flax (aligned)	PP	39	—	—	212	23	Dew retted, boiled, MAA-PP coupled
Hemp (aligned)	PP	46	—	—	127	11	Wrap spun, short hemp/PP hybrid yarn, CM
Kenaf selected (aligned)	PLA	~80	223	23	254	22	Emulsion PLA Prepare CM
Kenaf (aligned)	PLA	40	82	8	126	7	CM
Hemp (aligned)	PLA	30	77	10	101	7	Wrap spun alkali-treated short hemp hybrid yarn, CM
Hemp (biaxial)	PLA	45	62	7	124	9	Wrap spun bleached hemp hybrid yarn, CM

Source: Adapted from Ref. [59].

9.7.3 Flame-Retardant Properties of NFPCs

The eco-friendly and sustainable nature of natural fiber composites makes them a suitable candidate over conventional composites based on synthetic fibers. Natural fibers are used in diversified domains such as building materials [60], aerospace industry, and automotive industry [61]. Natural fibers are organic and are very sensitive as they tend to alter their properties if a flame is introduced to them. Flame retardancy is another aspect that has become greatly significant in order to fulfil safety measures taken while developing natural fiber composites.

The two most widely used metal hydroxide flame retardants are known to be aluminum hydroxide [$Al(OH_3)$] and magnesium hydroxide [$Mg(OH)_2$], which are purposefully added to polymers. The chemical reactions through which these two flame retardants decompose are as follows: Out of these two flame retardants, magnesium hydroxide displays better thermal stability compared to aluminum hydroxide since the temperature range given by the decomposition of magnesium hydroxide is nearly 300–320°C, which is much higher than the temperature range offered by aluminum hydroxide, which is only 200°C. For this reason, aluminum hydroxide is not considered thermally stable as it cannot be used for polyamides, polypropylene, or others, whereas magnesium hydroxide can be used [62].

Figure 9.17 shows two materials that are subjected to extreme heat conditions. The natural fiber composite is significantly less flammable than the material shown on the left, which shows that this composite has far superior thermal absorption as opposed to regular materials.

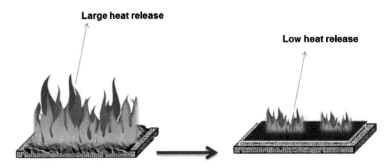

Figure 9.17 Natural fiber composite as opposed to a regular material [62].

9.7.4 Biodegradability of NFPCs

High-strength natural fiber composites are products of natural fiber reinforcement in polymers, which provide biodegradability, enhanced properties related to mechanical structure. At temperatures as high as 240°C, natural fibers start degrading whereas other fibers, with different levels of hemicelluloses, celluloses, and lignins, degrade at higher levels of temperatures, for example, lignin starts to decompose at 200°C, whereas at temperatures higher than this, other constituents will also degrade. Since the thermal stability of natural fibers is dependent on the structural factors of fibers, it can be improved if the structural factors or concentration levels are completely removed, such as hemicelluloses and lignin. With chemical treatments, this can be achieved. The degradation of natural fibers is an important aspect that must be considered during the development of materials and fibers. Natural fibers have very little environmental damage upon degradation in comparison to synthetic ones, which affect the environment due to pollution. Cellulose, hemicellulose, and lignin composition and concentrations affect thermal degradation features of lingo-cellulosic materials [63].

Although natural fibers are known for their exceptional and distinguished properties, they are known to perish over a short duration of time, as shown in Fig. 9.18.

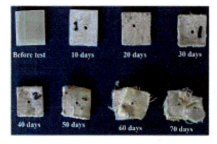

Figure 9.18 Biodegradability of a natural fiber composite (sisal) [63].

9.7.5 Energy Absorption of NFPCs

High strength, energy absorption, and stiffness are obtained by composite materials, which are widely used in automotive and motorsport sectors mainly due to the property of mass reduction. Enhanced energy absorption is evident from the increased volume fraction, which is possible only in the presence of low speed such as 2.5 m/s. On the other hand, at high speeds such as 300 m/s, similar performance is shown by flax, jute, and hemp, but jute showed brittleness and low strength of fibers. The potential of NFPCs, which is required for application in providing sustainable energy absorption, was investigated by Meredith et al. while keeping focus on motorsport [64]. Vacuum-assisted resin transfer molding (VARTM) manufacturing is used to test conical specimens of jute, hemp, and flax for their features and properties. The values showed by different kinds of materials were recorded to analyze specific energy absorption (SEA).

Figure 9.19 illustrates the energy absorbed by different fibers over a period of time. Energy absorbed is dependent on time. The energy absorbed is due to the load applied. Kenaf and coir show the highest energy absorbed, whereas sisal and ramie show less energy absorbed. All natural fibers undergo a time period of 250 h.

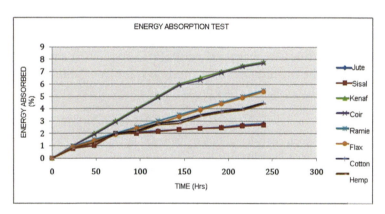

Figure 9.19 Energy absorption by fibers over time. Reprinted from Ref. [64], with permission from Elsevier.

9.7.6 Water Absorption Characteristics of NFPCs

The reinforcement of natural fibers in polymers works well. One of the main weaknesses exhibited in the application of natural fibers is their susceptibility to moisture. Mechanical properties of polymeric composites illustrate a high dependency on the interface adhesion between the polymer matrix and the fiber. Pectins, lignins, hemicelluloses, and celluloses present in natural fibers all have hydroxy 1 group, which makes natural fibers strongly polar and hydrophilic. Polymers, on the other hand, are hydrophobic. Due to this lack in suitability between the matrix and fibers, weaknesses in the interface region them results. When the bulk of the matrix is exposed to water, it tends to gradually decrease at the composite materials' outer layer. When a composite material absorbs a high rate of water, its causes an increment in its deflection, a conceivable decline in its strength, an increased weight of wet profiles, and causing pressure on nearby structures. These can cause destruction of mechanical characteristics of the composite materials, involving bigger possibility of their microbial inhabitation, warping, and buckling [65]. The moisture content of these various fibers is shown in Table 9.7.

The mercerization of OPF-sisal fiber-NR hybrid composites led to reduced water adsorption by the composite by improving the adhesive characteristics of the fiber surface and also providing a large surface area, which provides better mechanical interlocking. The chemical treatment is achieved using four types of reagents: acetic anhydride (Ac), maleic anhydride (MA), styrene (S), and acrylic acid (AA). The chemical treatment decreases the global diffusivity of water and also concludes that the water mobility in the fiber core is more than at the surface [66].

Table 9.7 The equilibrium moisture content of different natural fibers at 65% relative humidity (RH) and 21°C

Fiber	Equilibrium moisture content (%)
Sisal	11
Hemp	9
Jute	12
Flax	7
Abaca	15
Ramie	9
Pineapple	13
Coir	10
Bagasse	8.8
Bamboo	8.9

Source: Reprinted from Ref. [65], with permission from Elsevier.

9.8 Products and Applications of Plant Fiber–Reinforced Thermoplastics

Reinforced fiber composite materials based on thermoplastic materials are being increasingly used in many areas of technology. They are used in place of metallic materials as they promise a substantial reduction in weight. For that reason, besides the thermoplastic matrix, these composite materials include a fibrous component, which has a considerable influence on mechanical characteristics, particularly tensile and flexural strength as well as impact toughness of the composite material [67].

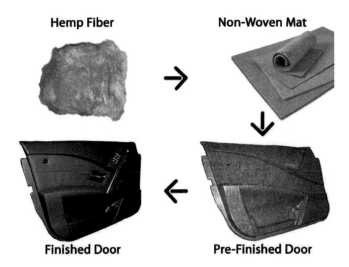

Figure 9.20   Application of natural fibers [68].

Figure 9.20 shows the application of natural fibers in the automotive sector. After several years of thorough research, the use of natural fibers in composites was found to exceed the high performance demand, required for strength and durability. Natural fiber composites are made of a mixture of 50% hemp and 50% polypropylene (PP), which are formed into fleece mats and are later formed into various components. A quick expanding application for flax fiber is as reinforcement and filler in the production of flax fiber composites. The binding materials range from thermoplastics such as polypropylene to thermoset resins such as polyester or polyurethane. Typical applications include automotive interior substrates, furniture, and other flax fiber–based consumer products [68].

Flax fiber composites are of interest to automotive and other applications due to the following features:

- Cost effective
- High tensile strength and stiffness
- Ideally suited for needle punched non-woven products
- Effective replacement for glass fiber
- Reduces molding time
- Weight reduction in finished part
- Easy to process and recycle
- Can be customized to meet a variety of specifications and different manufacturing systems

Most of the technologies developed for automotive applications can be used to make consumer products from flax fiber composites. It is possible to use compression molding, injection molding, and hybrid technologies to produce consumer goods from flax fiber composites. Such products include furniture, sporting goods, recreational products, luggage, musical instruments, and sound reinforcement gear. In most applications if the product uses glass fiber, then flax fiber most likely could be substituted as reinforcement in the product [69].

Figure 9.21 shows the use of flax fiber in the automotive interior. Natural fibers used in automotive composites instead of fiberglass result in both ecological and technological benefits. When it is compared to traditional fiberglass, natural fiber composites do not splinter on impact, use less energy to produce, have a lower material cost, and are recyclable.

In Fig. 9.22, flax fiber has been molded into a brief case and can also be used to produce mineral-based composites. The rising price of energy, particularly petroleum, is making these other reinforcing fibers more expensive and the excellent properties and cost of flax fiber are opening new applications every day. It is possible to use compression molding, injection molding, simple hand lay-ups, or hybrid technologies to produce consumer goods from flax fiber composites, such as furniture, sporting goods, recreational products, luggage (brief case), musical instruments, and sound reinforcement gear. In most applications if the product uses glass fiber, then flax fiber most likely could be substituted as reinforcement in the product.

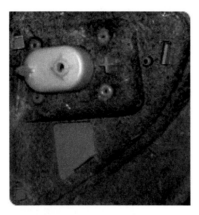

Figure 9.21 Flax fiber–based automotive interior trim part shown with flax fiber composite substrate and plastic inserts for fastening. Image taken from Ref. [70], copyright © 2006–2018 Stemergy. All rights reserved.

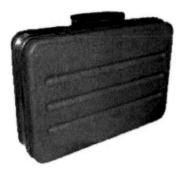

Figure 9.22 Flax fiber composite molded brief case made with flax fiber and polypropylene compression molded non-woven material. Image taken from Ref. [70], copyright © 2006–2018 Stemergy. All rights reserved.

9.9 Plant Fiber–Reinforced Thermoset Composites

Thermoplastics widely used for biofibers are polyethylene, polypropylene (PP), and polyvinyl chloride (PVC); here phenolic, polyester, and epoxy resins are mostly utilized thermosetting matrices. Different factors can affect the characteristics and performance of NFPCs. The hydrophilic nature of natural fibers and fiber loading have impacts on the composite properties [71]. Usually, a high fiber loading is needed to attain good properties of NFPCs. Generally, the rise in fiber content causes improved tensile properties of the composites. Another vital factor that considerably impacts the properties and surface characteristics of the composites is the process parameters utilized. For that reason, appropriate process techniques and parameters should be rigorously chosen in order to get the best characteristics of producing composite. The chemical composition of natural fibers also has a big effect on the characteristics of the composite represented by the percentage of cellulose, hemicellulose, lignin, and waxes. In Table 9.8, we see that flax alone is stronger (tensile strength 280 Mpa), whereas if you have flax yarn, it is weaker (tensile strength 133 Mpa). However, in thermoplastics, it is the other way around.

9.9.1 General Characteristics of NFPCs

The properties of natural fiber composite are different from each other because of the different kinds of fibers, sources, and moisture conditions. The performance of NFPCs relies on some factors, such as mechanical composition, microfibrillar angle, structure, defects, cell dimensions, physical properties, chemical properties, and also the interaction of a fiber with the matrix [72]. Since every product in the market has drawbacks, natural fiber–reinforced polymer composites also have drawbacks. The couplings between natural fiber and polymer matrix are problem taken into consideration, as a result of the difference in chemical structure between these two phases. This leads to unproductive stress transfer during the interface of the NFPCs. Thus, the chemical treatments for the natural fiber are necessary to achieve good interface properties. The reagent functional groups in the chemical treatments have the ability to react on the fiber structures and alter the fiber composition. Natural fibers include a functional group named hydroxyl group, which makes the fibers hydrophilic. During manufacturing of NFPCs, weaker interfacial bonding occurs between hydrophilic natural fiber

Table 9.8 Mechanical properties of thermosets

Fiber	Matrix	Fiber content (m%)	Tensile strength (MPa)	Stiffness/Young's modulus (GPa)	Flexural strength (MPa)	Flexural modulus (GPa)	Notes: Processing/length/treatment
Sisal (aligned)	Epoxy	~77	330	10	290	22	Untreated bundles CM/leaky mold
Flax (aligned)	Epoxy	46/54	280/279	35/39			Enzyme extracted RTM
Flax (yarn) (aligned)	Epoxy	45			311	25	Not stated
Hemp (aligned)	Epoxy	65	165	17	180	9	CM
Flax yarn (aligned)	Epoxy	45	133	28	218	18	Autoclave
Flax (woven)	Epoxy	~50	104	10			Sized and dried prior to pre-preg

Source: Reprinted from Ref. [73], with permission from Elsevier.

and hydrophobic polymer matrices due to the hydroxyl group in natural fibers. This could produce NFPCs with weak mechanical and physical properties.

Plant fiber–reinforced composites (PFRC) are emerging in a variety of industries due to their ability of affordability, environmentally friendly, and render relatively high specific mechanical properties compared to glass fiber–reinforced composites. Another advantage of using PFRC is that the light weight of PFRC can reduce the total weight mass of the desired application, thus reducing operation costs during utilization, which is a great contribution to sustain the environment [74].

In Fig. 9.23, natural fiber is used to make door panel. Many of the technologies established for automotive applications can be used to make consumer products from flax fiber composites. They have the ability to integrate fabric and leather coverings, natural fiber composite blends, and many more, which makes their door systems lighter, high-strength, and noise reducing.

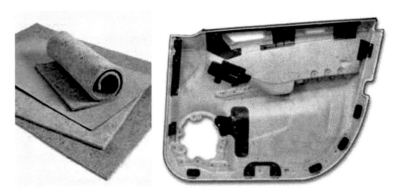

Figure 9.23 Reinforced door panel with natural fibers. Image source: © 2013 FlexForm Technologies. All Rights Reserved.

9.9.2 Vacuum-Assisted Resin Transfer Molding

Great quality and large-sized PFRCs are frequently fabricated by vacuum-assisted resin transfer molding (VARTM) process for its easy preparation and low cost [76], which will further reduce the production cost.

Plant Fiber–Reinforced Thermoset Composites | 253

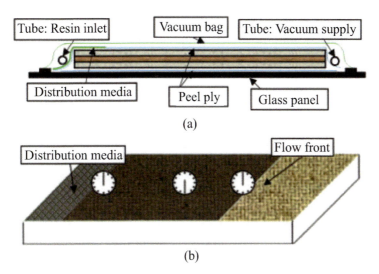

Figure 9.24 (a) Illustration of VARTM preparation and (b) scheme of the permeability measurement. Reprinted from Ref. [76], with permission from Elsevier.

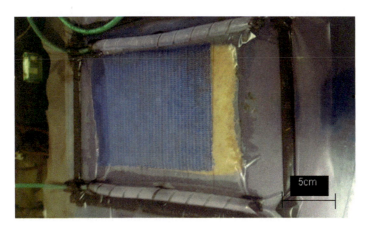

Figure 9.25 Kenaf fiber infusion.

During the VARTM process shown in Figs. 9.24 and 9.25, permeability of reinforcement is especially important for the composite to reach its maximum design properties. The process can be improved further with the use of distribution mats and pipes. Considering the same porosity, banana, kenaf, and sisal fiber mats possess higher permeability than those of glass fiber mats due to more direct channels for resin flow developed by plant fiber mats. This is applicable for design requirements where high strength-to-weight ratios are needed. Moreover, the rough twisted surface of plant fiber provides more tubular channels for the micro-flow of the resin, and the pressure generated by these channels is two or three times higher than that of synthetic fibers, especially in applications where internal strength and durability are desirable. The fluid absorption and swelling of plant fibers decrease their permeability to some extent. Lower permeability of reinforcements may lead to a higher void content inside composites and also a prolonged infusion time, especially with low pressure injection process. The mechanical properties of the composites may have been weakened by these methods. Improving the low permeability of one kind of reinforcement with another kind of reinforcement with high permeability may be an efficient way [77]. The addition of these high permeability materials usually has some detrimental effects on the mechanical properties of the manufactured composite, particularly for inter-laminar properties because of the weak interface between the two different materials. The mechanical properties of different plant fibers differ due to their different structures as they grow naturally. For instance, kenaf and sisal fiber possess better mechanical properties [78], owing to their smaller diameters and lumen sizes as opposed to the shorter banana fibers shown in Fig. 9.26. The permeability of these fabrics is relatively low due to their smaller flow channels. Different kinds of plant fibers have larger fiber diameters and lumen sizes such as kenaf and sisal fibers, which could lead to a high permeability of their fabrics. The mechanical properties of these fibers are not high enough due to the more existing defects caused by the larger fiber diameters. Therefore, combining these two types of plant fiber fabrics may lead to a reinforcing material for composites that possesses both high permeability and good mechanical properties.

9.9.3 Resin Transfer Molding

Resin transfer molding (RTM) produces high-volume, high-quality composite parts made of fiber-reinforced plastic (fiberglass). RTM uses a matched mold set to create a fixed cavity from which a part is prepared.

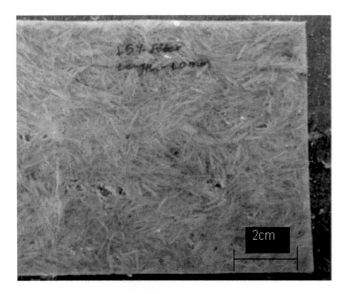

Figure 9.26 Fabricated short banana fiber–reinforced epoxy composites.

Figure 9.27 describes how the RTM process works. Simply, a fabric is laid onto the mold cavity. The mold is then closed, and resin is then injected into the mold cavity, impregnating the fiberglass. The mold is then opened and the part is removed, after the resin hardens.

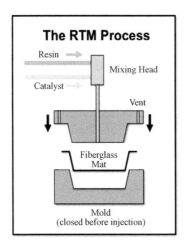

Figure 9.27 RTM process. Reprinted from Ref. [79], with permission from John Wiley and Sons.

Common materials used to build RTM molds are also known as tooling, include fiberglass, aluminum, and steel. The manufacturing process to build a fiberglass RTM mold is shown in Fig. 9.28. The material selected to build a specific mold is based on a variety of factors, such as quantity, size, finish quality, part complexity, and required cycle time. For high-volume production, molds are usually heated. Computerized control systems are incorporated to automate the entire molding process. Parts built with the RTM process are typically superior to conventional spray-up fiberglass in terms of structural properties such as water tightness and aesthetics. Since parts are made within a closed mold, part consistency is excellent. Parts have two smooth surfaces, and RTM allows the use of high-strength fabrics, encapsulation of core materials, and production of complicated part geometry.

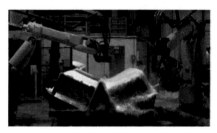

Figure 9.28 Manufacturing process fiber glass mat. Reprinted from Ref. [80], with permission from Springer Nature.

Closed-molding processes, such as RTM and vacuum infusion, allow for a nicer, cleaner working environment and are far more environment friendly than manual spray-up, which often produces 10 times more emissions than closed-molding. In fact, closed-molding is considered by the EPA to be such an ecologically friendly process that the MACT (Maximum Achievable Control Technology) standard for reinforced plastics does not involve the additional emissions controls that are required for open-molded processes.

9.9.4 Benefits of RTM

- Good surface quality
- Wide range of reinforcements
- Large, complex shapes
- Dimensional tolerances

- Low capital investment
- Less material wastage
- Tooling flexibility
- Low environmental impact
- Labor savings
- Ability to add inserts and reinforcements at a point of infusion for greater strength

9.9.5 Mechanical Properties of NFPCs

The mechanical properties of natural fibers can be enhanced in many ways, resulting in high strength and structure. Once the base structures are made strong, the polymers can be easily strengthened and improved. There are several aspects that effect composites, which are performance level or activities: (a) orientation of fiber, (b) strength of fibers, (c) physical properties of fibers, (d) interfacial adhesion property of fibers, and many more. The mechanical efficiency of NFPCs is dependent on the surface provided by fiber matrix along with the stress transfer function in which stress is transferred to fiber from matrix. This has been reported by many investigators in several researches. Characteristic components of natural fibers such as orientation, moisture absorption, impurities, physical properties, and volume fraction are such features that play a constitutive role in the determination of NFPCs mechanical properties. NFPCs show better mechanical properties than a pure matrix in cases where jute fibers are added in PLA (polylactic acid); in this case, 75.8% of PLA's tensile strength was improved; however, introduction or incorporation of flax fibers showed a negative impact on this addition. The addition of flax fibers resulted in 16% reduced tensile strength of the composites. The stiffness and stress transfer in composites increase with an increased or excessive addition of fibers, which provides a better loss modulus and also a better storage modulus [81].

9.9.6 Viscoelastic Behavior of NFPCs

Insights into the structure, morphology, and determination of the interface characteristics of natural fiber composite materials are provided by the dynamic mechanical measurements or the viscoelastic behavior over a range of temperatures. The maximum energy stored in the material during one cycle of oscillation is a measure of the storage modulus. The load-bearing capability and the stiffness behavior of natural fiber composite materials give an insight of the storage modulus. In a polymeric material, the degree of molecular mobility related to the loss modulus to the storage modulus is known as the mechanical damping coefficient ratio. On the other hand, loss modulus is proportional to the amount of energy dissipated as heat by the sample [82].

The corresponding viscoelastic properties were determined as a function of temperature and frequency when the measurements were executed in the tensile mode of the used equipment. At the temperature range of 30–140°C at 0.1, 1, and 10 Hz frequencies, respectively, the experiments executed the graphs plotted, as storage modulus versus temperature, as shown in Figs. 9.29 and 9.30.

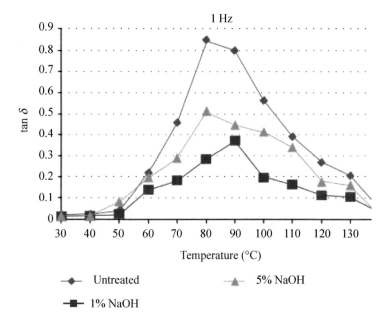

Figure 9.29 Versus temperature curves of the alkali-treated and untreated composites at 1 Hz frequency. Reprinted from Ref. [82], with permission from Elsevier.

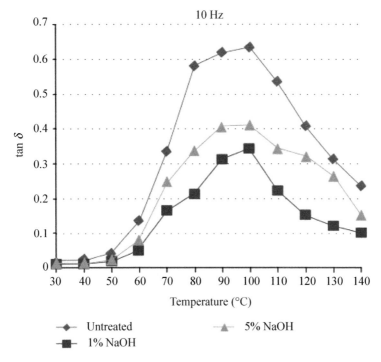

Figure 9.30 Versus temperature curves of alkali-treated and untreated composites. Reprinted from Ref. [82], with permission from Elsevier.

9.10 Applications of Natural Fiber Polymer Composites

Applications of NFPCs in engineering are increasing. The different kinds of natural fibers such as bamboo, oil palm, kenaf, hemp, and jute reinforced composites have been granted a great importance in construction, packing, automotive applications, and structural components [83]. NFPCs are finding way in aerospace, recreation, electrical and electronic industries, boats, machinery, office products, and so forth. NFPCs are used in polymer composites due to their properties, which include:

- Relatively high strength
- Totally biodegradable
- Resistance to corrosion and fatigue
- Improving the surface finish of molded part composites
- Relatively good mechanical properties
- Relatively low production cost
- Low specific weight
- Improving the surface finish of molded part composites
- Available and renewable sources

On the other hand, there are physical disadvantages of NFPCs such as moisture absorption, restricted processing temperature, and variable quality, and these disadvantages limiting their performance [84].

9.10.1 Natural Fiber Applications in the Industry

Other than the car industry, applications of NFPCs are found in [85]

- Ceilings
- Building and construction
- Aerospace
- Sports
- Office products
- Machinery

Biocomposites are considered one of the main green materials. They are applied in the building industry in two principle products: (1) structural biocomposites, which include bridge as well as roof structure, and (2) non-structural biocomposites, which include window, exterior construction, composites panels, and door frame [86]. Most of the applications of NFPCs are concentrated on no-load bearing indoor components in civil engineering because of their vulnerability to environmental attack. Green buildings need to be ecologically mindful, suitable, and healthy places to live and work [87]. Table 9.9 shows these applications.

Table 9.9 Various applications of cellulose fiber in industry, construction, and other industries

Fiber	Application
Hemp fiber	Construction products, textiles, cordage, geotextiles, paper and packaging, furniture, electrical, manufacture, bank notes, and manufacture of pipes
Oil palm fiber	Building materials such as windows, door frames, structural insulated panel, building systems, siding, fencing, roofing, decking, and other building materials
Wood fiber	Window frame, panels, door shutters, decking, railing systems, and fencing
Flax fiber	Window frame, panels, decking, railing systems, fencing, tennis racket, bicycle frame, fork, seat post, snowboarding, and laptop cases
Rice husk fiber	Building materials such as building panels, bricks, window frame, panels, decking, railing systems, and fencing
Bagasse fiber	Window frame, panels, decking, railing systems, and fencing
Sisal fiber	In construction industry such as panels, doors, shutting plate, and roofing sheets; also manufacturing of paper and pulp
Stalk fiber	Building panel, furniture panels, bricks, and constructing drains, and pipelines
Kenaf fiber	Packing material, mobile cases, bags, insulations, clothing-grade cloth, soilless potting mixes, animal bedding, and material that absorbs oil and liquids
Cotton fiber	Furniture industry, textile and yarn goods
Coir fibers	Building panels, flush door shutters, roofing sheets, storage tank, packing material, helmets and post boxes, mirror casing, paper weights, projector cover, voltage stabilizer cover, a filling material for the seat upholstery, brushes and brooms, ropes and yarns for nets, bags, and mats, as well as padding for mattresses, seat cushions
Ramie fiber	Use in products as industrial sewing thread, packing materials, fishing nets, and filter cloths. It is also made into fabrics for household furnishings (upholstery, canvas) and clothing, paper manufacture.
Jute fiber	Building panels, roofing sheets, door frames, door shutters, transport, packaging, geotextiles, and chip boards

Source: Ref. [88]

Table 9.9 illustrates the different types of fibers used in industry. Each fiber possesses a unique property in relevance to its desired application. Some of these natural fibers are scarce, while others are abundant, increasing the demand and supply of these fibers. Natural fibers are extracted without damaging the integrity of an ecosystem, thus making them a valuable entity. The huge variety of natural fibers justifies the need to incorporate this natural resource in more of our lives.

9.11 Rubber Composite Materials (Natural Fibers)

Rubber is synthesized organically or manufactured artificially in chemical plants. It has a huge variety of applications and is used in everyday life, but as civilization becomes more advanced, new design requirements such as low cost, lightweight, renewable character, high specific strength, and modulus are needed; the complexity of rubber becomes more understood leading to the development of rubber composites (infused with natural fibers). Not all natural fibers are suitable for developing rubber composites. Fibers chosen for the development of rubber composites are based on a variation of their properties, but the most significant being the cellulose content of the fiber. Cellulose is the main component of plant cell walls. Cellulose molecules give a plant its properties and is the basic building block for many textiles. In some rubber composites, cellulose is used as a reinforcing agent to enhance the properties of the rubber composite for its desired application. Fibers such as jute, hemp, and flax have attracted considerable scientific interest in the field of rubber composites due to their intrinsic low density as well as the high specific mechanical properties [89].

Figure 9.31 shows a rubber composite reinforced with a natural fiber; the applications of this material are in shutters, transport, packaging, and geotextiles.

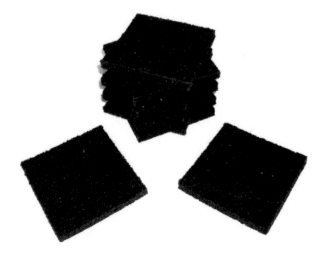

Figure 9.31 Natural fiber–reinforced rubber composite (© Castlewood, Castle Composites Ltd).

9.11.1 Properties of Rubber Composites

As rubber composites are suitable for most industries, their properties are generally distinguished on their specific applications, but most of these composites illustrate a similar direction in terms of properties [91].

- High availability
- Low specific weight, which results in a higher specific strength and stiffness
- Lightweight
- Renewable character
- Good processing characteristics

Table 9.10 shows the mechanical properties of rubber fiber composite. These fibers have been selected because they form an excellent candidate with rubber. Hemp composite is the most versatile and durable fiber that has the highest properties in comparison with other fibers listed. Jute and flax are suitable constituents, showing a high specific Young's modulus. All other fibers listed are best used to their desired application.

Table 9.10 Mechanical properties of rubber infused with natural fiber

Rubber and fiber composite	Density (g/cm³)	Tensile strength (MPa)	Young's modulus (GPa)	Elongation at break (%)	Specific tensile strength (MPa)	Specific Young's modulus (MPa)
Flax	3.5	1300–2200	38.6	2–4.5	457–950	26.25
Kenaf	2.9	900–1200	27.8	5	350–852	12–20
Sisal	3.1	1380–1400	18–22	7–12	480–667	12–19
Jute	2.89	1100–1600	32–38	3.89–5.66	485–911	22.82
Hemp	4.26	1050–1800	18–19	5.01–8.9	250–389	28.5–30.25
Coir	2.56	800–1000	8.89–11	32.33–40.56	50.1	8–15.62
Ramie	3.68	500–800	6.85–7.9	6.89–13	456–522	14.8–20.89

Source: Reprinted from Ref. [92], with permission from Elsevier.

9.11.2 Manufacturing Process of Rubber Composites

Due to the versatility of rubber and the adaptability of natural fibers, the manufacturing process of rubber composites ranges from many methods. Some include [93]

- Compression molding
- Injection molding
- Hot pressing
- Extrusion
- Curing

The preparation of materials for these processes is far longer as constituents and chemicals are extracted from the natural fiber and the rubber used.

9.11.3 Applications of Rubber Composites

Rubber composites are used in a variety of industries. Their properties are only limited to their design capabilities. Due to the low cost factor and other numerous abilities, these materials are suitable for [94]

- Aerospace industry
- Construction and tools
- Mechanical components
- Textile and clothing
- Medical community

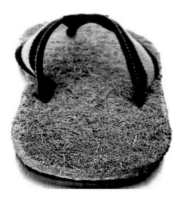

Figure 9.32 Cocoze coconut fibre flip-flops (Copyright Cocoze).

In Fig. 9.32, this shoe revolves around clear pending foot bed made of natural fiber and rubber. The foot beds gently exfoliate the soles of your feet, leaving them healthier and prettier.

9.12　Conclusion and Future Scope

In recent years, there is a paradigm shift in the field of material science in the usage of natural fibers. The improved interest is mainly due to environmental concerns, which have surfaced recently and also due to the low cost involved in obtaining these renewable resources, which is an ideal substitute for synthetic fibers, which are potentially toxic. Fibers such as flax, hemp, jute, and sisal have been stated to be ideal candidates for reinforcement in polymers by various researchers. Fibers such as flax and hemp have various applications and are used in a broad range of research. More research into other fibers that are available locally and are underutilized has to be undertaken. These fibers are renewable, carbon neutral, biodegradable, and also produce wastes that are either organic or can be used to generate electricity or make ecological housing material. Natural fibers in clothing allow fabric to breathe, reducing the risk of skin rashes and allergic reactions, and also insulate the wearer against hot and cold temperatures. Natural fiber composites are used in various applications and hold promising mechanical and physical properties. The cellulose extracted from natural fibers is used as a reinforcing agent in rubber composites, which hold a broad perspective in the scientific community. There are many methods to process natural fiber composites, such as injection and compression molding, resin transfer molding, vacuum-assisted resin transfer molding, and polymer solution casting. Thermoset polymers are an excellent substitute for regular materials as they possess enhanced properties and good aesthetics. These fibers can also replace synthetics in industrial materials, for example, in home insulation panels. Insulation made from wool or hemp rather than fiberglass draws moisture away from walls and timber, and is safer because wool is naturally fire resistant. The future scope for these materials holds promising applications and could improve the standard living of an individual.

Acknowledgements

The authors thank the Council of Industrial and Scientific Research (CSIR) South Africa "Biocomposites Centre of Competence" research project support (SIIGBC3.11214.02100.02170).

References

1. Lu, B., Zhang, L., and Zeng, J. (2005). Natural fibre reinforced composite, *J. Reinf. Plast. Compos*, **47**(2), pp. 502.
2. Fuqua, M. A., Huo, S., and Ulven, C. A. (2012). Natural fibre reinforced composites, *Polym. Rev.*, **52**(3), pp. 259-320.
3. Pandey, J. K., Ahn, S. H., Lee, C. S., Mohanty, A. K., and Misra, M. (2010). Recent advances in the application of natural fibre based composites, *Macromol. Mater. Eng.*, **295**(11), pp. 975-989.
4. Li, Y., Luo, Y., and Han, S. (2010). Multi-scale structures of natural fibres and their applications in making automobile parts, *J. Biobased Mater. Bioenergy*, **4**(2), pp. 164-171.
5. Umer, R., Bickerton, S., and Fernyhough, A. (2011). The effect of yarn length and diameter on permeability and compaction response of flax fibre mats, *Compos. A: Appl. Sci. Manuf.*, **42**(7), pp. 723-732.
6. Munikenche Gowda, T., Naidu, A., and Chhaya, R. (1999). Some mechanical properties of untreated jute fabric-reinforced polyester composites, *Compos. A: Appl. Sci. Manuf.*, **30**(3), pp. 277-284.
7. Mosier, N., Wyman, C., Dale, B., Elander, R., Lee, Y. Y., Holtzapple, M., and Ladisch, M. (2005). Features of promising technologies for pretreatment of lignocellulosic biomass, *Bioresour. Technol.*, **96**(6), pp. 673-686.
8. Gauvin, R., Trochu, F., Lemenn, Y., and Diallo, L. (1996). Permeability measurement and flow simulation through fibre reinforcement, *Polym. Compos.*, **17**(1), pp. 34-42.
9. Pitchumani, R. and Ramakrishnan, B. (1999). A fractal geometry model for evaluating permeabilities of porous preforms used in liquid composite molding, *Int. J. Heat Mass Transf.*, **42**(12), pp. 2219-2232.
10. Wiselogel, A., Tyson, S., and Johnson, D. (1996). Biomass feedstock resources and composition, In: *Handbook on Bioethanol: Production and Utilization*, Wyman, C. E. (Ed.), Taylor & Francis, pp. 105-118.
11. Ahmed, K. S., Vijayarangan, S., and Rajput, C. (2006). Mechanical behavior of isothalic polyester-based untreated woven jute and glass fabric hybrid composites, *J. Reinf. Plast. Compos.*, **25**(15), pp. 1549-1569.

12. Belgacem, M. N. and Gandini, A. (2005). The surface modification of cellulose fibres for use as reinforcing elements in composite materials, *Compos. Interface*, **12**(1-2), pp. 41–75.

13. Ratim, S., Bonnia, N. N., and Surip, S. N. (2012). The effect of woven and non-woven fibre structure on mechanical properties polyester composite reinforced kenaf, *AIP Conf. Proc.*, **1455**, 131; doi: http://dx.doi.org/10.1063/1.4732481.

14. Vernet, N., Ruiz, E., Advani, S., Alms, J. B., Aubert, M., Barburski, M., Barari, B., Beraud, J. M., Berg, D. C., Correia, N., Danzi, M., Delaviere, T., Dickert, M., Di Fratta, C., Endruweit, A., Ermanni, P., Francucci, G., Garcia, J. A., George, A., Hahn, C., Klunker, F., Lomov, S. V., Long, A., Louis, B., Maldonado, J., Meier, R., Michaud, V., Perrin, H., Pillai, K., Rodriguez, E., Trochu, F., Verheyden, S., Wietgrefe, M., Xiong, W., Zaremba, S., and Ziegmann, G. (2014). Experimental determination of the permeability of engineering textiles: Benchmark II, *Compos. A: Appl. Sci. Manuf.*, **61**, pp. 172–184.

15. Ku, H., Wang, H., Pattarachaiyakoop, N., and Trada, M. (2011). A review on the tensile properties of natural fibre reinforced polymer composites, *Compos. Part B*, **42**(4), pp. 856–873.

16. Aziz, S. H. and Ansell, M. P. (2004). The effect of alkalization and fiber alignment on the mechanical and thermal properties of kenaf and hemp bast fiber composites. Part 1. Polyester resin matrix, *Compos. Sci. Technol.*, **64**(9), 1219–1230.

17. Tawakkal, I. S. M. A., Cran, M. J., and Bigger, S. W. (2014). Effect of kenaf fibre loading and thymol concentration on the mechanical and thermal properties of PLA/kenaf/thymol composites, *Industrial Crops Products*, **61**, pp. 74–83.

18. Arsène, M. A., Bilba, K., Okwo, A. S., Soboyejo, A. B., and Soboyejo, W. O. (2007). Tensile strength of vegetable fibre effect of chemical and thermal treatments, *Mater. Manuf. Process.*, **22**(2), pp. 214–227.

19. Van de Weyenberg, I., Ivens, J., De Coster, A., Kino, B., Baetens, E., and Verpoest, I. (2003). Influence of processing and chemical treatment of flax fibres on their composites, *Composites Sci. Technol.*, **63**(9), pp. 1241–1246.

20. May-Pat, A., Valadez-González, A., and Herrera-Franco, P. J. (2013). Effect of fibre surface treatments on the essential work of fracture of HDPE-continuous henequen fibre-reinforced composites, *Polymer Testing*, **32**(6), pp. 1114–1122.

21. Holbery, J. and Houston, D. (2006). Natural-fibre-reinforced polymer composites in automotive applications, *JOM*, **58**(11), pp. 80–86.
22. Khristova, P., Kodsachia, O., Patt, R., Khider, T., and Karrar, I. (2002). Alkaline pulping with additives of kenaf from Sudan, *Industrial Crops Products*, **15**, pp. 229–235.
23. Smook, G. A. (1989). Overview of the pulp and paper industry from chemical industry, *J. Chem. Technol. Biotechnol.*, **45**, pp. 15–27.
24. Sun, R., Mark Lawther, J., and Banks, W. B. (1995). Influence of alkaline pre-treatment on cell-wall components of wheat straw, *Industrial Crops Products*, **4**, pp. 127–145.
25. Blankenhorn, P., Silsbee, M. R., Blankenhorn, B. D., and DiCola, M. (2001). Effects of fibre surface treatments on mechanical properties of wood fibre-cement composites, *Cement and Concrete Research*, **31**, pp. 1049–1055.
26. Garrote, G., Eugenio, M. E., Díaz, M. J., Ariza, J., and López, F. (2003). Hydrothermal and pulp processing of Eucalyptus, *Bioresour. Technol.*, **88**, pp. 61–68.
27. Araki, J., Wada, M., Kuga, S., and Okano, T. (1998). Flow properties of microcrystalline cellulose suspension prepared by acid treatment of native cellulose, *Colloid. Surf. A Physicochem. Eng. Aspects*, **142**, pp. 75–82.
28. Pouteau, C., Cathala, B., Dole, P., Kurek, B., and Monties, B. (2005). Structural modification of Kraft lignin after acid treatment: Characterisation of the apolar extracts and influence on the antioxidant properties in polypropylene, *Industrial Crops Products*, **21**, pp. 101–108.
29. Meon, M. S., Othman, M. F., Husain, H., Remeli, M. F., Syawal, M. S. M. (2012). Improving tensile properties of kenaf fibres treated with sodium hydroxide, *Proceedings of the International Symposium on Robotics and Intelligent Sensors 2012 (IRIS 2012), Kuching, Sarawak, Malaysia*, pp. 1587–1592.
30. Caballero, J. A., Marcilla, A., and Conesa, J. A. (1997). Thermogravimetric analysis of olive stones with sulphuric acid treatment, *J. Anal. Appl. Pyrolysis*, **44**, pp. 75–88.
31. Grohmann, K., Cameron, R. G., and Buslig, B. S. (1995). Fractionation and pretreatment of orange peel by dilute acid hydrolysis, *Bioresour. Technol.*, **54**(2), pp. 129–141.
32. Sun, Y. and Cheng, J. J. (2005). Dilute acid pretreatment of rye straw and Bermudagrass for ethanol production, *Bioresour. Technol.*, **96**(14), pp. 1599–1606.

33. Marcilla, A., Conesa, J. A., Asensio, M., and Garcia-Garcia, S. M. (2000). Thermal treatment and foaming of chars obtained from almond shells: kinetic study, *Fuel*, **79**(7), pp. 829–836.
34. Shafizadeh, F. (1982). Introduction to pyrolysis of biomass, *J. Anal. Appl. Pyrolysis*, **3**, pp. 283–305.
35. Várhegi, G., Antal Junior, M. J., Jakab, E., and Szabó, P. (1997). Kinetic modelling of biomass pyrolysis, *Journal of Analytical and Applied Pyrolysis*, **42**(1), pp. 73–87.
36. Capart, R., Khezami, L., and Burnham, A. K. (2004). Assessment of various kinetic models for the pyrolysis of microgranular cellulose, *Thermochimica Acta.*, **417**, pp. 79–89.
37. Tsujiyama, T. and Miyamori, A. (2000). Assignment of DSC thermograms of wood and its components, *Thermochimica Acta*, **351**, pp. 177–181.
38. Paris, O., Zollfrank, C., and Zickler, G. A. (2005). Decomposition and carbonisation of wood biopolymers: A microstructural study of softwood pyrolysis, *Carbon*, **43**, pp. 53–66.
39. Abou-Yousef, H., El-Sakhawy, M., and Kamel, S. (2004). Multi-stage bagasse pulping by using alkali/Caro's acid treatment, *Ind. Crops Products*, **21**(3), pp. 337–341.
40. Arkles, B. (1977). Tailoring surfaces with silanes, *CHEMTECH*, **7**, pp. 766–778.
41. Singleton, A. C. N., Baillie, C. A., Beaumont, P. W. R., and Peijs, T. (2003). On the mechanical properties, deformation and fracture of a natural fibre/polymer composite, *Compos B: Eng*, **34**, pp. 519.
42. Wielage, B., Lampke, T. H., Utschick, H., and Soergel, F. (2003). Processing of natural-fibre reinforced polymers and the resulting dynamic-mechanical properties, *J Mater Process Technol.* **139**, pp. 140.
43. Abu Bakar, M. S., Cheng, M. H. W., Tang, S. M., Yu, S. C., Liao, K., Tan, C. T., Khor, K. A., and Cheang, P. (2003). Tensile properties, tension-tension fatigue and biological response of hydroxyapatite composites for load-bearing orthopedic implants, *Biomaterials*, **24**, pp. 2245.
44. Mohanty, A. K., Wibowo, A., Misra, M., and Drzal, L. T. (2003). Effect of process engineering on the performance of natural fibre reinforced cellulose acetate biocomposites, *Compos A: Appl Sci Manuf*, **35**, 363.
45. Agrawal, R., Saxena, N. S., Sharma, K. B., Thomas, S., and Sreekala, M. S. (2000). Activation energy and crystallization kinetics of untreated and treated oil palm fibre reinforced phenol formaldehyde composites, *Mater Sci. Eng. A*, **277**, pp. 77.
46. Rout, J., Misra, M., Tripathy, S. S., Nayak, S. K., and Mohanty, A.K. (2001). The influence of fibre treatment on the performance of coir-polyester composites, *Compos. Sci. Technol.*, **61**(9), pp. 1303–1310.

47. Xue, L., Lope, G. T., and Satyanarayan, P. (2007). Chemical treatment of natural fibre for use in natural fibre-reinforced composites: A review, *J. Polym. Environ.*, **15**(1), pp. 25–33.
48. Li, Y. and Yuan, B. (2014). Nonlinear mechanical behavior of plant fibre reinforced composites, *J. Biobased Mater. Bioenergy*, **8**(2), pp. 240–245.
49. Dai, D. and Fan, M. (2014). Wood fibres as reinforcements in natural fibre composites: Structure, properties, processing and applications, In: *Natural Fibre Composites: Materials, Processes and Properties*, Woodhead Publishing, Cambridge, pp. 3–65.
50. Mishra, S., Tripathy, S. S., Misra, M., Mohanty, A. K., and Nayak, S. K. (2002). Novel eco-friendly biocomposites: Biofibre reinforced biodegradable polyester amide composites—fabrication and properties evaluation, *J. Reinf. Plast. Comp.*, **21**(1), pp. 55–70.
51. Bergthaller, W., Funke, U., Lindhauer, M. G., Radosta, S., Meister, F., and Taeger, E. (1999). Processing and characterization of biodegradable products based on starch and cellulose fibres, In: *Biopolymers: Utilizing Nature's Advanced Materials*, Imam, S. H., Greene, R. V., and Zaidi, B. R. (Eds.), vol. 723, American Chemical Society, pp. 14–38.
52. Cao, X., Jiang, M., and Yu, T. (1989). Controllable specific interaction and miscibility in polymer blends, hydrogen bonding and morphology, *Macromolecular Chem.*, **190**, pp. 117–1128.
53. Mallick, P. K. (1988). *Fibre Reinforced Composites: Materials, Manufacturing and Design*, New York: Marcel Dekker, pp. 13.
54. Garnier, M. (2004). In-line compounding and molding of long-fibre reinforced thermoplastics (D-LFT): Insight into a rapid growing technology, In: *Proceedings of ANTEC 2004*, Chicago, Illinois, pp. 3500–3503.
55. Truckenmuller, F. and Fritz, H. G. (1991). Injection molding of long fibre-reinforced thermoplastics: A comparison of extruded and pultruded materials with direct addition of roving strands, *Polym. Eng. Sci.*, **31**(18), pp. 1316–1329.
56. Franzen, B., Kalson, C., Kubat, J., and Kitano, T. (1989). Fibre degradation during processing of short fibre reinforced thermoplastics, *Composites*, **20**(1), pp. 65–76.
57. Samuel, O. D., Agbo, S., and Adekanye, T. A. (2012). Assessing mechanical properties of natural fibre reinforced composites for engineering applications, *J. Miner. Mater. Charact. Eng.*, **11**, pp. 780–784.
58. Gowthami, A., Ramanaiah, K., Prasad, A. V. R., Reddy, K. H. C., and Rao, K. M. (2012). Effect of thermal and mechanical properties of fibre reinforced composites, *J. Mater. Environ. Sci.*, **4**, pp. 199–204.

59. Mohanty, A. K., Misra, M., and Drzal, L. T. (2005). *Natural Fibers, Biopolymers, and Biocomposites*, CRC Press.
60. Gallo, E., Schartel, B., Acierno, D., Cimino, F., and Russo, P. (2013). Tailoring the flame retardant and mechanical performances of natural fibre-reinforced biopolymer by multi-component laminate, *Compos. Part B: Eng.*, **44**(1), pp. 112–119.
61. Komuraiah, A., Kumar, N., and Prasad, D. (2013). Determination of energy changes and length of micro cracks formed in cotton fibre reinforced natural composite laminate due to environmental degradation, *APCBEE*, pp. 120–125.
62. Chapple, S. and Anandjiwala, R. (2010). Flammability of natural fibre-reinforced composites and strategies for fire retardancy: a review, *Journal of Thermoplastic Composite Materials*, **23**, pp. 871–893.
63. Lunt, J. M. and Shortall, J. B. (1979). The effect of extrusion compounding on fibre degradation and strength properties in short glass-fibre reinforced nylon 66, *Plast Rubber Process*, **4**(4), pp. 108–114.
64. Silva, F., Njuguna, J., Sachse, S., Pielichowski, K., Leszczynska, A., and Giacomelli, M. (2012). The influence of multiscale fillers reinforcement into impact resistance and energy absorption properties of polyamide 6 and polypropylene nanocomposite structures, *Materials Design*, **50**, pp. 244–252.
65. Kakroodi, A. R., Kazemi, Y., and Rodrigue, D. (2013). Mechanical, rheological, morphological and water absorption properties, *Compos. Part B Eng.*, **51**, pp. 337–344.
66. Pan Y. and Zhong, Z. (2015). A micromechanical model for the mechanical degradation of natural fibre reinforced composites induced by moisture absorption, *Mechanics Mater.*, 85, pp. 7–15.
67. Eckert, C. H. (1999). Functional fillers for plastics: Outlook to the year 2005. *Proceedings of the Fifth International Conference on Woodfibre Plastic Composites*, Madison, May 26–28, **7263**, pp. 10–22.
68. Joseph, K., Mattoso, L. H. C., Toledo, R. D., Thomas, S., de Carvalho, L. H., Pothen, L., Kala, S., and James, B. (2000). Natural fibre reinforced thermoplastic composites, In: *Natural Polymers and Agrofibres Composites*, Frollini, E., Leao, A. L., and Mattoso, L. H. C. (Eds.), Embrapa Instrumentação Agropecuária, Sao Carlos, Brazil, pp. 159–201.
69. Oksman, K. and Selin, J. F. (2004). Plastics and composites from polylactic acid, In: *Natural Fibres, Plastics and Composites*, Wallenberger, F. T. and Weston, N. (Eds.), Springer US, pp. 149–166.

70. Stemergy Renewable Bio Fiber Products. Flax fiber composites for consumer product reinforcements. http://www.stemergy.com/products/flaxfibre/flaxfibercomposites/
71. Ing. Aková Eva. (2013). Development of natural fibre reinforced polymer composites, *Transfer Inovácií*, **25**.
72. Abdullah, A. K., Magniez, K., and Bronwyn, L.F. (2011). Effect of manufacturing process on the flexural, fracture toughness, and thermomechanical properties of bio-composites, *J. Compos.*, **42**, pp. 993–999.
73. Venkateshwaran, N., Elaya Perumal, A., and Arunsundaranayagam, D. (2013). Fiber surface treatment and its effect on mechanical and visco-elastic behaviour of banana/epoxy composite, *Mater. Des.*, **47**, pp. 151–159.
74. Francucci, G., Rodríguez, E. S., and Vázquez, A. (2010). Study of saturated and unsaturated permeability in natural fibre fabrics, *Compos. A: Appl. Sci. Manuf.*, **41**(1), pp. 16–21.
75. FlexForm Technologies. Products: One-step 3D moulding. http://www.flexformtech.com/Auto/
76. Li, Y., Xie, L., and Ma, H. (2015). Permeability and mechanical properties of plant fiber reinforced hybrid composites, 86, pp. 313–320.
77. Naik, N. K., Sirisha, M., and Inani, A. (2014). Permeability characterization of polymer matrix composites by RTM/VARTM, *Prog. Aerosp. Sci.*, **65**, pp. 22–40.
78. Francucci, G., Vázquez, A., Ruiz, E., and Rodríguez, E. S. (2012). Capillary effects in vacuum-assisted resin transfer molding with natural fibres, *Polym. Compos.*, **33**(9), pp. 1593–1602.
79. Rodriguez, E., Giacomelli, F., and Vazquez, A. (2004). Permeability-porosity relationship in RTM for different fibreglass and natural reinforcements, *J. Compos. Mater.*, **38**(3), pp. 259–268.
80. Nguyen, V. H., Lagardère, M., Park, C. H., and Panier, S. (2014). Permeability of natural fibre reinforcement for liquid composite molding processes, *J. Mater. Sci.*, **49**(18), pp. 6449–6458.
81. Ma, H., Li, Y., and Luo, Y. (2011). The effect of fibre twist on the mechanical properties of natural fibre reinforced composites, In: *18th International Conference on Composite Materials (ICCM-18)*, Jeju, South Korea, August 21–25, 2011.
82. George, G., Jose, E. T., Åkesson, D., Skrifvars, M., Nagarajan, E. R., and Joseph, K. (2012). Viscoelastic behaviour of novel commingled

biocomposites based on polypropylene/jute yarns, *Compos. Part A Appl. Sci. Manuf.*, **43**(6), pp. 893–902.
83. Shalwan, A. and Yousif, B. F. (2013). In state of art: Mechanical and tribological behaviour of polymeric composites based on natural fibres, *Mater. Design*, **48**, pp. 14–24.
84. Coutinho, F. B., Costa, T. H. S., Carvalho, D. L., Gorelova, M. M., and De Santa Maria, J. C. (1998). Thermal behaviour of modified wood fibres, *Polym. Testing.*, **17**, pp. 299–310.
85. Verma, D., Gope, P. C., Shandilya, A., Gupta, A., and Maheshwari, M. K. (2013). Coir fibre reinforcement and application in polymer composites: A review, *J. Mater. Environ. Sci.*, **4**, pp. 263–276.
86. Chadramohan, D. and Marimuthu, K. (2011). Tensile and hardness tests on natural fibre reinforced polymer composite material, *Int. J. Adv. Eng. Sci. Technol.*, **6**, pp. 97–104.
87. Drzal, L. T., Mohanty, A. K., and Misra, M. (2001). Bio-composite materials as alternatives to petroleum-based composites for automotive applications, *ACCE*.
88. Ticoalu, A., Aravinthan, T., and Cardona, F. (2010). A review of current development in natural fibre composites for structural and infrastructure applications, *Southern Region Engineering Conference*, pp. 1–5.
89. Raghavendra, S., Lingaraju, Shetty, P. B., and Mukunda, P. G. (2013). Mechanical properties of short banana fibre reinforced natural rubber composites, *Int. J. Innovative Res. Sci., Eng. Technol.*, **2**(5).
90. Castlewood. The Art of Composite Decking: Rubber Support Pads http://www.castlewooddecking.co.uk/rubber-support-pads
91. Barlow, F. W. (1993). *Rubber Compounding: Principles, Materials and Techniques*, 2nd edition, Marcel Dekker, Inc., New York.
92. Geethamma, V. G., Kalaprasad, G., Groeninckx, G., and Thomas, S. (2005). Dynamic mechanical behavior of short coir fibre reinforced natural rubber composites, *Compos. Part A*, **36**(11), pp. 1499–1506.
93. Navarro, F. J., Partal, P., Martínez-Boza, F. J., and Gallegos, C. (2010). Novel recycled polyethylene/ground tire rubber/bitumen blends for use in roofing applications: Thermo-mechanical properties, *Polym. Test.*, **29**(5), pp. 588–595.
94. Joseph, S., Jacob, M., and Thomas, S. (2005). Natural fibre–rubber composites and their applications, In: *Natural Fibres, Biopolymers, and Biocomposites*, Mohanty, A. K., Misra, M., and Drzal, L. T. (Eds.), CRC Press, Boca Raton, pp. 435–472.

Chapter 10

Multifaceted Applications of Nanoparticles and Nanocomposites Decorated with Biopolymers

Natarajan Kumari Ahila,[a] Arivalagan Pugazhendhi,[b]
Sutha Shobana,[c] Indira Karuppusamy,[d] Vijayan Sri Ramkumar,[e]
Ethiraj Kannapiran,[a] Periyasamy Sivagurunathan,[f] and
Gopalakrishnan Kumar[f]

[a]*Department of Animal Health and Management, Alagappa University, Karaikudi 630003, India*
[b]*Department of Environmental Engineering, Daegu University, Gyeongsangbuk-do 38453, South Korea*
[c]*Department of Chemistry and Research Centre, Aditanar College of Arts and Science, Tirchendur, Thoothukudi 628216, India*
[d]*Research Centre for Stratergic Materials, Corrosion Resistant Steel Group, National Institute for Materials Science (NIMS), Tsukuba, Ibaraki 305-0047, Japan*
[e]*Department of Environmental Biotechnology, Bharathidasan University, Tiruchirappalli 620024, India*
[f]*Center for Materials Cycles and Waste Management Research, National Institute for Environmental Studies (NIES), Tsukuba, Ibaraki 305-0053, Japan*
gopalakrishnanchml@gmail.com, kumar.gopal@nies.go.jp

Biopolymers and bionanocomposites are an exceptional group of materials with outstanding physical, chemical, and mechanical

Biocomposites: Biomedical and Environmental Applications
Edited by Shakeel Ahmed, Saiqa Ikram, Suvardhan Kanchi, and Krishna Bisetty
Copyright © 2018 Pan Stanford Publishing Pte. Ltd.
ISBN 978-981-4774-38-3 (Hardcover), 978-1-315-11080-6 (eBook)
www.panstanford.com

properties and are recognized as promising candidates for diverse field applications. Biopolymers are produced from plants, animals, and microorganisms, which include a long chain of amino acids or monosaccharides or nucleotides. These play a crucial role in many fields, ranging from medical to environmental and energy; especially, its role in nanomedicine is rewarding. A critical need in the field of bionanotechnology is the development of reliable and ecofriendly processes. The metallic nanoparticles encapsulated with biopolymers can be widely used in drug delivery, gene therapy, tissue engineering, therapeutic medicine, antimicrobial, biosensing, etc. Nanoparticles of noble metals such as silver, gold, and platinum, when conjugated with biopolymers, have showed higher efficiency for their antibacterial, antifungal, and antiviral activities. Here, we have provided a comprehensive overview of synthesis, processing, and developing methods of the most investigated biomaterials and nanoparticles in biological and biomedical contexts, including nanoparticles, nanocomposites, biopolymers, biopolymer-encapsulated nanoparticles and nanocomposites. In addition, the recent challenges and applications of these materials in various fields specific to biomedicine as well as for personalized medicinal benefits are considered and explained in detail.

10.1 Introduction

Nanotechnology has been a pullulating field for the past two decades, making a potential impact in all spheres of human life. This technology engineers the functional systems of matter at the atomic and molecular scales with at least one dimension sized from 1 to 100 nm, as miniaturization becomes more important in areas such as computing, sensors, and biomedical applications. In order to design and study modern devices, which are suitable for various possible commercial applications, a wide range of materials are required. In this context, nanomaterials play a vital role in recent technologies to reach high performance devices [1]. The nanosized materials exhibit completely new or improved or novel physical, chemical, and biological properties based on specific characteristics such as size distribution and morphology compared to their macroscale form of the same material [2]. Researchers have exploited many materials from organic to inorganic for wide application at their nanoregime. Among them, metallic nanoparticles are the most competent, as they hold incredible electromagnetic, optical, mechanical, catalytic, and antimicrobial properties [3]. Noble metals such as gold, silver, platinum, copper, and titanium were used mostly for the synthesis of stable dispersions of nanoparticles, which have multiple applications [4]. However, these solo nanoparticles have some lacunae such as insufficient stability, nanotoxicity, including environmental and health risks.

The hybrids of inorganic/organic nanoparticles are known as nanocomposites, which have been attracting a great deal of research attention that can overcome the latter issues of nanomaterials. These nanocomposite materials are of contemporary interest in interdisciplinary areas, which intersect biology, material science, and nanotechnology. These tailored composites of nanomaterials in the continuous phase of matrix have improved performance with novel structural, mechanical, optical, catalytic, sensing, and biomedical properties. Nanocomposites may be composed of either multiple nanoscale materials or a nanoscale material built in bulk material. In the recent years, many nano-techies exerted to synthesize metal nanoparticles of different sizes, shapes, composition, crystallinity, controlled dispersion, and improved stability to perk up the curious properties for their potential applications. This chapter deals with the synthesis and application of noble metal nanomaterials reinforced in the biopolymer matrix, the polymer matrix nanocomposites (PMNC).

The polymer matrix has several functions, including holding the bound reinforced material in place, transferring the external loads, and also protecting them from adverse effects. In addition, it can also act as a reducing and stabilizing agent for the nanoparticles. There are enormous synthetic and natural polymers formed by a single unit of monomers that have relatively high thermal stability, unique rheologic properties, high dielectric strength; they are chemically inert and processable, which provides means for fabrication of objects of desired form and dimensions. Two different composites can be formed: metal core nanoparticles covered with a polymer shell and metal nanoparticles embedded in the polymer matrix. Various methods have been employed for the synthesis of nanocomposites with amazing physical, chemical, electrochemical, and biological properties. The main challenges in preparing nanocomposites are the control of particle size, compatibility of different material components, and homogenous dispersion of metal nanoparticles in the polymer matrix to endow desirable and unique properties. Similarly, biodegradability plays a crucial role in biomedical applications. Different types of polymers such as synthetic, biodegradable synthetic polymers, and natural biopolymers are widely used. (This will be discussed later in this chapter.)

All the synthesizing methods are based on two different strategies: ex situ and in situ strategies. In the ex situ approach, polymerization of organic monomer and metal nanoparticles produced by soft chemistry is performed separately and then physically or mechanically mixed to form polymer–metal nanocomposites. In the latter approach, PMNC is generated inside the polymer matrix by the reduction of metal ions in the dispersed polymer matrix or in other words, polymerization of monomer dispersed with metal nanoparticles [5]. Simultaneous polymerization–reduction approach is also another version of the in situ synthesis. A few examples of the various methods employed for the synthesis of polymer–metal nanocomposites are vapor deposition, microwave irradiation, photochemical reduction, radiation induced and sonochemical methods, ultrasonication, solvent evaporation, coprecipitation, electrospinning, sol–gel process, film casting, dip coating, physically mixing, layer-by-layer assembly, ionotropic gelation, colloidal assembly, coprecipitation, covalent coupling, etc. The physical and chemical methods require high energy input, pressure, temperature, and expense; using more complex steps, hazardous chemicals, and bioaccumulation in the environment are uneconomical techniques. The greener method is cost effective, clean, non-toxic, and has sufficient material sources, mild reaction conditions, good dispersion of nanoparticles, mostly one-pot synthesis, and can also be easily scaled up for large-scale synthesis. Also, the development of polymer-immobilized metal nanoparticles using biological method reduces the chances of their appearance in the environment. This chapter precisely deals with the fabrication of PMNC from widely used natural biopolymers obtained from different biological sources and with its biomedical applications.

10.2 Biosynthesis of Metal Nanocomposites

Generally, biosynthetic methods have to be optimized on the basis of their modes of applications. Therefore, the compatibility of hybrid biopolymers and nanoparticles should be considered. Based on the literature, biopolymers are the main components in the synthesis of biocomposites. There are many techniques such as physical, chemical, electrochemical, or biological methods available to fabricate nanoparticles using biopolymers. Biologically synthesized nanoparticles hybrid with the biopolymers using several techniques. Microorganisms used as bio-factory, which produces biopolymers and simultaneously reduce nanoparticles, finally to composite. The overall scheme of this chapter can be seen in Fig. 10.1. Widely used biopolymers and their properties are elucidated in Table 10.1.

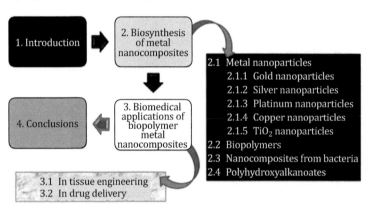

Figure 10.1 Overall scheme of the chapter.

10.2.1 Gold Nanoparticles

The noble metal gold has captivated humans for centuries and has been conceived as the precious metal occupying a premier position in the world economy, representing wealth and high value [6]. As a bulk metallic form, they have been used for monetary and jewelry applications, and over recent decades as an electrical conductor and chemically inert contact material in the electronics industry. Being

Table 10.1 Widely used biopolymers and their sources, properties, and applications

Biopolymers	Backbone structure	Source	Intrinsic properties	Applications
Gelatin	Partial hydrolysis of collagen	Skin, bones, tissues of animals	Hemostatic, pro-angiogenic, non-immunogenic, biodegradable, and biocompatible	Foods, cosmetics, and medicines
Starch	Semi-crystalline polymer with amylose and amylopectin monomers	Plants	Biodegradable, renewable	Synthetic additives in plastics, detergents, pharmaceutical tablets, pesticides, cosmetics, and even oil-drilling fluids
Cellulose	β-1,4-linked glucan chains	Bacteria, algae, tunicates, and higher plants	Various plasticizers, various thermal, mechanical, barrier, and physical properties, biodegradable and environmentally safe	Textiles and paper Biomedical field
Chitin and Chitosan	β-(1→4)-linked N-acetylglucosamine	Exoskeleton, or outer covering, of insects, crustaceans, and arachnids	Applicability, water sorptivity, oxygen permeability, blood-coagulating property, and cytokine induction (interleukin-8)	Fibroblast migration and proliferation; it is used as wound dressing material

Biopolymers	Backbone structure	Source	Intrinsic properties	Applications
Polylactic acid (PLA)	Aliphatic polyester	Renewable resources, such as corn starch, tapioca roots, chips, starch, or sugarcane, various bacteria	Biodegradable thermoplastic, weather resistance and workability	Biomedical applications
Poly(ε-caprolactone) (PCL)	Polyesters	Renewable resources	Intrinsic hydrophobic, biodegradable	Scaffolds for various tissue engineering applications, drug delivery, long-term implantable devices.
Collagen	Monomers of collagen	Bones, muscles, skin, and tendons,	Strength and structure	Healing and repairing of the body's tissues, Collagen dressings attract new skin cells to wound sites
Poly(3-hydroxybutyrate-co-3-hydroxyvalerate) PHBV	Linear aliphatic polyester	Bacteria	Biodegradable, non-toxic, and biocompatible plastic	Development of implanted medical devices for dental, orthopedic, hernioplastic, and skin surgery, potential medical devices like bioresorbable surgical sutures and biodegradable screws

nanosized, the innovative properties, including optical, magnetic, electronic, and structural properties, make nanosized particles (generally 1–100 nm) very promising for a wide range of biomedical applications such as in cellular imaging, molecular diagnosis, and targeted therapy depending on the structure, composition, and shape of the nanomaterials [7]. Among the nanosized noble metals, gold nanoparticles (Au NPs) are extensively explored in modern material science because of their enormous colloidal preparation methods that give rise to monodispersed particles with well-defined morphologies and stability. Functionalized Au NPs with controlled geometrical and optical properties are the subject of intensive studies and biomedical applications, including genomics, biosensors, immunoassays, clinical chemistry, laser phototherapy of cancer cells and tumors, the targeted delivery of drugs, DNA and antigens, optical bioimaging, and the monitoring of cells and tissues with the use of state-of-the-art detection systems. The Au NPs biosynthesized from *Dysosma pleiantha* rhizome could be used as a potential candidate in drug and gene delivery to metastatic cancer. The biosynthesized Au NPs were non-toxic to cell proliferation, and also they can inhibit the chemo-attractant cell migration of human fibrosarcoma cancer cell line HT-1080 by interfering the actin polymerization pathway. Recently, Shankar et al. [8] reviewed the biosynthesis process and the applications of Au NPs and silver nanoparticles (Ag NPs) in drug delivery and cancer treatment in detail.

10.2.2 Silver Nanoparticles

Among the noble metals, silver has the most efficient optical property because the surface plasmon resonance energy is located far from the interband transition energy [9]. Silver has been time-honored as an effective antimicrobial agent that is non-toxic to humans and other living beings [10]. Hence, it has been indiscriminately used as traditional medicines to culinary items. Therefore, the recent research advancement is to develop experimental processes to synthesis nanoparticles with different sizes, shapes, composition, crystallinity, controlled dispersion, and improved stability. All these factors play a vital role in controlling their physical, chemical, and biological properties to ameliorate their boundless applications.

The Ag NP is an effective antimicrobial agent against a number of pathogenic microorganisms. Recently, Ag NPs were found to have a considerable size-dependent interaction with HIV type 1, preferably via binding to gp120 glycoprotein knobs [11]. In addition, Ag NPs became a promising material for their potential use as an alternative bactericide to combat antibiotic-resistant strains as the microbes are unlikely to develop resistance against silver. The extremely large surface area of Ag NPs provides better contact with microorganisms, thus resulting in efficient antimicrobial property. Perhaps, the nanoparticles get attached to the cell membrane and also penetrate inside the bacteria and interact with these proteins in the cell as well as with phosphorus-containing compounds such as DNA. Finally, the nanoparticles release silver ions in the bacterial cells, which enhance their bactericidal activity [12]. Moreover, the antimicrobial activity of the silver bionanoparticles was performed by well-diffusion method against *Staphylococcus aureus*, *Pseudomonas aeruginosa*, *Escherichia coli*, and *Klebsiella pneumoniae*. The highest antimicrobial activity of Ag NPs synthesized by *Solanum tricobatum* and *Ocimum tenuiflorum* extracts was found to be against *S. aureus* (30 mm) and *E. coli* (30 mm), respectively [13].

10.2.3 Platinum Nanoparticles

Platinum is one of the rare and expensive among noble metals. Platinum is a useful biomaterial and has numerous industrial catalytic applications, including automotive catalytic converters and petrochemical cracking catalysts. It has high corrosion resistance and usually used in the form of colloid or suspension in a fluid. They are the subject of extensive research due to their antioxidant properties. This metal is also considered the best electrocatalyst for the four-electron reduction of oxygen to water in acidic environments as it provides the lowest over potential and the highest stability.

10.2.4 Copper Nanoparticles

Copper, which belongs to Block D elements, is a ductile metal with very high thermal and electrical conductivity. It is also an efficient catalyst in hydrogen production. Among various metal nanoparticles, copper nanoparticles (Cu NPs) are an important semiconductor with a band gap of 2.1 eV. They have received much attention in the recent years due to their intrinsic properties and wide potential applications in many fields such as photochemical catalysis, biosensing, gas sensor, electrochemical sensing, and solar/photovoltaic energy conversion [14]. Another important use of Cu NPs includes the fabrication of low electrical resistance materials due to their remarkable conductive properties. In addition, Cu NPs and their oxides show broad spectrum biocidal effects and the antimicrobial activity has been reported in the studies of growth inhibition of bacteria, fungus, and algae [15]. Copper is found to be too soft for some applications; hence, it is often combined with other metals to form numerous alloys, such as brass, which is a copper–zinc alloy. The Cu NPs are graded as highly flammable solid; therefore, they must be stored away from sources of ignition. They are also known to be very toxic to aquatic life.

10.2.5 Titanium Oxide Nanoparticles

Titanium is a strong, lustrous, and corrosion-resistant chemical element, which belongs to the transition metal group. It is the ninth most abundant element in the earth's crust, and it was once considered a rare metal, but nowadays it is one of the most important metals in industrial applications. Ti is always bonded to other elements in nature. Only 5% of the Ti mined today is used in its pure metal form and the remaining is used to manufacture titanium dioxide (TiO_2), an ingredient in paper, paints, plastics, and white food colorings. TiO_2 is the most common compound of Ti, widely used in biomedical, self-cleaning, and photocatalytic applications [16]. It is one of the most examined single-crystalline structures in the surface science of metal oxide. TiO_2 has three major crystalline phase structures: anatase, rutile, and brookite. Anatase and rutile phases play a major role in the application point of view [17]. The TiO_2 NPs have been microbially synthesized using bacteria such as *Lactobacillus* sp., *Aeromonas hydrophila*, *Bacillus subtilis*, and fungus such as *Fusarium oxysporum*, *Sachharomyces cerevisae*, and *Aspergillus tubingensis* [18]. TiO_2 NPs are promising as efficient nutrient source for plants to increase biomass production due to enhanced metabolic activities and utilization of native nutrients by promoting microbial activities. The biosynthesis of TiO_2 NPs is at low cost, an ecofriendly biological approach developed using a fungi, *Aspergillus flavus* TFR 7. Their effect on mung bean (*Vigna radiata* L) was evaluated. Figure 10.2 shows the photographic images of plant growth under various treatments, which showed that the synthesized TiO_2 NPs can be used as plant nutrient fertilizer to enhance crop production. Moreover, the biosynthesis of TiO_2 NPs was achieved by a novel, biodegradable, and convenient procedure using *Aspergillus flavus* as a reducing and capping agent. The fungus-mediated TiO_2 NPs were proved to be a good novel antibacterial material [19].

Ecofriendly synthesis of TiO_2 NPs using a highly efficient *Propionibacterium* species isolated from coal fly ash resulted in a well-dispersed uniform-sized anatase form of nanoparticles that are highly stable, biocompatible, and cost effective, thereby offering several advantages over conventional methods. The TiO_2 NPs provide enhanced wound-healing activity [20]. The TiO_2 NPs synthesized from *Aspergillus niger* have been used to detect the larvicidal activity against *Aedes aegypti*. The *A. niger* releases enzymes capable of synthesizing TiO_2 NPs, which can be suggested to develop safer and effective larvicide alternative to chemical methods of mosquito control. Indeed, these nanoparticles can be effectively used to control mosquito population [21].

10.3 Biopolymers

Biopolymers are macromolecules synthesized from living organisms. Some of the widely used biopolymers are gelatin, starch, cellulose, chitin and chitosan, PLA, PCL, PVA, polyvinyl acetate (PVAc), collagen, and poly(3-hydroxybutyrate-co-3-hydroxyvalerate) (PHBV). Biopolymers are classified into two major types: natural and synthetic biopolymers.

Natural biopolymers: Based on the range of compositions, chemical functionality, and nature of the repeating unit, three groups are classified: polysaccharides made of sugars, proteins made of amino acids, and nucleic acids made of nucleotides. These are commonly called "structural biopolymers or natural biopolymers," and the schematic representations of these are shown in Fig. 10.2. The most commonly known natural biopolymers are polysaccharides (starch, cellulose, alginate, dextran, chitosan, and pullulan), proteins (casein, gluten, vicilin, gelatin, albumin, lecithin, legumin). Polyhydroxyalkanotes and bacterial cellulose are produced by bacteria. Figure 10.2 provides the list of natural biopolymers that could be used for various applications.

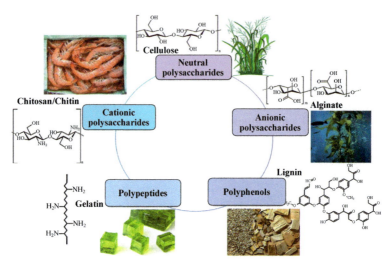

Figure 10.2 Schematic diagram of examples of structural or natural biopolymers (modified from https://schneppgroup.wordpress.com/research/biopolymers).

Synthetic biodegradable biopolymers: Another grouping is based on the backbone of polymers: polyesters, polysaccharides, polycarbonates, polyamides, and vinyl polymers. Based on the applications, biopolymers can be classified as bioplastics, biosurfactant, biodetergent, bioadhesive, bioflocculant, and so on. These kinds of polymers are known as synthetic biopolymers, which are synthesized using classical chemical synthesis with renewable bio-monomers, such as polylactic acid (PLA), poly(lactide-co-glycolide) (PLGA), polyanhydrides, poly-ε-caprolactone (PCL), poly-alkyl-cyanoacrylates, and polyphosphazene. Figure 10.3 shows the examples of synthetic biodegradable biopolymers (bioplastics).

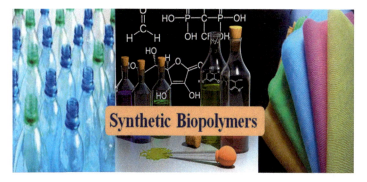

Figure 10.3 Examples of synthetic biodegradable biopolymers (bioplastics).

10.3.1 Nanocomposites from Bacteria

Cellulose is the most abundant natural polymer among renewable polymers. It is the basic unit in the cell wall of eukaryotic plants and algae, and also the major constituent of the fungal cell wall. Some of the bacterial genera can also secrete cellulose, including *Acetobacter, Rhizobium, Agrobacterium, Sarcina, Pseudomonas, Achromobacter, Alcaligenes, Aerobacter,* and *Azotobacter*. Bacterial cellulose (BC) is a promising, sustainable, and biodegradable nanofibrous material. The BC produced by rod-shaped aerobic gram-negative acetic acid bacteria *Gluconacetobacter xylinus* (earlier known as *Acetobacter xylinum*) has a linear β-1,4 glucose structure [22] and is the most exploited BC due to its high conceding ability. The BC has excellent and unique properties such as purity, hydrophilicity, high tensile strength and Young's modulus, high crystallinity, highly porous structure, environmental biodegradability, and excellent biocompatibility [15]. Bacteria efficiently synthesize BC in given optimum conditions such as pH, temperature, and with abundant carbon sources than nitrogen [23]. Several attempts have also been made by researchers to enhance BC production by bacteria. For instance, Siripong et al. [24] utilized ultraviolet (UV) radiation and/or N-methyl-N'-nitro-N-nitrosoguanidine (NTG) mutagenesis for strain improvement and obtained a high-yield strain for BC production. Strategies to improve the properties of BC have also been achieved by some modifications. For example, addition of nalidixic acids and chloramphenicol in the culture medium resulted in the formation of wider cellulose ribbons and increased Young's modulus of BC sheets. Acetylation, perpropionylation, and carbanilation of BC by using chemical reactions in ionic liquid 1-*N*-butyl-3-methylimidazolium chloride ensued the change of surface hydrophobicity and mechanical properties. Carboxymethylation, esterification, and other modifications could also enhance the properties of BC [22]. In 2003, Woodward and colleagues were the first to use nanocelluloses as template for synthesizing metal nanoparticles such as Pd, Au, and Ag precipitated from their metal precursors onto bacterial CNFs without the use of any external reducing agent [25].

10.3.2 Polyhydroxyalkanoates

Generally, bacteria grown under unfavorable growth conditions accumulate polyesters of various hydroxyalkanoate monomers in the cytoplasm as energy/carbon storage materials by granular inclusions. These granular particles consist of polyester, proteins, and lipids. They are branched into two groups based on the number of carbon atoms in the monomeric units: that is, short-chain-length (SCL) PHAs, which consist of 3–5 carbon atoms, and medium-chain-length (MCL) PHAs, which consist of 6–14 carbon atoms [26]. PHAs are biosynthesized by various gram-positive and gram-negative bacteria, and more than 300 different microorganisms are known to synthesize and accumulate PHAs intracellularly, including *Azotobacter*, *Pseudomonas*, *Bacillus*, and *Methylobacterium* sp. [27]. They are well recognized for their excellent biocompatibility, biodegradability, easier processability, and easily tunable properties by toning the process and molecular weight of the polymer composition. PHAs such as poly(3-hydroxybutyrate) (PHB) and related copolymers, mostly PHBV, are brittle; thus, their high crystalline nature has packaging and biomedical applications. Recently, Castro-Mayorga et al. [28] have successfully stabilized antimicrobial Ag NPs produced by chemical reduction in suspensions of an unpurified PHBV, which was previously obtained from mixed culture fermentation using synthetic medium mimicking fermented cheese whey. The synthesis of Ag NPs was carried out within the unpurified PHBV suspension (in situ), and physical mixing (mix) resulted in the stability of crystals for at least 40 days and spherical nanoparticles (11 ± 5.6 nm) obtained in situ.

10.3.3 Application of Biopolymer–Metal Nanocomposites

Metal nanoparticles with more distinguishing properties fabricated with biopolymers will definitely have enhanced properties that have multiple applications in various fields such as biomedicine, catalysis, sensors, environment, and energy resources. Applications of various nanocomposites are given in Table 10.2. It could be seen that most of the nanoparticles are gold and silver, which are noble metals and also bearing various unique features for usage in medical fields.

10.4 Biomedical Applications

10.4.1 Tissue Engineering

Tissue engineering is the application of biological, chemical, and engineering principles to restore, repair, or regenerate living tissue by combining biomaterials, cells, or tissue, or biologically active molecules and other factors of the tissue microenvironment [29]. Development of advanced biomaterials with controlled physical, chemical, electrical, and biological properties will, therefore, be beneficial to facilitate the formation of functional tissues. Some of the challenges in tissue engineering are biomimicking the complex tissue architecture and the natural cellular microenvironment for the formation of function tissues. Porosity is crucial as it enables the diffusion of cellular nutrients and waste and provides for cell movement. Biopolymer nanocomposites can overcome these challenges and effectively involve in the tissue engineering scaffold design. Some of biopolymer nanocomposites are discussed here. Polysaccharides such as alginate have natural polymeric sponge structure, which is more advantageous for the scaffold design. As the alginates are soft, scaffolds can be with hydroxyapatite (HAP)–polymer nanocomposites and have widespread applications. Composite membranes from HAP nanoparticles and chitosan/collagen sols have also been synthesized to study connective-tissue reactions [30]. Poly(ε-caprolactone) (PCL) is a biodegradable and non-toxic aliphatic polyester synthesized by the ring-opening

Table 10.2 Bacterial nanocellulose composites with noble metal nanoparticles and their applications in different fields

Metal NPs	Synthesized methods	Types of nanocellulose	Applications	References
Ag NPs	$AgNO_3$ (reduction by $NaBH_4$)	Bacteria CNFs	Antibacterial	[31]
Ag NPs	$AgNO_3$ (reduction by bacterial CNFs: 80°C, 4 h)	Bacteria CNFs	Antibacterial	[32]
Ag NPs	$AgNO_3$ (reduction by triethanolamine)	Bacteria CNFs (triethanolamine as complexing agent)	Antibacterial	[33]
Ag NPs	$AgNO_3$ (reduction by NH_2NH_2, NH_2OH, ascorbic acid)	Bacteria CNFs (polyvinylpyrrolidone) (PVP) and gelatin used as additional stabilizers	Antibacterial	[34]
Ag NPs	$AgNO_3$ (reduction by sodium citrate)	Bacteria CNFs (sodium citrate as additional stabilizer)	Substrate enhanced Raman scattering (SERS) substrates	[35]
Au NPs	$HAuCl_4$ (reduction by citrate ions and surface of CNFs)	Wood or bacteria CNFs	Security paper making: optical properties	[36]
Au NPs	$HAuCl_4$ (reduction by poly(ethyleneimine)]	Bacteria CNFs (heme proteins: horseradish peroxidase, hemoglobin, and myoglobin immobilized onto CNFs)	Electrocatalysis: reduction of H_2O_2	[37]
Cu-Pd NPs	$PdCl_2$ and $CuCl_2$ (reduction by KBH_4)	Bacteria CNFs	Water denitrification: nitrate reduction	[38]

CNFs: cellulose nanofibers
Source: Ref. [39].

polymerization of ε-caprolactone. It has a melting temperature of 61°C and a T_g of 60°C at which it converts to a rubbery state. In this state, it permits the diffusion of low–molecular weight species at body temperature, thus making PCL a promising candidate for controlled release and soft-tissue engineering. In addition, nanocomposite hydrogels containing metal nanoparticles are extensively used as conductive scaffolds. Such conductive scaffolds can be used to engineer tissues that require propagation of electrical signals to facilitate the formation of functional tissues. Biopolymeric nanocomposites are further exploited in bone grafting, vascular implants, etc. For example, BC-hydroxyapatite scaffolds for bone regeneration have been developed by immersing the BC gel in simulated body fluid or in both calcium and phosphate solutions, and BC-polyester and BC-PVA nanocomposites were developed for potential applications as vascular implants. PHA is yet another example with distinguished and advantageous characteristics such as biocompatibility and generation of mild foreign-body response, making it suitable for use in implants.

10.4.2 Drug-Delivery Systems

Nanoparticles decorated/fabricated with biopolymers have attracted the drug-/gene-delivery systems. Drug-delivery systems ameliorate the problems of conventional administration by enhancing drug solubility, prolonging duration time, reducing side effects, and retaining drug bioactivity. The nanosized particles can transverse cellular membrane to mediate the drug/gene delivery and the functional groups of biopolymers can help in targeting. Drug delivery is a multidisciplinary field, which constitutes knowledge from the field of chemistry, pharmaceutical sciences, medicine, and engineering. Nowadays, drug-delivery systems have enhanced bioavailability, improve the uptake, preserve drug concentration by controlling the rate of drug release, and reduce side effects by releasing the drugs at the target cell. For example, polyhydroxyalkanoates such as PHB and related copolymers, mostly PHBV, are widely used in drug-delivery systems.

10.5 Conclusion

Bionanocomposites provide a paradigm in developing an ecofriendly biosynthesis strategy with improved intrinsic properties of biopolymers and noble nanoparticles. They open a different direction for extensive applications in comprehensive fields such as biomedicine, biosensors, and industry. Additionally, the cost-effective method of synthesis via biological routes opens a window for large-scale applications and also commercialization. Developing new aspects of synthesizing methods in an efficient manner and applications in combined fields would provide more insights into the field and also maturation. Further, developments in the application of nanoparticles should be prospected toward success in the future.

References

1. Indira, K., Mudali, U. K., Nishimura, T., and Rajendran, N. (2015). A review on TiO_2 nanotubes: Influence of anodization parameters, formation mechanism, properties, corrosion behavior and biomedical applications, *J. Bio Tribo Corros.*, **1**, 28.
2. Tratnyek, P. G. and Johnson, R. L. (2006). Nanotechnologies for environmental cleanup, *Nano Today*, **1**, 44–48.
3. Gajbhiye, M., Kesharwani, J., Ingle, A., Gade, A., and Rai, M. (2009). Fungus-mediated synthesis of silver nanoparticles and their activity against pathogenic fungi in combination with fluconazole, *Nanomed. Nanotechnol.*, **5**, 382–386.
4. Ahmad, A., Senapati, S., Khan, M. I., Kumar, R., and Sastry, M. (2003). Extracellular biosynthesis of monodisperse gold nanoparticles by a novel extremophilic actinomycete, *Thermomonospora* sp., *Langmuir*, **19**, 3550–3553.
5. Zhang, T., Wang, W., Zhang, D., Zhang, X., Ma, Y., Zhou, Y., and Qi, L. (2010). Biotemplated synthesis of gold nanoparticle–bacteria cellulose nanofiber nanocomposites and their application in biosensing, *Adv. Funct. Mater.*, **20**, 1152–1160.
6. Pinto, R. J. B., Marques, P. A. A. P., Martins, M. A., Neto, C. P., and Trindade, T. (2007). Electrostatic assembly and growth of gold nanoparticles in cellulosic fibres, *J. Colloid Interf. Sci.*, **312**, 506–512.
7. Huang, X. and El-Sayed, M. A. (2010). Gold nanoparticles: Optical properties and implementations in cancer diagnosis and photothermal therapy, *J. Adv. Res.*, **1**, 13–28.

8. Shankar, P. D., Shobana, S., Karuppusamy, I., Pugazhendhi A, Ramkumar, V. S., Arvindnarayanan, S., and Kumar, G. (2016). A review on the biosynthesis of metallic nanoparticles (gold and silver) using bio-components of microalgae: Formation mechanism and applications, *Enzyme Microb. Technol.*, **95**, 28–44.

9. Kreibig, U. and Vollmer, M. (1995). *Optical Properties of Metal Clusters, Springer Series in Materials Science*, Springer, Berlin.

10. Jeong, S. H., Yeo, S. Y., and Yi, S. C. (2005). The effect of filler particle size on the antibacterial properties of compounded polymer/silver fibers, *J. Mater. Sci.*, **40**, 5407–5411.

11. Elechiguerra, J. L., Burt, J. L., Morones, J. R., Camacho-Bragado, A., Gao, X., Lara, H. H., and Yacaman, M. J. (2005). Interaction of silver nanoparticles with HIV-1, *J. Nanobiotechnol.*, **3**, 6.

12. Rai, M., Yadav, A., and Gade, A. (2009). Silver nanoparticles as a new generation of antimicrobials, *Biotechnol. Adv.*, **27**, 76–83.

13. Logeswari, P., Silambarasan, S., and Abraham, J. (2015). Synthesis of silver nanoparticles using plants extract and analysis of their antimicrobial property, *J. Saudi Chem. Soc.*, **19**, 311–317.

14. Alzahrani, E. and Ahmed, R. A. (2016). Synthesis of copper nanoparticles with various sizes and shapes: Application as a superior non-enzymatic sensor and antibacterial agent, *Int. J. Electrochem. Sci.*, **11**, 4712–4723.

15. Ebrahimi, F. (Ed.) (2012). *Nanocomposites: New Trends and Developments*, InTech. www.intechopen.com/books/nanocomposites-new-trends-and- developments.

16. Indira, K. (2015). Development of titanium nanotube arrays for orthopaedic applications. Dissertation, Anna University, http://shodhganga.inflibnet.ac.in/handle/10603/37614.

17. Diebold, U. (2003). The surface science of titanium dioxide, *Surf. Sci. Rep.*, **48**, 53–229.

18. Suriyaraj, S. P. and Selvakumar, R. (2014). Room temperature biosynthesis of crystalline TiO_2 nanoparticles using *Bacillus licheniformis* and studies on the effect of calcination on phasestructure and optical properties, *RSC Adv.*, **4**, 39619–39624.

19. Rajakumar, G., Rahuman, A. A., Roopan, S. M., Khanna, V. G., Elango, G., Kamaraj, C., Zahir, A. A., and Velayutham, K. (2012). Fungus-mediated biosynthesis and characterization of TiO_2 nanoparticles and their activity against pathogenic bacteria, *Spectrochim. Acta A*, **91**, 23–29.

20. Babitha, S. and Korrapati, P. S. (2013). Biosynthesis of titanium dioxide nanoparticles using a probiotic from coal fly ash effluent, *Mater. Res. Bull.*, **48**, 4738–4742.

21. Durairaj, B., Xavier, T., and Muthu, S. (2014). Fungal generated titanium dioxide nanoparticles: A potent mosquito (*Aedes aegypti*) larvicidal agent, *Sch. Acad. J. Biosci.*, **2**, 651–658.

22. Qiu, K. and Netravali, A. N. (2014). A review of fabrication and applications of bacterial cellulose based nanocomposites, *Polym. Rev.*, **54**, 598–626.

23. Ramana, K. V., Tomar, A., and Singh, L. (2000). Effect of various carbon and nitrogen sources on cellulose synthesis by *Acetobacter xylinum*, *World J. Microbiol. Biotechnol.*, **16**, 245–248.

24. Siripong, P., Chuleekorn, S., and Duangporn, P. (2012). Enhanced cellulose production by ultraviolet (UV) irradiation and N-methyl-N'-nitro-N-nitrosoguanidine (NTG) mutagenesis of an acetobacter species isolate, *Afr. J. Biotechnol.*, **11**, 1433–1442.

25. Evans, B. R., O'Neill, H. M., Malyvanh, V. P., Lee, I., and Woodward, J. (2003). Palladium-bacterial cellulose membranes for fuel cells, *Biosens. Bioelectron.*, **18**, 917–923.

26. Shrivastav, A., Hae-Yeong, K., and Young-Rok, K. (2013). Advances in the applications of polyhydroxyalkanoate nanoparticles for novel drug delivery system, *BioMed. Res. Int.*, **2013**, e581684.

27. Steinbuchel, A. and Fuchtenbusch, B. (1998). Bacterial and other biological systems for polyester production, *Trends Biotechnol.*, **16**, 419–427.

28. Castro-Mayorga, J. L., Martínez-Abad, A., Fabra, M. J., Olivera, C., Reis, M., and Lagarón, J. M. (2014). Stabilization of antimicrobial silver nanoparticles by a polyhydroxyalkanoate obtained from mixed bacterial culture, *Int. J. Biol. Macromolec.*, Special Issue: Biodegradable Biopolym., **71**, 103–110.

29. Kingsley, J. D., Ranjan, S., Dasgupta, N., and Saha, P. (2013). Nanotechnology for tissue engineering: Need, techniques and applications, *J. Pharm. Res.*, **7**, 200–204.

30. Hule, R. A. and Pochan, D. J. (2007). Polymer nanocomposites for biomedical applications, *MRS Bull.*, **32**, 354–358.

31. Yang, G., Xie, J., Hong, F., Cao, Z., and Yang, X. (2012a). Antimicrobial activity of silver nanoparticle impregnated bacterial cellulose membrane: Effect of fermentation carbon sources of bacterial cellulose, *Carbohydr. Polym.*, **87**, 839–845.

32. Yang, G., Xie, J., Deng, Y., Bian, Y., and Hong, F. (2012b). Hydrothermal synthesis of bacterial cellulose/AgNPs composite: A "green" route for antibacterial application, *Carbohydr. Polym.*, **87**, 2482–2487.

33. Barud, H. S., Regiani, T., Marques, R. F. C., Lustri, W. R., Messaddeq, Y., and Ribeiro, S. J. L. (2011). Antimicrobial bacterial cellulose-silver nanoparticles composite membranes, *J. Nanomater.*, **2011**, e721631.

34. Maria, L. C. S., Santos, A. L. C., Oliveira, P. C., Valle, A. S. S., Barud, H. S., Messaddeq, Y., and Ribeiro, S. J. L. (2010). Preparation and antibacterial activity of silver nanoparticles impregnated in bacterial cellulose, *Polímeros*, **20**, 72–77.

35. Marques, P. A. A. P., Nogueira, H. I. S., Pinto, R. J. B., Neto, C. P., and Trindade, T. (2008). Silver-bacterial cellulosic sponges as active SERS substrates, *J. Raman Spectrosc.*, **39**, 439–443.

36. Pinto, R. J. B., Neves, M. C., Neto, C. P., and Trindade, T. (2012). Composites of cellulose and metal nanoparticles, http://dx.doi.org/10.5772/50553.

37. Wang, W., Tai-Ji, Z., De-Wen, Z., Hong-Yi, L., Yu-Rong, M., Li-Min, Q., Ying-Lin, Z., and Xin-Xiang, Z. (2011). Amperometric hydrogen peroxide biosensor based on the immobilization of Heme proteins on gold nanoparticles–bacteria cellulose nanofibers nanocomposite, *Talanta*, **84**, 71–77.

38. Sun, D., Yang, J., Li, J., Yu, J., Xu, X., and Yang, X. (2010). Novel Pd-Cu/bacterial cellulose nanofibers: Preparation and excellent performance in catalytic denitrification, *Appl. Surf. Sci.*, **256**, 2241–2244.

39. Kaushik, M. and Moores, A. (2016). Review: Nanocelluloses as versatile supports for metal nanoparticles and their applications in catalysis, *Green Chem.*, **18**, 622–637.

Chapter 11

Bionanocomposites, Their Processing, and Environmental Applications

Sagar Roy and Chaudhery Mustansar Hussain

Department of Chemistry and Environmental Sciences,
New Jersey Institute of Technology, University Heights, Newark,
NJ 07102, USA
chaudhery.m.hussain@njit.edu

Recently, the use of renewable resources is gaining attention as an alternative to petroleum resources. On the other hand, reinforcement of biopolymers with nanoscale, in particular, has gained a massive attraction from the researchers in academia and industries, because of the exponential improvement in physical, mechanical, and thermal properties with smaller amount of incorporation. Particularly, the low cost of the raw material such as cellulosic particles as a reinforcing phase in nanocomposites has numerous well-known advantages, for example, low density, renewable nature, wide variety of filler availability, low energy consumption, modest abrasivity during processing, relatively reactive surface, and biodegradability. This chapter is intended to review the recent research activities in the area of nanocomposites using biopolymers

Biocomposites: Biomedical and Environmental Applications
Edited by Shakeel Ahmed, Saiqa Ikram, Suvardhan Kanchi, and Krishna Bisetty
Copyright © 2018 Pan Stanford Publishing Pte. Ltd.
ISBN 978-981-4774-38-3 (Hardcover), 978-1-315-11080-6 (eBook)
www.panstanford.com

as prime materials for environmental protection. Therefore, in this chapter, general preparation methods and biodegradability aspects of bionanocomposites with their possible environmental applications have been discussed.

11.1 Introduction: Biodegradable Polymers

Recently, a group of novel nanostructured hybrid materials, called bionanocomposites, signifies a promising area of research that bridges material science, nanotechnology, life and environmental sciences [1–3]. The term "bionanocomposite" deals with a class of nanocomposites involving naturally occurring biopolymers or synthetic biofunctional polymers, in which nanoscopic species of typically 1–100 nm in at least one dimension are dispersed in polymer matrices in order to enhance the overall performances of the composite systems. The presence of nanomaterials dramatically alters the properties of the pristine biopolymer, including improved strength and modulus, enhanced chemical and thermal resistance, superior barrier properties, ablation resistance, gas permeability, flame retardancy, etc. The distinctive properties of nanomaterials, such as size, mechanical, thermal, and surface properties can introduce unique combination with polymer matrix at very low concentration, which is extremely necessary to obtain the desired end product. The diverse application opportunities of these bionanocomposites make the nanomaterials ubiquitous in polymer systems. Since the instigation of nanocomposites, scientists are contributing enormous effort in this particular research field because of the outstanding attributes of these nanohybrids as structural or functional materials. In addition to all the benefits offered by nanocomposites materials, bionanocomposites exhibit biocompatibility and biodegradability. Moreover, the field of bionanocomposites has generated much interest as they can be synthesized and fabricated in the ways similar to that of conventional polymer composites.

Bionanocomposites are generally fabricated using a specific type of polymer matrices that degrade into natural by-products such as gases (CO_2, N_2), water, biomass, and inorganic salts after use. The end products of these "biodegradable" polymers are gradually absorbed or eliminated from the system. Biodegradation is a natural process, and the simple by-products are mineralized and redistributed through natural cycles. In a living system, this polymer matrix serves as a potential biological carrier and breaks down after completing its function via hydrolysis or chain scission caused by metabolic process [4, 5]. However, biodegradation of such polymers requires specific pH, humidity, oxygenation, and the presence of catalysts [4]. The presence of microorganisms in the biosphere also plays an important role in the degradation process. In 1990 and 1992, the confusion regarding true definition of "biodegradable" led to a lawsuit on deceptive and fraudulent environmental advertising. It was thus required to define the term more scientifically through common test methods and protocols [6]. A number of standard organizations have defined biodegradable polymers and a few of these are as follows:

- **ISO 472: 1988.** A plastic designed to undergo a significant change in its chemical structure under specific environmental conditions resulting in a loss of some properties that may vary as measured by standard test methods appropriate to the plastics and application in a period of time that determines its classification. The change in chemical structure results from the action of naturally occurring microorganisms.
- **ASTM sub-committee D20.96 proposal.** Degradable plastics are plastic materials that undergo bond scission in the backbone of a polymer through chemical, biological and/or physical forces in the environment at a rate which leads to fragmentation or disintegration of the plastics.
- **Japanese Biodegradable Plastic Society draft proposal.** Biodegradable plastics are polymeric materials which are changed into lower molecular weight compounds where at least one step in the degradation process is through metabolism in the presence of naturally occurring organisms.
- **DIN 103.2 working group on biodegradable polymers.** Biodegradation of a plastic material is a process leading to naturally occurring metabolic end products.

- **General definition of biodegradation.** It is a process whereby bacteria, fungi, yeasts, and their enzymes consume a substance as a food source so that its original form disappears. Under appropriate conditions of moisture, temperature, and oxygen availability, biodegradation is a relatively rapid process. Biodegradation for limited periods is a reasonable target for the complete assimilation and disappearance of an article, leaving no toxic or environmentally harmful residue.

- **CEN: Biodegradable plastics.** A degradable material in which the degradation results from the action of microorganisms and ultimately the material is converted to water, carbon dioxide and/or methane and a new cell biomass.

- **Biodegradation.** Biodegradation is a degradation caused by biological activity, especially by enzymatic action, leading to a significant change in the chemical structure of a material.

- **Inherent biodegradability.** The potential of a material to be biodegraded, established under laboratory conditions.

- **Ultimate biodegradability.** The breakdown of an organic chemical compound by microorganisms in the presence of oxygen to biodegradability carbon dioxide, water and mineral salts of any other elements present (mineralization) and new biomass or in the absence of oxygen to carbon dioxide, methane, mineral salts and new biomass.

11.2 Conventional Polymers versus Biodegradable Polymers

Conventional polymers are used widely in different fields because of their excellent properties such as high mechanical strength, low density (useful for transporting goods), and low cost due to manufacturing scale and process optimization, easy processability, versatility, and impermeability to water and microorganisms. The advancements of these traditional polymers are the results of decades of sincere research and developments. In terms of generation of carbon footprint, utilization of raw materials and release of waste, their fabrication is exceptionally resourceful. However, the inertness and durability of these polymers ensued in their accumulation in the ecosystem.

Like conventional polymers, biodegradable polymers possess same structural and functional properties; in addition, they degrade via microbial and environmental actions upon disposal without any undesirable ecological impact. The degradation of conventional plastics using burning process generates huge amount of toxic fumes that are potentially hazardous to people's health and the environment. On the other hand, burning biodegradable plastics releases very little, if any, toxic chemicals into the air. In recent times, a large amount of plastic fragments in the ocean was observed, which not only pollute the ocean but also destabilize the ocean ecosystems. Conversely, biodegradable plastics are decomposed by microorganisms and bacteria in the soil, which actually enhance the soil quality and make the ground more fertile.

The problems with traditional polymers arise from the shortage of landfill. This shortage and the demand for globally sensible consumption of resources are considered the main reasons for utilizing biodegradable materials. Many countries are now concerned about reducing waste and endeavor to protect the environment; they have made a start to accept biodegradable polymers. Although higher manufacturing cost restricts the usage of these ecofriendly polymers, many organizations and governments are working to make biodegradable polymers more of a reality. The increasing demands for materials that do not harm the planet and large commercial-scale production of these polymers will possibly propel the prices down.

11.3 Classification and Properties of Biodegradable Polymers

According to the origin and their chemical composition, synthesis procedures, processing techniques, applications, etc., biodegradable polymers can be classified in several categories based on their origin (such as natural polymers and synthetic polymers), chemical composition (such as polymers with carbon backbone, polymers with hydrolyzable backbones), etc.

11.3.1 Natural Biodegradable Polymers

11.3.1.1 Polysaccharides

The primary polysaccharides of interest are cellulose and starch. However, complex carbohydrate polymers, such as xanthan, curdlan, pullulan, and hyaluronic acid, produced by bacteria and fungi are also gaining attention. These complex carbohydrates comprise more than one type of carbohydrate unit and possess regularly arranged branched structures. The difference in their structure also leads to differentiate in the degradation mechanisms. Cellulose is the most abundant polymer found in nature, with an estimated annual natural production of 1.5×10^{12} tons. Isolation and application of cellulose have been known since more than 150 years ago. Cellulose is the main constituent of the lignocellulosic plant cell wall. Generally, cellulose content in lignocellulosic plant varies between 23% and 53% on a dry-weight basis; the amount of cellulose, however, depends on plant species, growing conditions, place, ultimate growth, and maturity. In most of the straw species, the amount of cellulose was ~35–45% of the dry substances. The polymer obtained from plant consists of very long macromolecular chains of "cellobiose" as repeating unit. It is composed of D-glucose unite linked by β-1,4 glycoside bonds. The structure is shown in Fig. 11.1. The orientation of the long chain includes planner chain conformation and parallel-chain packing. Due to the absence of any branches in the main backbone chain, efficient chain packing takes place, which eventually generates a native crystalline state, resulting in stiff and dimensionally stable natural fibers. The unique functional characteristics generated from the chemical structure of cellulose offer many useful properties.

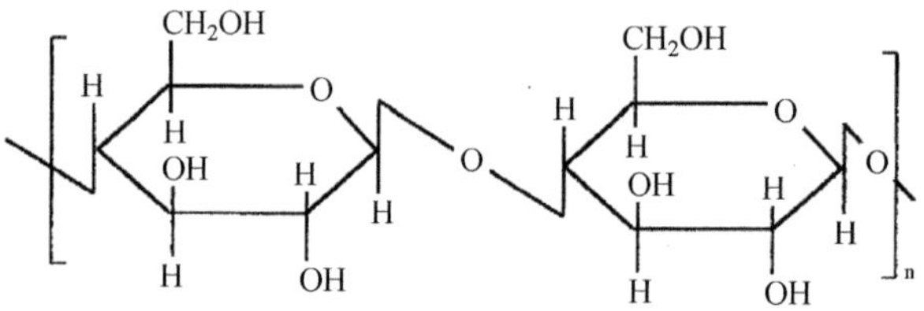

Figure 11.1 The structure of cellobiose as repeating unit and composed D-glucose unite linked by β-1,4 glycoside bonds.

Cellulose is highly resistant to strong alkali (17.5 wt%) but undergoes hydrolysis under acidic environment to water-soluble sugars. The stability of cellulose in the presence of oxidizing agents is also very high. In the presence of strong intra- or intermolecular hydrogen bonding, bundles of cellulose chains aggregate to form microfibrils, which are further assembled to fibrils and finally to cellulose fibers. Cellulose is an infusible and insoluble polymer with high tensile strength and needs to be transformed into a processable form via chemical modification. Important derivatives such as esters (cellulose acetate, carboxymethyl cellulose, and cellulose xanthate), ethers (methylcellulose, hydroxypropyl methyl cellulose, and hydroxyethyl cellulose), and acetals (especially the cyclic acetal formed between the C2 and C3 hydroxyl groups and butyraldehyde) can be synthesized by the reaction of hydroxyl groups present in the repeating units. Some of the commercially available cellulose derivatives are Tenite® (Eastman, USA), Bioceta® (Mazzucchelli, Italy), Fasal® (IFA, Austria), and Natureflex® (UCB, Germany).

Enzymatic oxidation with peroxidase secreted by fungi leads to biodegradation of cellulose. Cellulose has been used significantly in paper, wood product, textile, film, and fiber industries, and more recently as a source of biofuel production. Regenerated or mercerized cellulose (cellulose II, Rayon) is normally used as fiber material and film production. As a biodegradable polymer, cellulose and its derivatives have received significant attention than any other materials since they are prone to biodegradation when attacked by a variety of microorganisms. Although cellulose exists together with lignin and possesses a complicated chemical structures, cellulose does decompose readily via complex bioreactions. Biodegradation via fermentation of cellulose has been proposed as a synthesis route of several chemicals, such as ethanol and acetic acid; however, commercial importance is yet to be achieved.

11.3.1.2 Lignocellulosic complex (fibers)

Another class of biodegradable polymer complex is plant fibers, which are mainly composed of cellulose (30–50%), hemicellulose (20–50%), lignin (15–35%), pectin, and waxy substances. Approximately 50% of the global biomass is composed of these lignocellulosic complex. In this complex formation, cellulose fibrils are hydrogen bonded with hemicellulose and form reinforcing constituents for the fiber structure. On the other hand, lignin and pectin are connected with cellulose–hemicellulose grid as a bonding agent to fasten altogether a wide variety of engineering and daily usable products, such as paper, lumber, and starting material of various chemicals. Advanced materials, including biodegradable polymers, have been produced from these lignocellulosic materials. Pectin and high amylase starch blends produce high temperature stable (180°C), strong, flexible film. Further blending with poly(vinyl alcohol) (PVA) generates a water-soluble film, forming a material that can be used for the production of detergents and insecticides, pouches, flushable liners, and bags, and medical-delivery systems and devices [7].

11.3.1.3 Starch

Starch is another well-known variety of hydrocolloid biopolymer occurring widely in plants. This low-cost polysaccharide material is abundantly available in different natural resources, including potatoes, corn, wheat, and rice. The granule form of starch comprises two major variety of components: a liner crystalline, boiling water-soluble polymer, amylose (poly-α-1,4-D-glucopyranoside, 20 wt% of the granule), and the remaining is amylopectin (poly-α-1,4-D-glucopyranoside and α-1,6-D-glucopyranoside), a branched, amorphous, and boiling water-insoluble polymer. In this polymer, alternating amorphous and semi-crystalline layers of around 120–400 nm form the granules or growth rings. However, the relative amounts and molar masses of these components may vary with the starch source, yielding to materials of different physical, mechanical, and biodegradable properties. The physical and thermal stability of starch under stress is not very high. At 150°C, glucoside links start to break and above 250°C, the granules collapse. According to the Australian Academy of Science, "starch can be processed directly into a bioplastic, but because it is soluble in water, articles made from starch will swell and deform when exposed to moisture, limiting its use" [8]. In order to solve this issue, the polymer needs to blend with other stable polymer or modified chemically. The processing technology of starch is quite similar to the conventional plastic technologies such as injection molding, blow molding, film blowing, foaming, thermoforming, and extrusion [9]. Starch has been used as a raw material for film production extensively. The barrier property of this film exhibits very high water vapor and low water and oxygen permeability [10] and are thus efficient constituents for food packaging, disposable food service ware, purchase bags, composting bags, and loose fill products. It is also very useful to fabricate agricultural mulch films. It has been used as filler to various polymers, such as low density polyethylene (LDPE) to make it biodegradable. This porous film is readily attacked by microorganisms and rapidly saturated by oxygen, which synergistically enhance the biodegradation rate. Medical application as hygiene material is also known. Thermoplastic hydrogel based on starch–cellulose acetate blend has been used as bone cement or drug delivery. In starch, both fractions are readily hydrolyzed at the acetal link by enzymes. The α-1,4 link is attacked by amylases, while glucosidases attack the α-1,6 link. The biodegradation of starch generates non-toxic ecofriendly by-products.

11.3.1.4 Chitin and chitosan

Chitin is the second most abundant natural macromolecule, found in the shells of crabs, lobsters, crawfish, shrimps, and insects. This linear copolymer consists of N-acetylglucosamine and N-glucosamine connected through β-1,4 linkage. Depending on the processing technique, these co-monomer units are distributed randomly or as a block throughout the polymer backbone chain. The units resemble with cellulose having amino groups. Farming of fungi using fermentation technology can provide an alternative source of chitin [11].

Chitosan is synthesized via partial alkaline N-deacetylation process. The degree of deacetylation, ranging from 30% to 100%, depends on the preparation method and is measured by the ratio of glucosamine to acetyl glucosamine. The crystallinity, surface energy, and degradation rate of chitosan are highly dependent on the degree of deacetylation. The glucosamine units are usually predominant in chitosan.

The solubility of chitin in water is negligible in its native form; partly deacetylated form of chitosan makes it water soluble. Chitosan is also soluble in weekly acidic solutions and forms a cationic polymer with a high charge density, which develop polyelectrolyte complexes with various anionic polymers. Both biopolymers are found biocompatible and have antimicrobial activities. They showed the ability to absorb heavy metal ions. Chitosan is transformed into different forms such as gels, powders, fibers, and films, which find many applications in the area of drug encapsulation, membrane, contact lens materials, cell culture, blood coagulation inhibitor, etc. Artificial skin and absorbable sutures prepared from chitin fibers exhibit superior biocompatibility and efficiency in wound treatment. Its ability to hold water molecules has found applications in the cosmetic industry. It has also been used as a carrier in drug delivery for cancer therapy, is non-toxic after oral administration in humans, and is an FDA-approved food additive.

Chitosan can be degraded by enzymes such as chitosanase, lysozyme, and papain. In living organisms, chitosan is degraded primarily by lysozyme via hydrolysis of the acetylated residues. The lowest biodegradation in vivo was observed with higher deacetylated form that may last for several months.

11.3.1.5 Alginic acid

Alginic acid is a high–molecular weight (500 kDa) biopolymer found within the cell walls and intercellular spaces of marine plants such as brown algae. It has a linear, copolymer structure comprising (1-4) glycosidically linked β-D-mannuronic acid and α-L-guluronic acid monomers. The ratio of these monomers varies with sources. This polymer offers structural flexibility and strength to marine plants. With monovalent, low–molecular weight amines and quaternary ammonium compounds, alginic acid forms water-soluble salts and becomes gels upon the introduction of counterions. The presence of polyvalent cations such as Ca^{2+}, Be^{2+}, Cu^{2+}, Al^{3+}, and Fe^{3+} converts it into water-insoluble polymer. Several parameters such as pH, type of counterions, and the functional charge density control the degree of crosslinking.

This non-toxic biopolymer has been extensively used as a food additive and a thickener in salad dressings and ice creams. Control release drug-delivery system utilizes the advantages of alginate gels. Alginate is also found very useful in encapsulation of various herbicides, microorganisms, and cells.

11.3.2 Polypeptides of Natural Origin

Proteins are natural biopolymers that have found several applications in their native form, such as wool, silk, and collagen. The three-dimensional structure of these proteins is stabilized mainly by non-covalent interactions. The unit structure of proteins forms through regular arrangements of various types of amino acids. Structural heterogeneity, thermal sensitivity, and hydrophilic behavior of proteins control the functional properties of specific protein. The degradation of proteins by enzymes occurs via amide hydrolysis reaction. Various vegetable and animal proteins are commonly used as biodegradable polymers, some of which are as follows:

11.3.2.1 Collagen and gelatin

Collagen, a major component of animal connective tissues, is one of the most abundant proteins that support mechanical stress transferred to it. The basic components of the 22 different varieties (types I–IV) of collagen are glycine, proline, hydroxyproline, and lysine, which combine together to form polypeptide linkages. It is a rod-shaped, high–molecular weight (~300,000) polymer with a length of nearly 300 nm. Because of the presence of acidic, basic, and hydroxylated amino acid residues more than lipophilic residues, it is hydrophilic in nature. The polymer chain flexibility depends on the amount of glycine content. The biopolymer shows unique physicochemical, mechanical, and biological properties and has been extensively investigated for various biomedical applications. The acidic solution of collagen can be processed easily into different forms such as tubes, sheets, foams, sponges, powders, nanofibrous matrices, and fleeces. The collagen solution is quite viscous and suitable for injectable solutions and dispersions. Collagen undergoes degradation within an in vivo system in the presence of suitable enzymes such as collagenases and metalloproteinases, to yield the corresponding amino acids. The rate of degradation can be controlled significantly by enzymatic pretreatment or crosslinking.

Gelatine, another variety of high–molecular weight polypeptide, consists of 19 amino acids. It is produced by denaturation and/or physical–chemical degradation of collagen. The polymer is water soluble and possesses good film-forming abilities. However, amino acid composition and the molecular weight distribution and presence of other additives control the mechanical and barrier properties of these films. Blending with other natural and synthetic polymers, such as soy protein, oils and fatty acids, or certain polysaccharides, and grafting with methyl methacrylate and poly(ethyl acrylate) offer enhanced film and barrier properties. The polymer has been used widely in industrial, pharmaceutical, and biomedical applications. Coatings and microencapsulation of various drugs using this biodegradable hydrogel were found suitable for human body without any adverse effect after degradation. The degradation behavior is carried out via hydrolysis of the amide linkages in the presence of a variety of proteolytic enzymes, such as proteases.

11.3.2.2 Corn zein

Another variety of plant-based biopolymer is zein protein, mainly found in corn endosperm. The alcohol-soluble polymer can be easily extracted with aqueous alcohol solution and dried to granular powder form. Three major varieties of protein fractions, based on their solubility, are found in zein: α-zein, β-zein, and γ-zein. The water sorption of zein is extremely low; however, it becomes plasticized in the presence of high water content. Glycerol, glyceryl monoesters, polyethylene glycol, etc., are the common plasticizers of zein protein. Plasticization alters the rheological behavior and introduces flexibility toward the brittle polymer film. Zein film exhibits superior barrier toward oxygen and moisture barriers, used in the food-packaging industry. The polymer, blended with steric acid and wood resin, is used to coat vitamin and mineral-enriched rice to prevent loss of nutrients during cold water washing. Medicines are coated with zein for controlled drug release and protection.

11.3.2.3 Wheat gluten

Wheat gluten mainly consists of four different types of wheat storage protein: albumins, globulins, gliadins, and glutenins. While albumins and globulins are water and salt soluble, gliadins are alcohol soluble and glutenins are soluble or dispersible in dilute acid or alkali solutions. Gluten is obtained as an industrial by-product of wheat starch production via wet milling. This biopolymer forms a homogeneous, transparent, mechanically strong film, which is suitable for diverse applications such as postal envelope windows, plastic films for agricultural use, paper coatings, fertilizer bags, and cosmetics. At low humidity, the polymer film shows very high gas barrier properties, especially for O_2, CO_2, and ethylene.

11.3.2.4 Soy protein

Soy protein is an abundant and cheap biopolymer obtained as a coproduct during the processing of soybean oil. It consists of a complex mixture of proteins, mostly globulins (90%) with a molecular weight ranging from 200 to 600 kDa. The excellent fiber-forming property, along with adhesion, cohesion, and solubility, makes this biopolymer an outstanding candidate for various food applications. It is also used as a film-forming agent and produces edible and environment-friendly biodegradable films. The films show high mechanical strength and slight water resistance with excellent transparency.

11.3.2.5 Casein and caseinate

About 80% of milk protein consists of casein. It is a phosphoprotein. Depending on the molecular weight and 1°, 2°, and 3° structure, it can be separated into various electrophoretic fractions, such as αs1-casein, αs2-casein, β-casein, and κ-casein. All varieties of casein form stable micelles utilizing extensive electrostatic and hydrogen bonding, and hydrophobic interactions and exist with colloidal calcium phosphate. Casein is a water-insoluble biopolymer, but in the presence of alkali, caseinate becomes water soluble. The biodegradable polymer finds applications in the area of paper coatings, glues, paints, textile fibers, leather finishing, and plastics. The films produced from casein and caseinate not only improve the appearance of food products and protect them from their surrounding environment, but also label food items inserted into them. The high nutrition value of casein-based edible films makes it very attractive.

11.3.2.6 Whey proteins

Whey protein is another protein found in milk with casein. Addition of a coagulant (usually renin) to milk separates the curds (casein) and whey. This biopolymer is the water-soluble part of milk. It consists of mainly five different proteins: α-lactalbumins, β-lactoglobulins, bovine serum albumin, immunoglobulins, and proteose peptones. This biodegradable polymer possesses excellent film-forming properties. The produced film is colorless and odorless and has excellent nutritional value, which is useful for human food and animal feed and edible food packaging. The use of transparent flexible film from whey protein offers several environmental advantages because of its biodegradability and the ability to control moisture, carbon dioxide, oxygen, lipid, flavor, and aroma transfer.

11.3.3 Biopolymers Synthesized from Bio-derived and Synthetic Monomers

11.3.3.1 Poly(lactic acid) or polylactide

The aliphatic polyester class of biodegradable polymers has been studied extensively because of their synthetic versatility and diverse characteristics. The polymers are synthesized from renewable natural resources and possess very low or no toxicity. Poly(lactic acid) or polylactide (PLA) has two different optically active configurations: the L(+) and D(−) stereoisomers. The presence of methyl groups in the polymer backbone chain makes it hydrophobic and is observed to be more resistant to hydrolysis. PLA has high mechanical strength (32 MPa) and 30% elongation at break with a T_g of ~63.8°C. Plasticization with different oligomeric acid and PEG can improve the chain mobility and alters other physical properties. Poly(L-lactide) (PLLA) is a semi-crystalline polymer. It exhibits high mechanical strength and low extension, which is suitable for load-bearing applications such as orthopedic fixation devices. Its application in food-packaging industry is approved by the FDA. Polylactides undergo hydrolytic degradation via breakdown of the ester backbone. The degradation product is lactic acid, a normal human metabolic by-product, which is further disintegrated into water and carbon dioxide via the citric acid cycle.

11.3.3.2 Poly(glycolic acid)

Poly(glycolic acid) (PGA) is the simplest linear aliphatic polyester synthesized via ring-opening polymerization techniques of glycolide, a cyclic lactone. Due to its high crystallinity (45–55%), the polymer is insoluble in most organic solvent and water. However, with decreasing molecular weight, solubility increases. Similar to other aliphatic polyesters, this polymer has excellent mechanical properties and the melting point is also very high (220–225°C). PGA fibers demonstrate high strength and modulus (7 GPa). The presence of ester linkages makes the polymer susceptible to hydrolytic attack.

The non-toxic nature of PGA has led to its application in biomedical fields, and implantable apparatuses for medical use have been already manufactured. These includes plates, rods, screws, pins, and anastomosis rings. Scaffolds fabricated from PGA in the form of non-woven meshes have been applied in tissue engineering. High–molecular weight PGA has been already commercialized for food-packaging applications and as barrier material. On the other hand, low–molecular weight PGA has been found suitable in oil and gas applications.

11.3.3.3 Poly(ε-caprolactone)

Poly(ε-caprolactone) (PCL) is an aliphatic polyester consisting of "ε-caprolactone" as a monomer unit. The semi-crystalline linear polymer is synthesized via a ring-opening polymerization technique in the presence of tin octoate as catalyst. The semi-rigid polymer, with a low tensile strength of 23 MPa and a high elongation to break, possesses very low glass transition temperature (T_g) (–60°C) and melting temperature (60–65°C). Because of its low T_g, PCL is often utilized as a compatibilizer or as a soft block in various polymer formulations. The high processability and solubility in a wide variety of solvents make it highly attractive for several applications. Another interesting property exhibited by this polymer is its high thermal stability. PCL undergoes thermal decomposition at 350°C. The labile ester linkage undergoes a very slow hydrolytic degradation. The non-toxic biocompatible polymer has been used as long-term drug/vaccine delivery vehicle and as scaffolds for tissue engineering because of its slow degradation rate (~2–3 years) and high permeability to many drugs.

11.3.3.4 Poly(butylene succinate) and its copolymer

Poly(butylene succinate) (PBS) and its copolymers belong to the poly(alkenedicarboxylate) category, which are synthesized from the reaction between glycols (such as ethylene glycol and 1,4-butanediol) and dicarboxylic acids (such as succinic and adipic acid) via polycondensation reaction mechanism. PBS and several other polymers such as poly(ethylene succinate) (PES) and copolymer, that is, poly(butylene succinate-co-adipate) (PBSA) have been already commercialized. The molecular weight of these polymers varies between 10 and 100 kDa. The nature of the monomer units influences their physical and chemical properties, and also their biodegradability.

The crystalline polymer has a melting point of 90–120°C, and T_g ranges from −45°C to −10°C. The mechanical property of this thermoplastic is similar to that of PE and PP, having tensile strength 330 kg/cm^2 and EAB 330%. The polymer exhibits better processability than PLA or PGA biopolymer and finds wide application in stretched blown bottles and as foams. The polymer can be processed via injection, extrusion, or blow molding and is suitable for fabrication of containers, bags, cutlery, packaging film, mulch film, and flushable hygiene products. The polymer exhibits lower biocompatibility, which may improve via surface modification through plasma treatment. The biodegradation rate is much slower, which can be enhanced via blending and copolymerization with other polymers.

11.3.3.5 Poly(*p*-dioxanone)

Poly(*p*-dioxanone) (PPDO) belongs to the family of aliphatic polyester and is synthesized by ring-opening polymerization of *p*-dioxanone. The properties of this semi-crystalline polymer depend on the chain length. PPDO exhibits low T_g (−10°C to 0°C), and a shear thinning rheology. With increase in molecular weight, tensile strength, modulus, and thermal stability of the polymer increase. The polymer is highly biocompatible and degradable by many microorganisms.

11.3.3.6 Poly(hydroxyalcanoate)

Poly(hydroxyalkanoates) (PHAs) are produced by many bacteria as intracellular carbon and energy-storage granules. The molecular weight of these intracellular biopolymers depends on several factors, including carbon source, bacterial growth and growth conditions, and may vary from 10 to 110 kDa. These polymers produce highly biodegradable and biocompatible thermoplastic materials and can replace conventional non-degradable polyethylene (PE) and polypropylene (PP). It has attracted great attention in food packaging.

11.3.4 Other Important Biodegradable Polymers

11.3.4.1 Bacterial cellulose

Bacterial cellulose is a specific product of primary metabolism with the formula $(C_6H_{10}O_5)_n$, produced by certain types of bacteria belonging to the genera *Acetobacter, Rhizobium, Agrobacterium*, and *Sarcina*. The chemical structure of bacterial cellulose is similar to that of plant cellulose, but its macromolecular structure and properties are quite different. The chemical purity of bacterial cellulose and ultrafine reticulated microstructure makes it appropriate for several applications, including paper and textile and in cosmetic and medicine.

11.3.4.2 Poly (vinyl alcohol) and Poly (vinyl acetate)

Among all vinyl polymers, the most readily biodegradable and largest synthetic water-soluble polymer produced in the world is poly(vinyl alcohol) (PVOH). The polymer is synthesized via partial or complete hydrolysis of poly(vinyl acetate) (PVAc). The molecular weight ranges from 26 to 30 kDa, with a 86.5–89% hydrolysis. The polymer is odorless, translucent, and water soluble and finds uses in food-packaging industries, protective coatings for food supplement tablets and dry foods. PVOH exhibits superior film-forming properties as well as emulsifier and adhesive. It is also highly resistant to various organic solvents, oil, and grease. The PVOH film shows high mechanical strength, along with oxygen and aroma barrier properties.

PVOH is completely degradable, and the reaction takes place in two steps: oxidation of hydroxyl group followed by hydrolysis. It is also easily disintegrated in waste water–activated sludges. The degradation via microorganism and by secondary alcohol peroxidases isolated from soil bacteria of the *Pseudomonas* strain has been studied thoroughly. The film-forming properties, along with biocompatibility and non-toxicity, makes PVOH suitable for disposable plastic substitutes and as a base material in agriculture and water treatment areas, for example, as a flocculant, metal-ion remover, and excipient for controlled release systems of drugs in biomedical field.

PVAc is a rubbery thermoplastic polymer, synthesized via radical polymerization reaction of vinyl acetate monomer. The biodegradation of PVAc is much slower compared to PVOH. However, a controlled hydrolyzed product would produce a biodegradable material with a wide range of properties and biodegradability. This has been widely used as glue material and paper coatings, paint ingredients, as binder in filter paper, sanitary napkins, and in textile applications.

11.3.4.3 Poly(carbonate)

Several varieties of polycarbonates prepared from different monomers are of great interest. Trimethylene carbonate is used as the monomer during the synthesis of poly(trimethylene carbonate) (PTMC) via ring-opening polymerization technique in the presence of diethylzinc as the reaction catalyst. The polymer alone exhibits very poor mechanical properties, thus copolymerized with several other monomers, such as glycolide and dioxanone, to obtain the desired characteristics. Another variety of polycarbonate is poly(propylene carbonate) (PPC), synthesized via copolymerization of propylene oxide and carbon dioxide. The polymer enhances compatibility and impact resistance. However, biodegradability is quite poor and can be improved through blending with other suitable polymers. Introduction of other polymers may decrease crystallinity, which enhances its susceptibility to enzymatic and microbial attacks.

11.3.4.4 Polyurethanes

Polyurethane (PU) is synthesized from the reaction between diisocyanate, a chain extender, and a polyol. Common isocyanates are toxic in nature, so aliphatic biocompatible diisocyanates have been chosen for the synthesis of PU. Diisocyanate forms the hard chain segment, whereas polyol provides the soft flexible segment. Depending on the segments, PU offers a wide variety of mechanical and chemical properties and is used in diversified fields such as protective coatings, thermoplastic elastomer, adhesives, fibers, and PU foams. PUs are resistant to biodegradation; however, incorporation of polyester-based polyol makes it readily biodegradable. Replacing polyols with vegetable oils, a renewable source, generates waterborne PU. Water-borne PU has received significant attention due to its environment-friendly application process, and its biodegradation is much faster than regular PU. The biodegradable polymer exhibits fair mechanical properties (tensile strength 9.3 MPa and 500% EAB).

11.3.4.5 Polyamide and poly(ester-amide)

Polyamides are characterized by amide (–CO–NH–) linkages, similar to that present in protein. Due to the presence of intermolecular H-bonding, they form high crystallinity, which hinders the biodegradation rate. Biodegradation by enzymes and microorganisms disintegrate the long-chain polymer into small oligomers. Incorporation of other monomers and functional groups (esters) could lead to faster biodegradation. Copolymer synthesized from 1.6-hexanediol, glycine, and diacids or 1,2-ethanediol, adipic acid, and amino acids, including glycine and phenylalanine, shows adequate enzymatic degradation. The polymers exhibit very good mechanical and thermal stability, similar to that of non-biodegradable polyethylene.

11.3.4.6 Polyanhydrides

Polyanhydrides are synthesized using anhydrides, diacids, or diacid esters with diacyl chlorides via several polymerization techniques, including melt condensation, ring opening, interfacial condensation, etc. Owing to two hydrolyzable sites in the main polymer backbone chain, polyanhydrides have become one of the most significant biodegradable materials. The presence of aromatic groups in the backbone resists the biodegradation rate compared to aliphatic polyanhydrides. Aliphatic homopolymers, such as poly(sebacic anhydride), exhibit high crystallinity, which hinders its practical applications. The fast biodegradation rate may be controlled by the use of hydrophobic groups in the diacid building block. Biomaterials produced from carboxyphenoxypropane have been thoroughly studied. The products formed after biodegradation are non-toxic and biocompatible. Copolymerization with other monomers improved the desired properties of polyanhydrides. Combination with imide enhances mechanical properties suitable for specific medical applications.

11.4 Nanofillers for Bionanocomposites

At the International Conference on Precision Engineering (ICPE) (Taniguchi 1974), the term "nanotechnology" was first coined by Norio Taniguchi and was defined as "production technology to get extra high accuracy and ultra-fine dimensions, that is, the preciseness and fineness on the order of 1 nm (nanometer), 10−9 m in length." Among several definitions suggested for nanotechnology, NASA recently proposed the most comprehensive description: "The creation of functional materials, devices and systems through control of matter on the nanometer length scale (1–100 nm), and exploitation of novel phenomena and properties (physical, chemical, biological) at that length scale." In the early 1990s, Nylon-6 nanocomposite was first reported by Toyota Research Laboratories in Japan and since then the journey into the nanosphere began. It has been observed that incorporation of very small amount of nanofiller resulted in distinct enhancement in thermal and mechanical properties of the base polymers. The interfacial contact between the nanofiller and the polymer offers superior performances. The conventional polymer nanocomposites (PNCs) possess environmental threat due to their inherent hazard.

Recently, a number of environment-friendly biopolymers have been developed, which reduce the dependence on fossil-based resources. The properties of these biodegradable polymers are somewhat inferior to those of conventional polymers; thus, bionanocomposites of such biopolymers have been developed to improve performances. The incorporation of nanofillers not only improves the physical and chemical properties, biodegradation of these bionanocomposites has also been observed to enhance, which make them a high-value material for the future. Bionanocomposites based on several nanofillers are found to be useful for a broad range of applications as these can be processed by similar techniques used for conventional polymer processing.

Nanofillers are extremely small in size, having at least one dimension 100 nm or less. It is nanoscale in one dimension, such as films, membranes, coatings; two dimensions, such as fibers or strands; or three dimensions, such as particles. Common types of nanostructures include quantum dots, nanocrystals, dendrimers, clusters, nanofibers, and nanotubes and can be classified as zero-dimensional, one-dimensional, two dimensional, and three-dimensional nanostructures. Among these nanofillers, cellulose-based nanofillers, carbon nanotubes (CNTs), and functional nanofillers are widely used to fabricate bionanocomposites.

11.4.1 Cellulose-Based Nanofillers

Cellulose is one of the most abundant biopolymers in nature. This biodegradable polymer can be synthesized by bacteria, such as *Acetobacter*, and also found naturally in a very high crystalline form in the cell walls of Valonia and Microdicyon, a variety of algae. The nanofillers synthesized from cellulose can be utilized as reinforcement fillers in combination with other conventional polymers or as matrix in fabrication of nanocomposites [12–14]. The high aspect ratio of the cellulose nanofillers not only provides excellent mechanical strength, but also promotes their thermal and barrier properties. The cellulose particles isolated from natural resources varied from one other depending on their size, surface-to-volume ratio, crystallinity, and crystal morphology. Cellulose nanofillers can be divided into several categories, including cellulose microcrystalline (MCC), microfibrillated cellulose (MFC), nanofibrillated cellulose (NFC), cellulose nanocrystals (CNC), bacterial cellulose (BC), and algae cellulose (AC).

Microcrystalline cellulose (MCC) is a highly crystalline structure of fine powder with particle sizes ranging between 10 and 50 μm in diameter, which forms through the formation of intermolecular hydrogen bonds between bundles of multi-sized cellulose microfibril aggregates. It has been used for pharmaceutical and food industry applications and also as reinforcing material. Microfibrillated cellulose (MFC) is 10–100 nm wide and 0.5–10 mm in length and possesses maximum aspect ratio. MFC has been widely used as a thickening agent in food and cosmetic industries. Nanofibrillated cellulose (NFC) is produced during the mechanical refining of cellulosic resources. NFCs are finer cellulose fibrils that contain both crystalline and amorphous regions and possess very high aspect ratio. The fibrils are 4–20 nm wide and 500–2000 nm in length. Cellulose nanocrystals (CNCs) (3–5 nm wide, 50–500 nm in length) are produced from wood fibers, microcrystalline cellulose, and microfibrillated cellulose by acid hydrolysis. In the crystalline region of cellulose fibrils, rod- or whisker-shaped CNC particles are found. The ribbon-shaped CNCs synthesized from tunicates exhibit the highest aspect ratio among other forms of cellulose.

11.4.2 Carbon Nanotubes

CNTs consist of a graphitic sheet of sp^2 hybridized carbon atoms rolled into a tubular array. Based on the number of graphene sheets that design them, carbon nanotubes are termed single-walled, double-walled, or multiwalled (SWNTs, DWNTs, or MWNTs, respectively). CNTs are most widely used as one-dimensional nanofillers. The diameter of CNTs varies from 1 nm to >30 nm, and the aspect ratios range from 102 to 106. CNTs are considered the most significant material in the nanoworld due to their exceptional mechanical, thermal, and electrical properties. Incorporation of a small amount of CNTs can significantly improve the physicochemical properties of the end product. The presence of strong C–C bond in CNTs makes it stiffer and stronger than any known substance. It has been observed that thin sheets of nanotubes are much lighter than steel but at least 250 times stronger. The distinctive nature of CNTs displays a remarkable response under large transverse deformations. CNTs have been found suitable for various applications as structural, electromagnetic, electroacoustic, chemical additives, medical, sensor device materials.

11.4.3 Nanoclays

Nanoclay has been investigated thoroughly as nanofillers. Natural clay (bentonite) generally forms by in situ alteration of volcanic ash. Nanoclay mainly contains montmorillonite and other constituents such as glass, illite, kaolinite, quartz, and zeolite. Montmorillonite clays primarily contain silica and partly alumina, having a structural formula of $Na_{1/3}(Al_{5/3}Mg^{1/3})Si_4O_{10}(OH)_2$. These nanofillers form sheet structure consisting of three layers containing two tetrahedral silicate layers and one octahedral alumina layer of thickness ~0.96 nm. The extremely fine-grained structure of montmorillonite does not produce any macroscopic crystals and swell in the presence of water or organic liquids. The moist clay, in its finest form, exhibits properties similar to colloid, with uniform particle size, tackiness, and plasticity. Nanoclay particles have been utilized long as flow modifiers in paints, inks, greases, and cosmetics and as carriers in drug-delivery systems. Recently, in the manufacturing of polymer–clay nanocomposites, it is being used largely. These inorganic–organic combinations display improved physical, thermal, and gas barrier properties. The usefulness of clay in pollution control and water treatment has also been investigated.

11.5 Processing Aspects of Bionanocomposites

Materials stemmed from natural resources are now being extensively studied as the demand for environmental sustainability has increased significantly. Synthesis of novel bionanocomposites has gained exclusive attention and is expected to open green areas for applications in food packaging, biomedical sphere, composites, electronics, automotive sector, construction, and other areas. It has been observed that introduction of a small amount of nanofillers into the polymer matrix radically enhances the properties of the base polymer. However, dispersion of the nanofillers in the polymer matrix is the main difficulty without degradation of the biopolymer or the filler phase. By the application of suitable processing technologies and through improvement in specific interactions between nanofillers and the polymer matrix, this problem can be potentially solved.

11.5.1 Conventional Manufacturing Techniques

The choice of a suitable fabrication method is the first and basic step for the manufacturing of nanobiocomposites. Some of the useful widely used conventional techniques are wet lay-up, pultrusion, resin transfer molding (RTM), vacuum-assisted resin transfer molding (VARTM), autoclave processing, resin film infusion (RFI), prepreg method, filament winding, automated fiber placement (AFP) technology, etc. [15].

In the wet lay-up method, the polymer resin is applied only in the mold. Although this method is quite simple, but the quality and performance of the finished product are much inferior and not uniform. In the pultrusion molding process, the reinforcing fibers are continuously soaked with liquid polymer resin and then carefully molded and extruded through a heated die. Although the process is not costly, the product contains voids and material accumulation can disrupt the fabrication process. RTM is commonly used to mold liquid composites with large surface areas, complex shapes, and smooth surface finishes. In RTM, the chemical reaction is much slower and supplied from the fiber mat or preform and mold wall. The slow reaction rate allows the resin a longer time to fill the mold. In RTM, the flow of the binder and fiber wet-out are major issues. VARTM is a modified form of RTM using vacuum. This technique offers high volume productivity at relatively low price. The application of vacuum ensures complete filling of the mold of complex shapes with superior surface smoothness. However, RTM and VARTM only deal with the polymer possessing low viscosity and high flow. The presence of nanofillers may change the rheological behavior and curing characteristics of the polymer matrix, which could hinder the flow pattern resulting in uneven distribution and defects.

Polymer nanocomposite processing using autoclave is a promising technique, mainly used to manufacture materials for new-generation aerospace application. This technology produces complex shapes with uniform distribution and minimum porosity. In RFI, dry fabrics are laid up interweaved with layers of thin film or sheet of solid resin supplied on a release paper. It was then heated to allow the resin to melt and flow into the fabrics and cured under pressure. In this technique, high fiber volumes can be accurately achieved with low void contents.

Filament winding is another fabrication process mainly utilized to fabricate circular and oval sectioned hollow components. These fiber tows are passed through a resin bath, and the resin-impregnated fibers are wrapped over a mandrel at the same or different winding angles to form the component part. This technique eliminates the viscosity-related flow problems and is widely used to manufacture complicated cylindrical parts for storage and transportation. AFP is one of the fastest evolving automation systems in composites manufacturing, where prepregged carbon fiber tows are mechanically and automatically placed on a tool to build a complex composite laminate. This process is industrialized as a coherent blending of filament winding and automated tape placement technique to reduce many of the restraints of nanocomposite fabrication techniques. AFP offers a repeatable and consistent manufacturing process, which is very unique in composites fabrication.

11.5.2 In Situ Intercalative Polymerization

In situ polymerization technique is often used to synthesize polymer–nanofiller composites, especially with the nanoclay-reinforced composite materials. The polymer usually forms in the gallery located between the silicate layers. The process involves penetration of liquid monomer into the silicate layer followed by heat- or radiation-initiated polymerization. This polymerization technique has been successfully applied for various polymer–clay composite fabrication systems, including manufacturing of nylon–montmorillonite nanocomposite and other thermoplastics. Modified montmorillonite (MMT) by bis(2-hydroxyethyl) methyl hydrogenated tallow alkyl ammonium cation has been successfully incorporated into diglycidyl ether of bisphenol A (DGEBA) matrix [16]. The tethering effect of in situ polymerization technique helps the chemically modified nanoclay's surface, such as with 12-aminododecanoic acid (ADA), to connect with nylon-6 polymer chains during polymerization. However, this technique is not applicable for all types of polymers and often the reaction remains incomplete.

11.5.3 Exfoliation–Adsorption

The exfoliation–adsorption technique is used to achieve exfoliation of the layered silicate into single layers employing a suitable solvent. The choice of solvent is very important as the polymer or pre-polymer needs to be soluble and the silicate layers are swellable. The layered silicate, such as montmorillonite, is well known to be swollen in an adequate solvent such as water, acetone, chloroform, or toluene, as the solvent easily overcomes the weak forces that stack the layers together. The dissolved polymer then adsorbs onto the delaminated sheets and finally the sheets sandwich the polymer and form intercalated multilayer structure upon drying the solvent. This technique is mainly applied to synthesize nanocomposites with water-soluble polymers, such as PVA and poly(ethylene oxide), and also fabricate epoxy–clay nanocomposites. The technique is not suitable for hydrophobic polymers such as polystyrene and poly(methyl methacrylate) due to the lack of compatibility, and the removal of the solvent is also an issue.

11.5.4 Melt Intercalation

Melt intercalation is an environment-friendly process that does not require any solvent, and the nanofillers are mixed into the polymer matrix in the molten state. Usually, thermoplastic polymers, with strong polar groups, such as polyamide-6 and ethylene vinyl acetate are mixed with nanofillers mechanically by conventional methods such as extrusion and injection molding. The process has been employed for the synthesis of recycled high-impact polystyrene (PS)/organoclay nanocomposites and for poly(ε-caprolactone) (PCL)/organo-modified montmorillonite (MMT) nanocomposites. Preparation of PCL–multiwalled carbon nanotubes (MWCNTs) mixture via melt blending followed by the synthesis of polycarbonate/ε-PCL–MWCNT nanocomposite has also been reported [17]. The functional groups present on the surface of the nanofillers are then intercalated with the polymer chain to form nanocomposites. The melt intercalation process is usually recommended for polymers that are not suitable for in situ polymerization or adsorption methods.

11.5.5 Foam Processing Using Supercritical CO_2

Foams are defined as materials containing gaseous voids surrounded by a denser matrix, which is usually a liquid or solid. Foams have been widely used in a variety of applications: insulation, cushion, absorbents, and weight-bearing structures. Recently, nanocomposite foam fabricated from polycarbonate (PC)-layered silicate and PC/SMA (polycarbonate/polystyrene-co-maleic anhydride) blend has been processed using supercritical CO_2 as a foaming agent. The prepared composite foam displays the most energetically stable polygon closed-cell structures having pentagonal and hexagonal faces. The cell size and larger cell density were obtained with the PC/SMA/MAE1 ($2C_{12}C_{18}$-fluorohectrite)-organoclay (1 wt%) composite signifying the dispersed clay particles as nucleating sites for cell formation and the lowering of d-spacing in the presence of nanoclay.

Polymeric foams are widely used in various applications, including aerospace, automotive, packaging, and cushioning.

11.5.6 Template Synthesis

The template synthesis process is quite different from other fabrication techniques. This method follows basic sol–gel procedures. An aqueous solution (or gel) of the water-soluble biopolymers and silicate-building blocks has been used to synthesize the clay within the polymer matrix. The polymer plays as the template that helps the nucleation and growth of silicate crystals. This technique allows the dispersion of the silicate layers into the polymer matrix in a single-step process. Template synthesis is extensively utilized to fabricate heterogeneous nanostructured composites.

The biopolymer nanocomposites show immense business potential as an alternative for current composites. However, development of suitable manufacturing processing technologies appropriate for commercialization is one of the biggest challenges. The primary concern is to disperse the nanofillers or its compatibility with the polymer matrix. Due to the strong tendency of fine nanofillers to agglomerate, it is observed that generation of a homogeneous dispersion of nanoparticles is extremely difficult using the traditional fabrication technique. Again, application of external forces may destroy the nanostructures. The poor rheological behavior of nanofiller-incorporated polymers or its viscous solution creates defects in the composite, which initiates crack, and failure of specimen can take place under low strains. The formation of particular alignment in the presence of nanofillers can be unfavorable to exploit unidirectional properties such as mechanical strength, modulus, and toughness. The presence of nanofillers also affects the degradation behavior of the biopolymers.

11.6 Environmental Applications of Bionanocomposites

Environmental applications of bionanocomposites have been known since ancient Rome. Clays and soil were combined with decaying urine to produce enhanced efficiency in laundry processes. As these are an abundant, low-cost, and non-toxic natural resource, these are very attractive for environmental protection in reducing hazardous species. For example, the possibility of combining adsorbent properties and ion-exchange capacity in bionanocomposites has been profited for the recovery of dyes and heavy metal ions.

Bionanocomposites are called super-absorbents because they show extremely high adsorption capacity when used with water. Recently, these super-absorbents have been successfully applied for the control of relative humidity in places requiring specific environmental conditions (museums, galleries), where these proved to have high moisture-absorption capacity and fast response to humidity changes [18, 19].

Bionanocomposites can also be of interest for developing other functional materials for uses in environmental remediation. This is the case of palygorskite bionanocomposites in which the presence of negatively charged sites in the modified cellulose chain allows their application in the removal of heavy metal ions such as Pb(II). In a similar way, the presence of protonated amino groups in chitosan-g-PAA/palygorskite bionanocomposites confers to these super-absorbents the possibility of being applied in removal of cationic pollutants in water as for instance Cu(II), Hg(II), or cationic dyes, such as methylene blue. In this last case, it is worthy to mention the high desorption of the dye at pH 2.0, allowing the regeneration and reuse of those clay composites, making them of potential interest for dye removal. Similarly, chitosan-g-PAA/palygorskite bionanocomposites prepared via in situ copolymerization in aqueous solution showed high efficacy for removing NH_4^+ ions in synthetic wastewater. These are promising results considering the ever-increasing global environmental problem in view of ammonium nitrogen coming from disposal of nutrients (N and P) of water plants or indirectly from agriculture and leaching from sludge deposited in landfill and field. These materials are partially degradable, showing slow release properties that can be applied in agriculture, contributing to alleviate environmental pollution [18–21].

One of the promising and interesting usages of bionanocomposites is that they promote the green chemistry of future materials. As a result, bionanocomposites have been used in several applications such as mirror housings in vehicles, door handles, door panels, trunk liners, instrument panels, parcel shelves, head rests, roofs, upholstery and engine covers, and intake manifolds and timing belt covers. Other applications currently being considered include impellers and blades for vacuum cleaners, power tool housings, mower hoods, and covers for portable electronic equipment such as mobile phones and pagers. Honeywell developed commercial clay–nylon-6 nanocomposite products for drink packaging applications. Starch-based resin is a biodegradable and compostable resin based on a blend of thermoplastic starch. The basic applications of starch-based resin are in making compostable bags and meat liners [20, 21].

11.7 Conclusion

This chapter discussed the present trend in the applications of bionanocomposites in the environmental direction. This is an exciting and rapidly developing research discipline. Right now, bionanocomposites are considered alternatives to synthetic, petroleum-based polymers for the modern society. Also bionanocomposites are renewable resources that can provide a basis for sustainable economic development and environment friendliness. It is believed that bionanocomposites will allow us to avoid problems caused by synthetic polymers. A wide variety of sources of biological origin are available for making bionanocomposites. They are highly versatile and have a broad range of physical properties suitable for diverse applications.

However, the main obstacle is the strong aggregation and pronounced tendency of agglomeration of nanoparticles owing to their very high surface and surface energy. Bionanocomposites are still a loosely defined family of nanomaterials. Apart from their environmental applications, they are successfully used as scaffolds and implants, drug-delivery systems, diagnostics, and biomedical devices. Moreover, biocompatibility makes them appropriate for cosmetics and biotechnology. In general, it is anticipated that bionanocomposites will substitute for the current materials very soon not only at the lab scale but also at the industrial scale, which are in contact with living beings.

References

1. Ozin G. and Arsenault A. *Nanochemistry: A Chemical Approach to Nanomaterials*, Royal Society of Chemistry, Cambridge, UK, 2005, Ch. 10.

2. Dujardin E. and Mann S. Bio-inspired materials chemistry. *Adv. Mater.*, 2002, **14**, 775.

3. Ruiz-Hitzky, E. and Darder, M. (Eds.) Special issue on trends in bio-hybrid nanostructured materials. *Curr. Nanosci.*, 2006, **2**, 153–294.

4. Drumright, R. E., Gruber, P. R., and Henton, D. E. Polylactide acid technology. *Adv. Mater.*, 2000, **12**, 1841–1846.

5. Hule, R. A. and Pochan, D. J. Polymer nanocomposites for biomedical applications. *MRS Bull.*, 2007, **32**, 354–358.

6. ASTM Standards, Vol. 08.01. 1998. D883-96: Standard Terminology Relating To Plastics. New York, NY.: ASTM

7. Tharanathan, R. N. Biodegradable films and composite coatings: Past, present and future. *Trends Food Sci. Technol.*, 2003, **14**, 71–78.

8. http://www.iopp.org/files/public/BerkeschShellieMSUBiodegradablePlastic.pdf, Shellie Berkesch, Michigan State University, March 2005.

9. Mohanty, A. K., Misra, M., and Hinrichsen, G. Biofibres, biodegradable polymers and biocomposites: An overview. *Macromol. Mater. Eng.*, 2000, **276–277**, 1–24.

10. Pedroso, A. G. and Rosa, D. S. Mechanical, thermal and morphological characterization of recycled LDPE/corn starch blends. *Carbohydr. Polym.*, 2005, **59**, 1–9.

11. Teng, W. L., Khor, E., Tan, T. K., Lim, L. Y., and Tan, S. C. Concurrent production of chitin from shrimp shells and fungi. *Carbohydr. Res.*, 2001, **332**, 305–316.

12. Iwatake, A., Nogi, M., and Yano, H. Cellulose nanofiber-reinforced polylactic acid. *Composites Sci. Technol.*, 2008, **68**, 2103–2106.

13. Lin, N., Chen, G., Huang, J., Dufresne, A., and Chang, P. R. Structure and mechanical properties of poly(lactic acid): A case of cellulose whisker-graft-polycaprolactone. *J. Appl. Polym. Sci.*, 2009, **113**, 3417–3425.

14. Babaee, M., Jonoobi, M., Hamzeh, Y., and Ashori, A. Biodegradability and mechanical properties of reinforced starch nanocomposites using cellulose nanofibers. *Carbohydr. Polym.*, 2015, **132**, 1–8.

15. Mazumder, S. K. (Ed.) *Composites Manufacturing, Materials, Product and Process Engineering*, CRC Taylor & Francis, 2002, ISBN 0-8493-0585-3.
16. Messermith, P. B. and Giannelis, E. P. Synthesis and characterization of layered silicate epoxy nanocomposites. *Chem. Mater.*, 1994, **6**, 1719–1725.
17. Maiti, S., Suin, S., Shrivastava, N. K., and Khatua, B. B. Low percolation threshold and high electrical conductivity in melt-blended polycarbonate/multiwall carbon nanotube nanocomposites in the presence of poly(ε-caprolactone). *Polym. Eng. Sci.*, 2014, **54**, 646–659.
18. Dasan, Y. K., Bhat, A. H., and Ahmad, F. Polymer blend of PLA/PHBV based bionanocomposites reinforced with nanocrystalline cellulose for potential application as packaging material. *Carbohydr. Polym.*, 2017, **157**, 1323–1332.
19. Zafar, R., Zia, K. M., Tabasum, S., Jabeen, F., Noreen, A., and Zuber, M. Polysaccharide based bionanocomposites, properties and applications: A review. *Int. J. Biol. Macromol.*, 2016, **92**, 1012–1024.
20. Reddy, M. M., Vivekanandhan, S., Misra, M., Bhatia, S. K., and Mohanty, A. K. Biobased plastics and bionanocomposites: Current status and future opportunities. *Prog. Polym. Sci.*, 2013, **38**(11), 1653–1689.
21. Ruiz-Hitzky, E., Darder, M., Fernandes, F. M., Wicklein, B., Alcântara, A. C. S., and Aranda, P. Fibrous clays based bionanocomposites. *Prog. Polym. Sci.*, 2013, **38**(11), 1392–1414.

Chapter 12

Bionanocomposites in Water and Wastewater Treatment

Gulshan Singh,[a] Deepali Sharma,[b] and Thor Axel Stenström[a]

[a]*SARChI Chair, Institute for Water and Wastewater Technology (IWWT), Durban University of Technology, PO Box 1334, Durban 4000, South Africa*
[b]*Department of Pharmaceutical Sciences, College of Health Sciences, University of KwaZulu-Natal, Durban 4001, South Africa*
gsingh.gulshan@gmail.com

The usage of water has increased more than three times the world's population increase, leading to worldwide deterioration in human health and limiting economic and agricultural development. The treatment of wastewater, to convert it into reusable form, is highly essential for future demands. Different methods have been used to treat wastewater, and a combination of advanced nanotechnology-oriented approach with the conventional methods offered interesting benefits. Moreover, the application of nanocomposite in wastewater treatment has proven to have better selectivity and stability and more efficient adsorption abilities than nanoparticles. In this chapter, important biopolymer-based bionanocomposites, for example, polymer-based bionanocomposites such as chitosan-based polymer

---

Biocomposites: Biomedical and Environmental Applications
Edited by Shakeel Ahmed, Saiqa Ikram, Suvardhan Kanchi, and Krishna Bisetty
Copyright © 2018 Pan Stanford Publishing Pte. Ltd.
ISBN 978-981-4774-38-3 (Hardcover), 978-1-315-11080-6 (eBook)
www.panstanford.com

bionanocomposites, clay nanocomposites, gum polysaccharide-based bionanocomposites, cellulosic nanocomposites, and their applications in wastewater treatment, have been described. The chapter also highlights the fact that multidirectional research is required to accelerate the application of bionanocomposites at a large scale for the efficient removal of different types of pollutants in wastewater.

12.1 Introduction

To meet the demands of potable and recreational water, especially for domestic and irrigation purposes, treatment of wastewater and converting it into a reusable form are essential for future demands. The increasing expenditure on wastewater disposal and stringent discharge policies have made wastewater treatment a very critical and important issue.

Various methods have been used for water treatment, but the use of composites and nanocomposites is gaining a lot of attention. A composite is a combination of two or more materials with distinct physical and chemical properties; the materials, when merged, result in a completely new material with different properties from those of the individual components [1].

These composites consist of two phases: (i) the continuous phase (matrix) and (ii) the dispersed phase (reinforced materials). There are various benefits of this conjugation, for example, high strength, stiffness, corrosion resistance, and thermal insulation. The composites in which one or more phase is derived from a biological material are termed "biocomposites." The first, that is, "continuous phase" normally consists of recycled wood fibers, waste paper, and plant fibers such as hemp, flex, and cotton. The second dispersed phase consists of natural and synthetic polymers, thermoplastics, and fossil-derived polymers [1]. The application of nanotechnology in different areas such as biological sciences, drug-delivery systems, and wastewater treatment has revolutionized the development of different nanomaterials, especially nanocomposites. Different nanoparticles, for example, ferric oxides, titanium oxides, magnesium oxides, aluminum oxides, and cerium oxides, have been used in the removal of contaminants from wastewater [2, 3].

It has been proved that nanocomposites have better selectivity and stability and more efficient adsorption abilities than nanoparticles. Nanocomposites are a combination of two phases in which one phase, at least, shows nanometer (1–100 nm) dimensions. Nanoparticles, in nanocomposites, are combined with different functionalized materials such as reduced graphene oxide, polymer matrices, carbon nanotubes (CNTs), and multiwalled CNTs (MWCNTs). Nanocomposite materials have emerged as suitable alternatives to overcome limitations of conventional composites due to their design uniqueness and property combinations [4]. These nanocomposites are unique in terms of high surface-area-to-volume ratio, nanosize range, minimized internal diffusion resistance, and a specific affinity for wastewater contaminants. Different types of nanocomposites have now been employed for the treatment of wastewater and drinking water [2, 5]. For example, magnetic nanocomposites exhibiting the properties of magnetic separation techniques as well as nanosized materials form a very efficient class of nanocomposite capable of removing different pollutants from wastewater [6].

The choice of nanocomposites depends on the type and concentration of the contaminant (microbial or chemical contaminants) present in wastewater. The ratio of nanocomposite efficiency to the cost involved also plays a major role in choosing and designing nanocomposites. When selecting nanocomposite as adsorbent (the preferred technique over precipitation) for pollutants in wastewater, the following considerations should be addressed: (i) the nanocomposite (adsorbent) should be highly selective for the pollutant, as we are dealing with large volumes and complex type of water; (ii) it should be easily available and recoverable from filters, and should be non-toxic and inexpensive.

Based on the matrix materials, nanocomposites can be classified into three groups: (i) metal matrix nanocomposites (MMNC), (ii) polymer matrix nanocomposites (PMNC), and (iii) ceramic matrix nanocomposites (CMNC) [7]. Although nanocomposites provide a lot of advantages in comparison to conventional composites, they face a few challenges in their fabrication. These limitations have given rise to the application of bionanocomposites, a hybrid of natural entity (especially biopolymers) and nanomaterials in treatment of wastewater (Fig. 12.1).

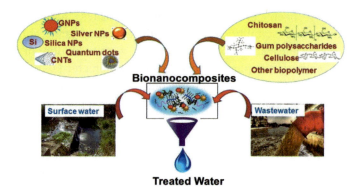

Figure 12.1 Schematic representation of application of bionanocomposites in wastewater treatment.

There are different types of bionanocomposites based on (i) type of matrix used, (ii) origin, (iii) shape, and (iv) size of reinforcements. For example, bionanocomposites can be classified into elongated particle, particulate, and layered structures based on the shape of the particle reinforcements [7]. The important factor that describes the ability of a nanofiller in augmenting composite attributes is the aspect ratio (ratio of particle length to thickness). Figure 12.2 gives the schematic classification on the basis of the shape of the particle reinforcement.

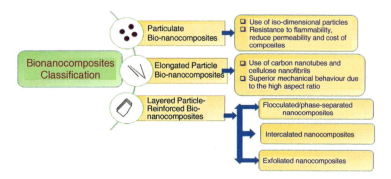

Figure 12.2 Classification of bionanocomposites based on the shape of particle reinforcements.

Bionanocomposites are further divided on the basis of the biopolymer used. In this chapter, we will discuss the important biopolymer-based bionanocomposites, for example, polymer-based bionanocomposites such as chitosan-based polymer bionanocomposites, clay nanocomposites, gum polysaccharide-based bionanocomposites, cellulosic nanocomposites, and their applications in wastewater treatment.

12.2 Polymer Bionanocomposites

With increasing awareness of using green products, biological sources are being exploited for the synthesis of traditional polymers. Advances in biotechnologies have led to the commercialization of many polymers that are otherwise obtained from petroleum feedstocks. Some of the new bio-based polymers that have been commercialized are bio-poly(butylene succinate) (PBS), bio-poly(trimethylene terephthalate) (PPT), bio-polyethylene (PE), bio-polypropylene (PP), and bio-polyethylene terephthalate (PET). Agro-based polymer includes starch, cellulose, chitosan, and proteins [8].

Bionanocomposites are formed by electrostatic interactions between the exfoliated nanoparticles and chitosan macromolecules. Chitosan is the second most abundant biopolymer on earth after cellulose. Shchipunov et al. [9] synthesized a bionanocomposite by combining clay nanoparticles with chitosan in aqueous solution. The clay nanoparticles were homogeneously dispersed in the polymer matrix due to progressive crosslinking, and the nanocomposite was biocompatible [9].

Polymer bionanocomposites have attracted much attention in various fields, including biosensing [10]. The main focus is due to the following properties: (i) Polymer matrix possessing functionalities can entrap nanoparticles and biomolecules; (ii) biocompatible nanoparticles can adsorb in or on the polymeric nanocomposites providing various sites on the nanocomposites for the binding of biomolecules, thereby retaining their bioactivity; (iii) incorporation of nanoparticles can give different functionalities to polymeric nanocomposites for the development of bio-devices, involving catalysis, electronics, optics, and magnetics; (iv) polymeric nanocomposites are cost effective, stable, and feasible to prepare. Polymeric bionanocomposites consisting of polydopamine (PDA), glucose oxidase (GOx), Pt and Au nanoparticles (NPs), have been designed and reported to entrap enzyme at high load/activity for highly sensitive glucose biosensing. Au nanoparticles are highly dispersed on PDA-PtNPs-GOx for efficient adsorption of antibody.

Polymeric bionanocomposites exhibited high load and activity of the enzyme label immobilized on the surface of nanomaterial, as well as high load of antibody on the surface for significant immunorecognition efficiency [11].

Poly(ether ether ketone) (PEEK) is an organic thermoplastic polymer used extensively as a biomaterial for medical applications owing to its high chemical and hydrolysis resistance, stability against UV radiation, biocompatibility, bioactivity, and superior mechanical properties [12].

The performance of bionanocomposite is dependent on the properties of the filler, such as shape, size, surface characteristics, and interfacial interaction with the host matrix. A homogenous dispersion of the filler particles (nanoparticles) is the key to the enhanced properties of bionanocomposites. ZnO nanoparticles have received much attention and have been an extensive area of research because of their low cost, easy availability, possibility for surface modifications with different functional groups, and biocompatibility. Novel poly(ether ether ketone) (PEEK)-based nanocomposites with different concentration of silane-modified ZnO nanoparticles have been prepared by cryogenic ball-milling, followed by compression molding. The nanoparticles were modified by silane to improve the dispersion and interfacial adhesion within the matrix. The bionanocomposites possessed excellent antibacterial property and thermal stability [13].

Polymer bionanocomposites have an ability to remove pollutants from wastewater. Hexavalent chromium (Cr^{6+}) is water soluble, mobile, and toxic to all living organisms. They can easily penetrate living cells and produce reactive oxygen species (ROS) and cause oxidant injury to cells. In humans, Cr^{6+} causes dermatitis and aggressive reaction in lungs and nasal septums. Therefore, many remedies and techniques are employed for its effective removal from wastewater. But these have drawbacks such as incomplete reduction of chromium. Recent studies have been carried out where magnetic nanoparticles, Fe_3O_4, are coated with microporous silica ($mSiO_2$), which is biocompatible and has highly reactive surface. To improve the adsorption process, the surface of silica is modified with amine groups and 4,4-azo-bis(4-cyanopentanoicchloride)

(ABPCA), an active radical initiator. Encapsulation of Fe_3O_4@ $mSiO_2$ was carried out using the polymer 4-vinyl pyridine (VP) and N-(methacryloyloxy)-succinimide (SMA) via polymerization. The fabricated bionanocomposite was attached to the surface of bacteria through the coupling reaction between the polymer and the amine group of the bacterial cells (Fig. 12.3). This system was effective in the rapid and complete reduction of hexavalent chromium and magnetic separation of bacteria [14].

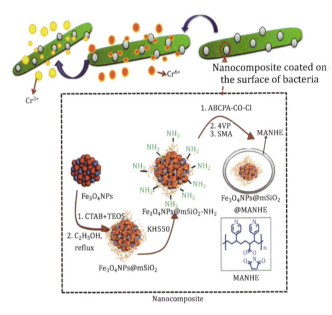

Figure 12.3 Illustration of the procedure for the reduction of Cr(VI) to Cr(III) in the presence of nanocomposite adsorbed on the surface of bacteria.

In another study, Fe_3O_4 nanoparticles modified with SiO_2 are coated with highly hydrophobic and crosslinked polymer, poly(lauryl methacrylate) (PLMA), for application in wastewater purification. It was observed that the adsorption of pollutants on the composite surface was driven by the hydrophobic interaction as well as the size of the pollutants [15].

Depending on the biopolymers, bionanocomposites are of two main types (Fig. 12.4): (i) polysaccharide-based bionanocomposites and (ii) protein-based bionanocomposites.

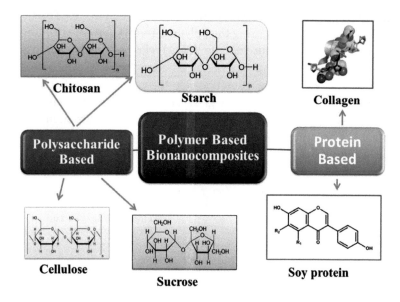

Figure 12.4 Types of polymer-based bionanocomposites.

12.2.1 Polysaccharide-Based Bionanocomposites

Among the family of renewable source–derived polymers, starch is an inexpensive and abundant natural polymeric carbohydrate material. This polysaccharide is produced by most green plants as a storehouse of energy. Thermoplastic starch (TPS)-clay bionanocomposites have been synthesized by an innovative methodology using a combination of methodologies commonly used in the composites and nanocomposites preparations. The bionanocomposites show that the addition of the cloisite-Na^+ clay reduces the surface hydrophilicity of the nanocomposites, thus increasing their use in industrial applications [16]. In one of the studies, modified potato starch is used as a matrix with water and sorbitol as plasticizers and cellulose nanowhiskers or layered silicates (LS) (synthetic hectorite) as reinforcements. The bionanocomposites exhibited improvement in tensile strength compared to pure matrix [17].

Poly(lactic acid) (PLA) is a biodegradable polymer that has become the most industrialized bio-sourced synthetic polyester. It is a linear, aliphatic, thermoplastic polyester produced either from

L-lactic acid or D-lactic acid monomers for many applications. It is commercially available and approved by the US Food and Drug Administration (FDA). Despite many applications, its tensile strength and ductility are compromised with the conventional polymers such as PET. Till date, many strategies have been developed to improve properties such as (i) polymer blending with organic or inorganic fillers and (ii) addition of plasticizers. Addition of nanosized biofillers to the PLA matrix to produce bionanocomposites has come up as an effective alternative way.

The matrix properties can be manipulated with the addition of nanosized fillers. Sucrose palmitate (SP), an ecofriendly filler, has been incorporated into the PLA matrix to fabricate bionanocomposites. Hydrogen bonding and intermolecular interaction were reported to exist between matrix and reinforcing agent [18].

12.2.1.1 Chitosan-based polymer bionanocomposites

Chitosan is one of the most widely exploited renewable natural polymer due to its unique biological chemical and structural properties. Chitosan is obtained by the commercial deacetylation of chitin, which is a component obtained from the shells of crab, shrimp, and krill. Chitosan-based bionanocomposites have gained a lot of attention due to their intrinsic properties such as biodegradability, non-toxicity, and enhanced functional and structural characteristics [19].

Different nanofiller reinforcements have been incorporated to chitosan to get promising bionanocomposites. The biocompatibility, biodegradability, antimicrobial property, non-toxicity, ease of chemical modification, and excellent film-forming ability of chitosan-based bionanocomposites have showed immense potential to overcome the drawbacks of conventional biopolymers [20]. Due to its different unique structural and physicochemical properties, chitosan bionanocomposites have found applications in different sectors of biotechnology, food and water industry, textiles, medicines, and agriculture. These materials have also been used in biomedical fields and different short-term applications, such as packaging, agriculture, and hygiene devices.

Chitosan has also demonstrated its suitability for the development of enzyme biosensors for the detection of proteins, metallic elements, and lipids. Chitosan-derived nanocomposites with nanorange reinforcements offer a stable and robust material than their conventional counterparts. The percentage of chitosan is kept high in comparison to the reinforcing material to highlight the chitosan properties (biocompatibility and bioactivity) in the final composite materials.

Chitosan–biopolymer clay bionanocomposite: Clays and other modified forms have been used as absorbent of metal ions and organic micropollutants from water medium due to their low cost involved and availability than other available adsorbents [21]. The disadvantage that restricts the use of neat clay minerals from their wide application in the removal of micro-contaminants in water, is their efficiency. The reduced efficiency is contributed by their low surface area and poor affinity for organic materials.

Montmorillonite (MMT), a hydrosilicate clay mineral, is extensively applied due to its permanent negative charge and cation exchange capacity [22] but faces poor adsorption of anionic organic compounds. Chitosan, along with its derivatives, has been used extensively as an adsorbent for the removal of dyes, proteins, and heavy metals from various aqueous media [23]. However, its application at low pH was restricted as it dissolves in acidic media. This further aggravates the need to couple this biopolymer with a supporting material for enhancing its functionality at low pH [24]. Chitosan clay bionanocomposites developed by blending chitosan and clay particles present a new class of bionanocomposites that can overcome the disadvantages associated with the use of clay without any modification in the removal of contaminants from wastewater. The cationic biopolymer, chitosan intercalates with MMT clay through cationic exchange and hydrogen bonding method, which results in nanocomposites with improved structural and functional properties. The developed bionanocomposite showed unique properties in terms of cost and efficiency in treating wastewater. There are investigations reported on the removal of micro-pollutants from water using chitosan nanoparticles with clays such as bentonite, kaolinite, and MMT [25, 26].

Nanoparticles-reinforced chitosan bionanocomposite: Chitin and chitosan derivatives have been extensively investigated as adsorbents for the removal of metal ions from water and wastewater. Chitosan nanocomposites have been prepared by reinforcing different nanomaterials such as TiO_2 (titanium dioxide), ZnO (zinc oxide), Fe_3O_4 (iron oxide), and MgO (magnesium oxide). The synergistic attributes of chitosan and nanoparticles enhance the overall value of bionanocomposites in terms of antimicrobial, magnetic property, and UV blocking. Due to its good photocatalytic property and stability in acidic and alkaline solvents, TiO_2 has been extensively used for the preparation of bionanocomposites. MgO nanoparticles also exhibit various properties such as electrical and thermal insulation, biocompatibility, non-toxicity, large surface-to-volume ratio, photocatalytic and antimicrobial activity [27]. Due to these special features, MgO nanoparticles have found their applications in diverse fields such as toxic waste remediation, refractory material and insulator, as a catalyst, and in ceramic materials [27].

In a recent study, a chitosan–magnetite nanocomposite strip was prepared to remove chromium ions from an aqueous solution [28]. The study revealed that the heavy metal removal efficiency of the chitosan–magnetite nanocomposite strip was found to be higher (92.33%) than the chitosan strip (29.39%) alone. For the removal of permethrin pesticide from water, chitosan–ZnO nanoparticle (CS–ZnONPs) composite was prepared and characterized by X-ray powder diffraction (XRD), scanning electron microscopy (SEM), spectroscopy, and infrared spectroscopy [29]. It was found that the 0.5 g of the developed bionanocomposite could remove 99% of the pesticide from the permethrin solution, proving that chitosan–magnetite nanocomposite could act as a potential adsorbent in water treatment applications.

Application of chitosan bionanocomposites in the removal of different types of contaminants from wastewater: The antimicrobial property of ZnO nanoparticles–reinforced chitosan bionanocomposites was explored by Rahman et al. [30]. The concentration of NaOH varied, keeping quantities of chitosan and zinc acetate dehydrate constant, resulting in the formation of three different composites. The characterization of composite was done by UV–visible spectra, XRD, and Fourier transform infrared spectroscopy (FTIR), and immobilization of ZnO nanoparticles on chitosan matrix was analyzed by SEM. It was observed that the final bionanocomposite exhibits a higher antimicrobial activity against gram-negative and gram-positive bacteria (*Escherichia coli* and *Staphylococcus aureus*) than chitosan itself. The study reported that the developed bionanocomposite can be used as a photocatalytic and natural antimicrobial agent.

Three different chitosan/cobalt–silica (Co-MCM) nanocomposites were synthesized varying the concentrations of Co-MCM to form chitosan/Co-MCM-5, chitosan/Co-MCM-15, and chitosan/Co-MCM-25 [31]. Different nanocomposites were characterized by FESEM, EDS, X-ray crystallography, IR spectrophotometer and were tested for absorption of dyes. The bioactivity and adsorption potential of chitosan/Co-MCM-15 was found to be higher than other bionanocomposites. Furthermore, a strong antimicrobial potential of chitosan/Co-MCM-15 against various gram-positive, gram-negative, and drug-resistant bacteria was also found. It was suggested that the improved adsorption and biological performance of chitosan/Co-MCM-15 chitosan/Co-MCM-15 might be due to the ideal dispersion of Co-MCM within the polymer chitosan [31].

For the efficient removal of toxic chromium (Cr), a glutaraldehyde crosslinked silica gel/chitosan-*g*-poly(butyl acrylate) nanocomposite, as a sorbent, was developed [32]. The characterization of the formed nanosorbent was carried out by different techniques such as FTIR, XRD, DLS, SEM, BET, and theoretical modeling was adopted to define isotherm constants. The study concluded that the developed nanocomposite could serve as an excellent biosorbent and could be considered for its practical implementation in the efficient removal of chromium ions from water and wastewater in the future. Chitosan bionanocomposites reinforced with gold and silver nanoparticles have been applied for the removal of Cu(II) ions from aqueous media [25].

Three hybrid nanocomposites—chitosan–clay, chitosan AgNP–clay, and chitosan AuNP–clay—were prepared and characterized by XRD, FTIR, and SEM techniques. The absorption of Cu(II) ions was analyzed, and it was found that chitosan AgNPs–clay and chitosan AuNP–clay hybrid composites have higher adsorbance of Cu(II) ions from aqueous solution than the individual chitosan (Ch)/clay composite, proving the potential role of metal nanoparticles in the adsorption of Cu(II) ions from aqueous medium. The chitosan AgNPs–clay composites showed the highest adsorption of Cu(II) ions among the tested reinforced bionanocomposites.

In a recent study, for the removal of methylene blue (a cationic dye) from aqueous solution, a magnetic bionanocomposite constituted by magnetic nanoparticles and clay reinforced in chitosan beads was prepared [33]. It was shown that the electrostatic interaction between the positively charged dye and the permanent negative charges of the tested clay drives the adsorption of the dye within a wide pH range. Some representative examples of chitosan bionanocomposites and their application in wastewater are summarized in Table 12.1.

12.2.1.2 Gum polysaccharide–based bionanocomposites

Polysaccharides are natural products produced as structural biopolymers or as energy storage by plants, animals, and microbes. Polysaccharide-based biopolymers consist of a branched structure in which a linear chain of a monosaccharide unit is attached to the side chains of other different monosaccharide units at certain positions.

Polysaccharides, in general, can swell in water to double their original size and can be used further for the development of nanocomposites. Graft copolymerization is one of the major techniques used to modify different polysaccharides chemically and forms more stable hydrocolloids.

In response to different types of stress, such as physical injury or fungal attack, plants produce exudate gum polysaccharides. Among these gums, ghatti, gum Arabic, gum karaya, and gum tragacanth have been used in various pharmaceutical and food applications. These gum polysaccharides that originate from plants generally have a high content of glucuronic or galacturonic acid residues (up to 40%).

Gum ghatti is an amorphous translucent exudate and has gained a lot of attention in recent years. The polysaccharide is an exudate of *Anogeissus latifolia* (family *Combretaceae*). It contains the monosaccharides L-arabinose, D-galactose, D-mannose, D-xylose, and D-glucuronic acid in a ratio of 10:6:2:1:2, with traces of 6-deoxyhexose. The functional properties of gum ghatti includes the following: (i) it does not readily dissolve in water but instead form dispersions (show non-Newtonian flow behavior); (ii) it acts as a superb emulsifier and has been used extensively to replace gum Arabic in more complex systems. The graft copolymer gum ghatti

Table 12.1 Examples of chitosan bionanocomposites and their application in wastewater treatment

Bionanocomposites	Characterization*	Contaminants	Activity	Reference
Chitosan, acrylic acid, and amine-functionalized nanosilica	FTIR, SEM, TGA	Co^{2+}, Cu^{2+}, Pb^{2+}, and Zn^2	Adsorption	[34]
Chitosan–ZnO nanoparticles (CS–ZnONPs)	SEM, XRD, FTIR	Permethrin pesticide	Adsorption	[29]
Glutaraldehyde crosslinked silica gel/chitosan-g-poly(butyl acrylate) (Cs-g-PBA/SG) nanocomposite	FTIR, XRD, DLS, SEM, BET isotherm	Toxic chromium ion	Adsorption	[32]
Chitosan–silica hybrid nanocomposite	DTA, CHN, SEM, FTIR	V(V), Mo(VI), and Cr(VI) oxo anions	Adsorption	[35]
Electrospun $H_4SiW_{12}O_{40}$ (SiW_{12})/chitosan (CS)/polycaprolactam (PA6) sandwich nanofibrous membrane (SNM)	XPS analysis	Cr(VI) and methyl orange (MO)	Adsorption and photocatalysis	[36]
Chitosan–silica nanoparticles–glutaraldehyde composite	SEM, FTIR-ATR, CAS	Oil	Separation of oil/water mixtures	[37]

Bionanocomposites	Characterization*	Contaminants	Activity	Reference
Hydroxyapatite/chitosan nanocomposite (nHApCs)	TEM, EDAX, XRD, FTIR, Zeta potential	Lead ions from aqueous lead-containing solutions	Removal by adsorption	[38]
Chitosan–ZnO bionanocomposite	UV-visible spectra, XRD, FTIR, SEM	*Escherichia coli* and *Staphylococcus aureus*	Antimicrobial activity	[30]
Chitosan/cobalt-silica (Co-MCM) nanocomposites	FESEM, EDS, X-ray crystallography, and IR spectrophotometer	Adsorption of dyes	Absorption	[31]
Zirconium-immobilized crosslinked chitosan (Zr-CCS) zinc oxide	FTIR, XRD, and SEM	Fluoride	Adsorption	[39]
ZnO and chitosan/ZnO composite (CZC)	DRS, FTIR, SEM, EDAX, XRD	Rhodamine B dye	Degradation	[40]

*FTIR: Fourier transform infrared spectroscopy; XRD: X-ray powder diffraction (XRD); DLS: dynamic light scattering; SEM: scanning electron microscopy; BET: Brunauer–Emmett–Teller; DTA: differential thermal analyses; CHN: carbon, hydrogen, and nitrogen (CHN) elemental analysis; CA: contact angles; TGA: thermal gravimetric analysis; DRS: diffuse reflectance spectra; EDAX: energy dispersive X-ray analysis have found its application as flocculants for wastewater treatment [41] and as a superb absorbent for crude oil recovery in the petroleum industry [42].

Gum Arabic is the exudate of Acacia tree bark and has a complex structure. The main chain of this polysaccharides consists of (1→3) and (1→6)-linked β-D-galactopyranosyl units along with (1→6)-linked β-D-glucopyranosyl uronic acid units. Gum Arabic is highly soluble in water and with low viscosity as compared to other exudate gums. The complex branched structure and low molecular weight contribute to different attributes of this polysaccharide, such as being surface active and with a capability to stabilize oil-in-water emulsion.

Gum Arabic has been used as stabilizer, emulsifier, and flavor encapsulation agent in the beverage and confectionary industries. Furthermore, the covalent association with a protein moiety adds unique features to the application of gum Arabic polysaccharides in various fields such as textiles and paper manufacturing. Gum Arabic has also been used as a "green stabilizer" for different nanocomposites, for example, poly(aniline) nanocomposites [43]. The effect of gum Arabic treatment on the dispersion of MWCNTs–epoxy nanocomposites in aqueous solution and the tensile characteristics were shown to be enhanced as compared to unmodified or acid-treated solutions [44].

Guar gum is a galactomannan polysaccharide where each unit is composed of two 1→4-linked β-D-mannopyranosyl subunits, with one unit of α-D-galactopyranosyl residue linked by 1→6-linkage as a side chain. Graft copolymerization of guar gum with application in different sectors of industries (e.g., printing, enzyme immobilization, preparation of hydrogels) has been reported. Guar gum has been modified with magnetic iron oxide nanoparticles, carbon nanotubes polyacrylamide or silica for the efficient removal of neutral, red, and methylene blue dyes as well as Cr(VI) and Cd(II) from aqueous medium [45–47]. Guar gum has been used to modify MMT to form polymer–clay bionanocomposites for potential pharmaceutical applications. The copolymer, developed by grafting partially carboxymethylated guar gum with 2-acrylamidoglycolic acid, was used for the adsorption of Ni^{2+}, Pb^{2+}, and Zn^{2+} ions [48].

Gum karaya is an anionic polysaccharide exudate from trees such as *Sterculia urens* (family *Sterculiaceae*). This polysaccharide is highly branched and consists of D-galacturonic acid, D-galactose, L-rhamnose, and D-glucuronic acid. Gum karaya is poorly soluble in water but can swell considerably and provide dispersions.

Gum karaya has found applications as a stabilizer in dairy products and used in salad dressings, in whipped creams, cheese spreads, and frozen desserts and also serves as a water-binding agent in processed meats and pasta. Different types of gum polysaccharides and their origin are mentioned in Table 12.2.

Table 12.2 Different gum polysaccharides and their origin

Gum polysaccharides	Origin	Solubility in water
Gum Arabic (plant)	*Acacia Senegal/Acacia seyal* (dry exudate)	Highly soluble
Gum karaya (plant)	*Sterculia urens* of *Sterculiaceae* family.	Solubility is very low, but it swells many times of its original weight to give dispersion
Gum tragacanth (plant)	*Astragalus gummifer* or other Asiatic species of *Astragalus* genus	Tragacanthin: water soluble; tragacanthic acid: water insoluble
Gum xanthan (microorganism)	*Xanthomonas campestris* (fermentation process)	Highly soluble
Gum gellan (microorganism)	*Aeromonas elodea*	Soluble
Guar gum (plant)	Seed of the plant *Cyamopsis tetragonoloba*	Soluble
Locust bean gum (plant)	Seeds of the carob tree of the *Ceretonia siliqua* family	A small proportion of locust bean gum is soluble in cold water; therefore, it forms a highly viscous solution with water.
Gum ghatti	An exudate of the *Anogeissus latifolia* tree belonging to the family *Combretaceae*	Variation in solubility and viscosity

Applications of gum polysaccharides-based bionanocomposites in the removal of contaminants from wastewater: Gum polysaccharides have been used extensively in developing nanocomposites for the removal of contaminants from wastewater. Polyacrylamide chains were grafted on the backbone of guar gum to develop a novel bionanocomposite by microwave irradiation, followed by in situ nanotized-silica integration on the surface of the guar gum backbone [49].

Guar gum promotes silica polymerization and probably acts as a template for nanoscale silica formation [49]. The application of the composite material in flocculation was investigated both in laboratory as well as in pilot scale. The flocculation kinetics and mechanism were explained on the basis of the pH of the suspension and flocculant dosage. It was suggested that because of strong matrix–nanofiller interactions as well as enhanced molecular weight and hydrodynamic radius, the modified biopolymer-based nanocomposite provides excellent potential as a flocculant for the treatment of various synthetic and industrial effluents through a green disposal technique [49].

Gum karaya-grafted poly(acrylamide-co-acrylic acid) with incorporated iron oxide magnetic nanoparticles (Fe_3O_4 MNPs) hydrogel nanocomposite was developed by graft copolymerization for the efficient removal of Cr^{2+}, Pb^{2+}, Ni^{2+} [50] and characterized by XRD, FTIR, TEM, and SEM. The nanocomposite showed 100% removal of contaminants within 5 min. Hence, the synthesized hydrogel nanocomposite proved to be a good flocculant and adsorbent for the efficient removal of heavy metal ions and suspended particles and had the potential to improve mine effluents water quality [50].

In another study, removal of malachite green from an aqueous solution was observed utilizing gum xanthan/Fe_3O_4 magnetic nanoparticles (MNPs) filled hydrogel nanocomposites [51]. Five isotherm models—Langmuir, Flory–Huggins, Temkin, Freundlich, and Dubinin–Kaganer–Radushkevich—were used to analyze the adsorption isotherm, and the Langmuir isotherm gave the best fit with a maximum adsorption efficiency of 497.15 mg/g at neutral pH. The developed hydrogel nanocomposite could readily be used for the adsorption of malachite green from aqueous solution [52].

Gum ghatti was used to crosslink poly(acrylic acid-co-acrylamide) reinforced with iron oxide magnetic nanoparticles to develop a nanocomposite for the removal of Rhodamine B [42]. The characterization of developed nanocomposite was performed by multiple techniques: BET, FTIR, XRD, SEM-EDX, TGA, and TEM. Different isotherm models (Langmuir, Freundlich, and Dubinin–Kaganer–Radushkevich) were used to study the adsorption isothermal data. It was found that the developed nanocomposite was able to efficiently adsorb Rhodamine B [42].

Guar gum–ZnO nanoparticle-based bionanocomposite was developed for the efficient removal of Cr(VI) from aqueous solution [45]. Four isotherm models (Langmuir, Freundlich, Dubinin–Kaganer–Radushkevich, and Temin) were used to study isotherm pattern. The guar gum–ZnO bionanocomposite showed an enhanced adsorption capacity for Cr(VI) and can serve as an ecofriendly and economical option for the removal of Cr(VI) from contaminated water.

12.2.1.3 Cellulose nanocomposites

Cellulose, the most abundant, renewable, and biodegradable polymer in nature, is a linear chain of ringed glucose molecules and has a flat ribbon-like structure with $\beta(1\rightarrow4)$ linkage. The repeat unit is composed of two anhydrous glucose rings $(C_6H_{10}O_5)_n$, where n = 10,000–15,000, linked via covalently bonded oxygen atom [52]. The intra-chain hydrogen bonding between hydroxyl groups and oxygen of the adjoining ring molecule stabilizes the linkage, thereby resulting in the linear configuration of the cellulose chain [53].

Research on cellulose nanocomposites started already in the mid-1990s. The first paper on cellulose nanocomposites was published by Chanzy and Cavaille group in Grenoble, France [54]. They extracted microfibrils or whiskers from a sea animal, which were monocrystals of cellulose with an aspect ratio of around 100 and an average diameter of 20 nm [54]. By 2000, many research groups had entered the field of cellulose nanocomposites. Nanocellulose nanocomposites have become the new-generation materials with a wide range of applications in pharmacology and medicine, tissue engineering, biosensors, and drug delivery [55].

Natural fibers are composed mainly of cellulose, lignin, and hemicellulose and, therefore, are also referred to as cellulosic or lignocellulosic fibers. Table 12.3 exemplifies the chemical composition of some of the lignocellulosic fibers [56].

Table 12.3 Chemical composition of lignocellulosic fibers

Name of the fiber	Cellulose (wt%)	Hemi-cellulose (wt%)	Lignin (wt%)	Ash (wt%)	Pectin (wt%)	Waxes (wt%)	Ref.
Sugarcane bagasse	55.3–55.2	16.8–29.7	24.3–25.3	1.1	10	—	[57]
Jute	67	16	9	1	0.2	0.5	[58]
Cotton	89	4	0.75	—	6	0.6	[59]
Hemp	77.5	10.0	6.8	—	2.9	0.9	[60]
Flax	70.5	16.5	2.5	—	0.9	1.7	[61]

Source: Table modified from Refs. [56, 62].

With the expanding concept of bio-based nanocomposites (bionanocomposites), cellulose nanoparticles (whiskers) are used as reinforcement materials because of their known advantages, such as their renewable nature, low density, wide availability, low energy consumption, reactive surface, high specific properties, and biodegradability [52]. There are different methods reported in the literature for the isolation of cellulose nanoparticles, including mechanical treatment, acid hydrolysis, and enzymatic hydrolysis. Excellent mechanical properties are achieved by addition of cellulose nanocrystals in low amounts in the polymer matrix [63]. Recyclable cellulose nanofiber membranes have also been synthesized using suspensions of cellulose nanofibers, silica nanoparticles (with size around 22 nm), and polyamide-amine-epichlorohydrin (PAE) via filtration. Silica nanoparticles act as spacers to control the pore size of the nanofiber network, whereas PAE is added to improve the wet strength of the membrane [64].

Nanoparticle-embedded cellulose membrane composites: Nanocomposites have wide applications due to the combined synergistic effects of the components. In one of the studies, cellulose was isolated from the citrus peel waste and was converted into value-added ZnO nanocomposite by impregnating ZnO nanoparticles into cellulose by coprecipitation method (Fig. 12.5). The nanocomposite was found to exhibit significant antibacterial and photocatalytic activity (degradation of methylene blue dye) [65].

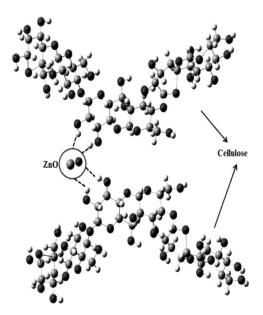

Figure 12.5 Proposed structure of ZnO nanoparticles impregnated into cellulose.

Doping cellulose and derivatives with nanoparticles leads to the formation of hybrid (organic/inorganic) nanocomposites with additional functionalities and superior thermal, mechanical, electrical, and optical properties, thereby expanding the area of applicability of cellulose-based materials. One of the widely used inorganic nanomaterials is TiO_2 with wide applications in catalysis, solar cells, pigments, corrosion protection, or optical coatings. It is used as a photocatalyst in the degradation of organic or inorganic contaminants in wastewater due to its high chemical stability, low toxicity, and low cost [66].

A wide range of cellulose-based nanocomposites doped with TiO_2 have been fabricated with applications as high-porosity nanohybrid membranes, self-cleansing materials, and nanocomposites with high photocatalytic activity. TiO_2-doped porous cellular membranes have also been synthesized with direct applications in water purification or self-cleaning surfaces [67].

Cellulose fiber–based membranes embedded with Ag nanoparticles have been developed using the force spinning (FS) technique followed by alkaline hydrolysis treatment [68]. This method utilizes centrifugal forces to produce fine fibers with significantly high yield. Since cellulose is a hydrophilic material, it can effectively absorb wound exudates and thus can be applied as a suitable wound-dressing material for the treatment of large wounds [69]. As cellulose is insoluble in typical solvents and lack melting point, it is directly spun from a cellulose solution. The fibers are regenerated by the alkaline hydrolysis of spun cellulose acetate (CA) fibers. Ag nanoparticles are embedded in these fibers as Ag has strong antimicrobial activity. The nanocomposite has been reported to have high water-retention capability, thus providing a prolonged moist microenvironment on wound, benefitting the re-epithelialization of the wound and preventing the formation of a scab [70].

Nanoparticle-embedded cellulose nanofiber films act as renewable ecofriendly catalysts. It is difficult to obtain individual cellulose nanofibers as cellulose is tightly packed sheet structure due to inter-fibril hydrogen bonds. The reaction mediated by 2,2,6,6-tetramethylpiperidine-1-oxyl radical (TEMPO) is reported to produce a single cellulose nanofibril by allowing the selective oxidation of C6 primary hydroxyl group of cellulose to a carboxylate group [71]. The impregnation of metal nanoparticles in TEMPO-oxidized cellulose nanofiber (TOCNF) network leads to improved magnetic, photocatalytic, antibacterial, electroconductive, deodorizing, and photoluminescent properties. Cu nanoparticle–loaded TOCNFs have excellent catalytic activity for the reduction of 4-nitrophenol, which is one of the most toxic and hazardous pollutants in wastewater generated from industrial and agricultural processes. It is observed that the reduction of 4-nitrophenol by $NaBH_4$ takes place appreciably in the presence of Cu nanoparticle-loaded TOCNF film, which serves as electron relay for an oxidant and reductant. The electron transfer is facilitated by metal nanoparticles. $NaBH_4$, which is nucleophilic in nature, donates electrons to metal nanoparticles. An electrophile (4-nitrophenol) captures electrons from nanoparticles. Thus, BH_4 ions and 4-nitrophenol are simultaneously adsorbed on the surface of Cu nanoparticles [72].

Removal of heavy metals such as lead, manganese, cadmium, and chromium, which are toxic to human and aquatic life, is one of the environmental challenges. There is a need for the designing of efficient environment-friendly adsorbents. Recently, Luo et al. fabricated millimeter-scale magnetic cellulose-based beads with micro- and nanopore structure. The composite beads were incorporated with carboxyl-decorated magnetite nanoparticles and nitric acid–modified activated carbon. The nanocomposite was based on sensitive magnetic response and was highly effective in the removal of heavy metal ions [73]. Polysaccharides have the capability to interact with various molecules via physical and chemical interactions. Since cellulose has many hydroxyl groups, which could be employed for coupling reactions and other functional modifications, it is considered to be promising as material for the adsorption and removal of contaminants from the water.

Surface adsorption mechanism in removing pollutants from wastewater: The industrial and agricultural wastes are increasing the concentration of contaminants (heavy metals, pesticides, toxic chemicals) in water. Therefore, there is an urgent call to develop new technologies for wastewater treatment. Adsorption is a simple and efficient method to remove organic or inorganic pollutants from water. Cellulose nanocomposites have emerged as efficient and effective alternative for the removal of contaminants in wastewater (Fig. 12.6).

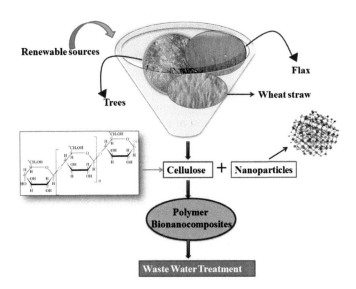

Figure 12.6 Polymer bionanocomposites in wastewater treatment.

Polysaccharides, such as maltodextrins, are another important type of chiral selectors used for the separation of enantiomers of chiral drugs. Depending on the adsorbed nature of binding, adsorption process can be classified as chemisorption and physisorption. Chemisorption involves covalent interaction between the adsorbates and the adsorbents, whereas physisorption involves non-covalent interactions. Most of the polymer composites take into account physisorption either by redox reactions or molecular interactions such as van der Waals forces, hydrophobic effects, $\pi-\pi$ interactions, hydrogen bonding, and electrostatic interactions. The driving force for adsorption phenomenon is the reduction of the interfacial energy between the adsorbate and the adsorbents and this is influenced by the pore size, surface area, and surface affinity or wettability [74].

The possible mechanism predicted for the adsorption of metal ions on the surface of nanocomposite is electrostatic interactions, ion exchange, micro-precipitation, or interaction followed by nucleation effects [75]. The incorporation of inorganic nanoparticles in the cellulose beads facilitates the transport of the pollutant from the solution to the inner nanoparticle–cellulose bead, which is a porous material. The adsorption process is estimated by adsorption isotherms. Langmuir isotherm is expressed as:

$$q_e = Q_{max}bC_e/(1 + bC_e) \quad (12.1)$$

Freundlich is represented as:

$$q_e = K_f C_e^{1/n} \quad (12.2)$$

where q_e (mg/g) is the equilibrium adsorption capacity, C_e (mg/L) is the equilibrium concentration of ions in solution, Q_{max} (mg/g) is the maximum adsorption capacity per gram of sorbent, b (L/mg) is the Langmuir constant related to the energy of adsorption, K_f (mg/g) and n are Freundlich constants related to adsorption capacity and heterogeneity factor, respectively [76].

The adsorption kinetics describe the metal uptake rate, which helps in understanding the adsorption property of heavy metal ions on the nanoparticle–cellulose beads. Cellulose nanocomposites increase the binding affinity of the pollutants due to the presence of the easily functionalizable surface [77].

12.2.2 Protein-Based Bionanocomposites

Most of the proteins consist of linear polymers built from the 20 different L-α-amino acids. The constituents are linked by the amide bonds. Proteins are amphoteric molecules; therefore, they can spontaneously migrate into an air–water interface or an oil–water interface. Once at the interface, proteins have the ability to interact with the neighboring molecules, thereby forming cohesive films that can withstand thermal and mechanical motions. Thus, proteins are used in adhesives and as edible films/coatings [78].

Protein-based bionanocomposites have found applications traditionally in the field of adhesives and as edible films/coatings. Swain et al. prepared soy protein–based nanocomposites via solution intercalation with the incorporation of organoclay with different concentrations without the use of any plasticizers [79]. The bionanocomposites possessed improved oxygen barrier function with higher thermal resistance, making them applicable as ideal food-packaging materials. With the incorporation of organoclay, the crystallinity of the bionanocomposites changed [79]. The application of protein-based bionanocomposites in wastewater treatment is not extensive but applied to remove oil spills from marine water.

Used or spent oils are toxic to the microflora present in the marine environment as well as effluent-treatment plants. Oil spill in waterbodies is a major environmental concern all over the world. A stable nanocomposite based on collagen and superparamagnetic nanoparticles has been prepared by a process utilizing protein wastes from the leather industry. A selective oil adsorption and magnetic tracking ability were exhibited by the nanocomposite for the removal of oil [80].

12.3 Conclusion and Future Perspectives

Inexorable industrialization and increase in population have challenged access to safe water globally. The treatment of wastewater and its utilization as an alternative source for irrigation and other vital usage have been proved to be a viable alternative to circumvent water scarcity. Different methods have been used to treat wastewater and coupling of advanced nanotechnology-oriented approach with the conventional methods offer interesting benefits.

The bionanocomposites developed by combining different natural polymers and nanomaterials have been applied in different fields such as drug-delivery systems, UV protection gels, anti-corrosion barrier coatings and paints, lubricants, fire-retardant materials, new scratch/abrasion-resistant materials, and film formation. In wastewater treatment, these bionanocomposites have been used successfully in the adsorption of micropollutants such as organic dyes and heavy metal ions and their antimicrobial potential has also been explored. Although bionanocomposites have key applications in numerous industrial fields, a number of technical and economic hurdles restrict their widespread commercialization. The problems associated with poor adhesion of matrix and fiber, orientation of the fiber, achievement of nanosize range, and achievement of actual renewable polymers need extensive research.

The technical issues, including overall impact performance, cost involved, investment in state-of-the-art equipment, are another bottleneck to develop ground-breaking technologies on nanocomposites.

Further, water industries are promoting sustainable development and trying to develop low-cost and simplified systems to explore different means to treat wastewater. Hence, large-scale developments of biopolymer-based bionanocomposites and their successful implication in the near future are possible.

Future trends include the coupling of nanotechnology potential with different polymer systems, where the improvement of new compatibility strategies would likely to be a prerequisite. There are advancement in the production of bio-PET nanocomposites, but extensive research and overall assessment of the technology developed are needed to overcome the existing challenges. The reinforcement of clay nanocomposites by glass fiber is also gaining a lot of attention, and the development of electrically conducting clay nanocomposites is in process. Multidirectional research is needed to promote the large-scale use of bionanocomposites for the effective removal of different types of pollutants from wastewater.

Acknowledgments

The support from the South African Research Chair Initiative of the Department of Science and Technology and National Research Foundation of South Africa is sincerely acknowledged.

References

1. Fowler, P. A., J. M. Hughes, and R. M. Elias, Biocomposites: Technology, environmental credentials and market forces. *Journal of the Science of Food and Agriculture*, 2006, **86**(12): 1781–1789.

2. Amin, M. T., A. A. Alazba, and U. Manzoor, A review of removal of pollutants from water/wastewater using different types of nanomaterials. *Advances in Materials Science and Engineering*, 2014: 24.

3. Nashaat, N. N., The application of nanoparticles for wastewater remediation, In *Applications of Nanomaterials for Water Quality*, 2013, Future Science Ltd., 52–65.

4. Camargo, P. H. C., K. G. Satyanarayana, and F. Wypych, Nanocomposites: Synthesis, structure, properties and new application opportunities. *Materials Research*, 2009, **12**: 1–39.

5. Simeonidis, K., et al., Inorganic engineered nanoparticles in drinking water treatment: A critical review. *Environmental Science: Water Research & Technology*, 2016, **2**(1): 43–70.

6. Horst, M. F., M. Alvarez, and V. L. Lassalle, Removal of heavy metals from wastewater using magnetic nanocomposites: Analysis of the experimental conditions. *Separation Science and Technology*, 2016, **51**(3): 550–563.

7. Zafar, R., et al., Polysaccharide based bionanocomposites, properties and applications: A review. *International Journal of Biological Macromolecules*, 2016, **92**: 1012–1024.

8. Reddy, M. M., et al., Biobased plastics and bionanocomposites: Current status and future opportunities. *Progress in Polymer Science*, 2013, **38**(10–11): 1653–1689.

9. Shchipunov, Y., N. Ivanova, and V. Silant'ev, Bionanocomposites formed by in situ charged chitosan with clay. *Green Chemistry*, 2009, **11**(11): 1758–1761.

10. Gangopadhyay, R. and A. De, Conducting polymer nanocomposites: A brief overview. *Chemistry of Materials*, 2000, **12**(3): 608–622.

11. Fu, Y., et al., Chemical/Biochemical preparation of new polymeric bionanocomposites with enzyme labels immobilized at high load and activity for high-performance electrochemical immunoassay. *The Journal of Physical Chemistry C*, 2010, **114**(3): 1472–1480.

12. Kurtz, S. M. and J. N. Devine, PEEK biomaterials in trauma, orthopedic, and spinal implants. *Biomaterials*, 2007, **28**(32): 4845–4869.

13. Diez-Pascual, A. M., C. Xu, and R. Luque, Development and characterization of novel poly(ether ether ketone)/ZnO bionanocomposites. *Journal of Materials Chemistry B*, 2014, **2**(20): 3065–3078.

14. Zhong, Y., et al., Fabrication of unique magnetic bionanocomposite for highly efficient removal of hexavalent chromium from water. *Scientific Reports*, 2016, **6**: 31090.

15. Shabnam, R. and H. Ahmad, Hydrophobic poly(lauryl methacrylate)-coated magnetic nano-composite particles for removal of organic pollutants. *Polymers for Advanced Technologies*, 2015, **26**(4): 408–413.

16. Aouada, F. A., L. H. C. Mattoso, and E. Longo, Enhanced bulk and superficial hydrophobicities of starch-based bionanocomposites by addition of clay. *Industrial Crops and Products*, 2013, **50**: 449–455.

17. Kvien, I., et al., Characterization of starch based nanocomposites. *Journal of Materials Science*, 2007, **42**(19): 8163–8171.

18. Valapa, R. B., G. Pugazhenthi, and V. Katiyar, Fabrication and characterization of sucrose palmitate reinforced poly(lactic acid) bionanocomposite films. *Journal of Applied Polymer Science*, 2015, **132**(3): doi: 10.1002/app.41320.

19. Fardioui, M., et al., Bionanocomposite materials based on chitosan reinforced with nanocrystalline cellulose and organo-modified montmorillonite, in *Nanoclay Reinforced Polymer Composites: Nanocomposites and Bionanocomposites*, M. Jawaid, A. E. K. Qaiss, and R. Bouhfid (Eds.), 2016, Springer Singapore: Singapore. pp. 167–194.

20. Depan, D. and R. P. Singh, Preparation and characterization of novel hybrid of bio-assisted mineralized Zn-Al layered double hydroxides using chitosan as a template. *Journal of Applied Polymer Science*, 2010, **115**(6): 3636–3644.

21. Unuabonah, E. I. and A. Taubert, Clay–polymer nanocomposites (CPNs): Adsorbents of the future for water treatment. *Applied Clay Science*, 2014, **99**: 83–92.

22. Babel, S. and T. A. Kurniawan, Low-cost adsorbents for heavy metals uptake from contaminated water: A review. *Journal of Hazardous Materials*, 2003, **97**(1–3): 219–243.

23. Liu, C. and R. Bai, Recent advances in chitosan and its derivatives as adsorbents for removal of pollutants from water and wastewater. *Current Opinion in Chemical Engineering*, 2014, **4**: 62–70.

24. Keng, P.-S., et al., Removal of hazardous heavy metals from aqueous environment by low-cost adsorption materials. *Environmental Chemistry Letters*, 2014, **12**(1): 15–25.

25. Azzam, E. M., et al., Preparation and characterization of chitosan-clay nanocomposites for the removal of Cu(II) from aqueous solution. *International Journal of Biological Macromolecules*, 2016, **89**: 507–517.

26. Wang, L., J. Zhang, and A. Wang, Removal of methylene blue from aqueous solution using chitosan-g-poly(acrylic acid)/montmorillonite superadsorbent nanocomposite. *Colloids and Surfaces A: Physicochemical and Engineering Aspects*, 2008, **322**(1–3): 47–53.

27. Salehifar, N., Z. Zarghami, and M. Ramezani, A facile, novel and low-temperature synthesis of MgO nanorods via thermal decomposition using new starting reagent and its photocatalytic activity evaluation. *Materials Letters*, 2016, **167**: 226–229.

28. Sureshkumar, V., et al., Fabrication of chitosan-magnetite nanocomposite strip for chromium removal. *Applied Nanoscience*, 2016, **6**(2): 277–285.

29. Moradi Dehaghi, S., et al., Removal of permethrin pesticide from water by chitosan–zinc oxide nanoparticles composite as an adsorbent. *Journal of Saudi Chemical Society*, 2014, **18**(4): 348–355.

30. Mujeeb Rahman, P., K. Muraleedaran, and V. M. Abdul Mujeeb, Applications of chitosan powder with in situ synthesized nano ZnO particles as an antimicrobial agent. *International Journal of Biological Macromolecules*, 2015, **77**: 266–272.

31. Khan, S. A., et al., Antibacterial nanocomposites based on chitosan/ Co-MCM as a selective and efficient adsorbent for organic dyes. *International Journal of Biological Macromolecules*, 2016, **91**: 744–751.

32. Nithya, R., et al., Removal of Cr(VI) from aqueous solution using chitosan-g-poly(butyl acrylate)/silica gel nanocomposite. *International Journal of Biological Macromolecules*, 2016, **87**: 545–554.

33. Bée, A., et al., Magnetic chitosan/clay beads: A magsorbent for the removal of cationic dye from water. *Journal of Magnetism and Magnetic Materials*, 2017, **421**: 59–64.

34. Pourjavadi, A., et al., Hydrogel nanocomposite based on chitosan-g-acrylic acid and modified nanosilica with high adsorption capacity for heavy metal ion removal. *Iranian Polymer Journal*, 2015, **24**(9): 725–734.

35. Budnyak, T. M., et al., Synthesis and adsorption properties of chitosan-silica nanocomposite prepared by sol-gel method. *Nanoscale Research Letters*, 2015, **10**(1): 87.

36. Cui, X., et al., Electrospun $H_4SiW_{12}O_{40}$/chitosan/polycaprolactam sandwich nanofibrous membrane with excellent dual-function:

Adsorption and photocatalysis. *RSC Advances*, 2016, **6**(98): 96237–96244.

37. Liu, J., et al., Superhydrophilic and underwater superoleophobic modified chitosan-coated mesh for oil/water separation. *Surface and Coatings Technology*, 2016, **307**, Part A: 171–176.

38. Mohammad, A. M., et al., Efficient treatment of lead-containing wastewater by hydroxyapatite/chitosan nanostructures. *Arabian Journal of Chemistry*, 2015.

39. Liu, Q., et al., Removal of fluoride from aqueous solution using Zr(IV) immobilized cross-linked chitosan. *International Journal of Biological Macromolecules*, 2015, **77**: 15–23.

40. Farzana, M. H. and S. Meenakshi, Facile synthesis of chitosan/ZnO composite for the photodegradation of Rhodamine B dye. *Journal of Chitin and Chitosan Science*, 2015, **3**(1): 21–31.

41. Rani, P., et al., Microwave assisted synthesis of polyacrylamide grafted gum ghatti and its application as flocculant. *Carbohydrate Polymers*, 2012, **89**(1): 275–281.

42. Mittal, H., et al., Flocculation characteristics and biodegradation studies of gum ghatti based hydrogels. *International Journal of Biological Macromolecules*, 2013, **58**: 37–46.

43. Quintanilha, R. C., et al., The use of gum Arabic as "Green" stabilizer of poly(aniline) nanocomposites: A comprehensive study of spectroscopic, morphological and electrochemical properties. *Journal of Colloid and Interface Science*, 2014, **434**: 18–27.

44. Kim, M. T., et al., Carbon nanotube modification using gum Arabic and its effect on the dispersion and tensile properties of carbon nanotubes/epoxy nanocomposites. *Journal of Nanoscience and Nanotechnology*, 2011, **11**(8): 7369–7373.

45. Khan, T. A., et al., Removal of chromium(VI) from aqueous solution using guar gum–nano zinc oxide biocomposite adsorbent. *Arabian Journal of Chemistry*, 2013.

46. Singh, V., et al., Removal of chromium (VI) using poly(methylacrylate) functionalized guar gum. *Bioresource Technology*, 2009, **100**(6): 1977–1982.

47. Singh, V., et al., Removal of cadmium from aqueous solutions by adsorption using poly(acrylamide) modified guar gum–silica nanocomposites. *Separation and Purification Technology*, 2009, **67**(3): 251–261.

48. Sand Arpit, et al., Studies on graft copolymerization of 2-acrylamidoglycolic acid on to partially carboxymethylated guar gum and physico-chemical properties. *Carbohydrate Polymers*, 2011, **83**: 14–21.

49. Pal, S., et al., Modified guar gum/SiO_2: Development and application of a novel hybrid nanocomposite as a flocculant for the treatment of wastewater. *Environmental Science: Water Research & Technology*, 2015, **1**(1): 84–95.

50. Fosso-Kankeu, E., et al., Preparation and characterization of gum karaya hydrogel nanocomposite flocculant for metal ions removal from mine effluents. *International Journal of Environmental Science and Technology*, 2016, **13**(2): 711–724.

51. Mittal, H., et al., Fe_3O_4 MNPs and gum xanthan based hydrogels nanocomposites for the efficient capture of malachite green from aqueous solution. *Chemical Engineering Journal*, 2014, **255**: 471–482.

52. Azizi Samir, M. A., F. Alloin, and A. Dufresne, Review of recent research into cellulosic whiskers, their properties and their application in nanocomposite field. *Biomacromolecules*, 2005, **6**(2): 612–626.

53. Moon, R. J., et al., Cellulose nanomaterials review: Structure, properties and nanocomposites. *Chemical Society Reviews*, 2011, **40**(7): 3941–3994.

54. Favier, V., et al., Nanocomposite materials from latex and cellulose whiskers. *Polymers for Advanced Technologies*, 1995, **6**(5): 351–355.

55. Galkina, O. L., et al., Cellulose nanofiber-titania nanocomposites as potential drug delivery systems for dermal applications. *Journal of Materials Chemistry B*, 2015, **3**(8): 1688–1698.

56. Siqueira, G., J. Bras, and A. Dufresne, Cellulosic bionanocomposites: A review of preparation, properties and applications. *Polymers*, 2010, **2**(4): 728.

57. Mwaikambo, L. Y. and M. P. Ansell, Mechanical properties of alkali treated plant fibres and their potential as reinforcement materials. I. Hemp fibres. *Journal of Materials Science*, 2006, **41**(8): 2483–2496.

58. Ramamoorthy, S. K., M. Skrifvars, and A. Persson, A review of natural fibers used in biocomposites: Plant, animal and regenerated cellulose fibers. *Polymer Reviews*, 2015, **55**(1): 107–162.

59. Faruk, O., et al., Biocomposites reinforced with natural fibers: 2000–2010. *Progress in Polymer Science*, 2012, **37**(11): 1552–1596.

60. Mohanty, A. K., M. Misra, and G. Hinrichsen, Biofibres, biodegradable polymers and biocomposites: An overview. *Macromolecular Materials and Engineering*, 2000, **276-277**(1): 1–24.

61. Bledzki, A. K., S. Reihmane, and J. Gassan, Properties and modification methods for vegetable fibers for natural fiber composites. *Journal of Applied Polymer Science*, 1996, **59**(8): 1329–1336.

62. Komuraiah, A., N. S. Kumar, and B. D. Prasad, Chemical composition of natural fibers and its influence on their mechanical properties. *Mechanics of Composite Materials*, 2014, **50**(3): 359–376.

63. Mariano, M., N. El Kissi, and A. Dufresne, Cellulose nanocrystals and related nanocomposites: Review of some properties and challenges. *Journal of Polymer Science Part B: Polymer Physics*, 2014, **52**(12): 791–806.

64. Varanasi, S., Z.-X. Low, and W. Batchelor, Cellulose nanofibre composite membranes: Biodegradable and recyclable UF membranes. *Chemical Engineering Journal*, 2015, **265**: 138–146.

65. Ali, A., et al., Zinc impregnated cellulose nanocomposites: Synthesis, characterization and applications. *Journal of Physics and Chemistry of Solids*, 2016, **98**: 174–182.

66. Turki, A., et al., Phenol photocatalytic degradation over anisotropic TiO_2 nanomaterials: Kinetic study, adsorption isotherms and formal mechanisms. *Applied Catalysis B: Environmental*, 2015, **163**: 404–414.

67. Wittmar, A., D. Vorat, and M. Ulbricht, Two step and one step preparation of porous nanocomposite cellulose membranes doped with TiO_2. *RSC Advances*, 2015, **5**(107): 88070–88078.

68. Xu, F., et al., Fabrication of cellulose fine fiber based membranes embedded with silver nanoparticles via Forcespinning, *Journal of Polymer Engineering*, 2016. Available at: https://doi.org/10.1515/polyeng-2015-0092

69. Czaja, W., et al., Microbial cellulose: The natural power to heal wounds. *Biomaterials*, 2006, **27**(2): 145–151.

70. Li, H., et al., Superabsorbent polysaccharide hydrogels based on pullulan derivate as antibacterial release wound dressing. *Journal of Biomedical Materials Research Part A*, 2011, **98**(1): 31–39.

71. Saito, T., et al., Individualization of nano-sized plant cellulose fibrils by direct surface carboxylation using TEMPO catalyst under neutral conditions. *Biomacromolecules*, 2009, **10**(7): 1992–1996.

72. Bendi, R. and T. Imae, Renewable catalyst with Cu nanoparticles embedded into cellulose nano-fiber film. *RSC Advances*, 2013, **3**(37): 16279–16282.

73. Luo, X., et al., Removal of heavy metal ions from water by magnetic cellulose-based beads with embedded chemically modified magnetite nanoparticles and activated carbon. *ACS Sustainable Chemistry & Engineering*, 2016, **4**(7): 3960–3969.

74. Huang, Y., et al., Applications of conjugated polymer based composites in wastewater purification. *RSC Advances*, 2014, **4**(107): 62160–62178.

75. Karim, Z., et al., High-flux affinity membranes based on cellulose nanocomposites for removal of heavy metal ions from industrial effluents. *RSC Advances*, 2016, **6**(25): 20644–20653.

76. Yu, X., et al., One-pot synthesis of porous magnetic cellulose beads for the removal of metal ions. *RSC Advances*, 2014, **4**(59): 31362–31369.

77. Carpenter, A. W., C. F. de Lannoy, and M. R. Wiesner, Cellulose nanomaterials in water treatment technologies. *Environmental Science & Technology*, 2015, **49**(9): 5277–5287.

78. Zhao, R., P. Torley, and P. J. Halley, Emerging biodegradable materials: Starch- and protein-based bio-nanocomposites. *Journal of Materials Science*, 2008, **43**(9): 3058–3071.

79. Swain, S. K., P. P. Priyadarshini, and S. K. Patra, Soy protein/clay bionanocomposites as ideal packaging materials. *Polymer-Plastics Technology and Engineering*, 2012, **51**(12): 1282–1287.

80. Thanikaivelan, P., et al., Collagen based magnetic nanocomposites for oil removal applications. *Scientific Reports*, 2012, **2**: 230.

Chapter 13

Gamma Radiation Studies on Thermoplastic Polyurethane/Nanosilica Composites

Abitha V. K.,[a] Rane Ajay Vasudeo,[b] Krishnan Kanny,[b]
Sabu Thomas,[a] Niji M. R.,[c] and K. Rajkumar[d]
[a]*School of Chemical Sciences, Mahatma Gandhi University, Kottayam 686560, India*
[b]*Composites Research Group, Department of Mechanical Engineering, Durban University of Technology, Durban 4000, South Africa.*
[c]*Department of Polymer Science and Rubber Technology, Cochin University of Science and Technology, Kochi 682022, India*
[d]*Indian Rubbers Manufacturers Research Association, Thane 400604, India*
ajayrane2008@gmail.com

Thermoplastic polyurethane (TPU) provides opportunities to the modern industry by its outstanding versatility, by improving the performance of any product from shoe soles to seals, films, conveyor belts, and cables. TPUs have high elongation and tensile strength, elasticity, and ability to resist oils, greases, solvents, chemicals, and abrasion. TPUs are classified as polyether-based and polyester-based, and they have the following characteristics within them. Polyester TPUs are unaffected by oils and chemicals, provide excellent

---

Biocomposites: Biomedical and Environmental Applications
Edited by Shakeel Ahmed, Saiqa Ikram, Suvardhan Kanchi, and Krishna Bisetty
Copyright © 2018 Pan Stanford Publishing Pte. Ltd.
ISBN 978-981-4774-38-3 (Hardcover), 978-1-315-11080-6 (eBook)
www.panstanford.com

abrasion resistance, offer a good balance of physical properties, and are perfect for use in polyblends. On the other hand, polyester TPUs are slightly lower in specific gravity than polyester TPUs and offer low temperature flexibility, good abrasion and tear resilience. They are also durable against microbial attack and provide excellent hydrolysis resistance, making them suitable for applications where water is a consideration. The mentioned work deals with preparation of composites based on TPU (polyester) and nanosilica via melt-blending process in a laboratory mixer. The prepared nanocomposites were tested for mechanical/thermal/electrical properties, and also irradiation properties were determined.

13.1 Introduction

Thermoplastic polyurethane provides opportunities to the modern industry by its outstanding versatility by improving the performance of any product from shoe soles to seals, films, conveyor belts, and cables. TPUs have high elongation and tensile strength, elasticity, and ability to resist oils, greases, solvents, chemicals, and abrasion. TPUs are classified in to polyester based and polyester based, which have the following characteristics. Polyester TPUs are unaffected by oils and chemicals, provide excellent abrasion resistance, offer a good balance of physical properties, and are perfect for use in polyblends. On the other hand, polyester TPUs are slightly lower in specific gravity than polyester TPUs and offer low temperature flexibility, good abrasion and tear resilience. They are also durable against microbial attack and provide excellent hydrolysis resistance, making them suitable for applications where water is a consideration. The mentioned work deals with the preparation of composites based on TPU (polyester) and nanosilica via the melt-blending process in a laboratory mixer. The prepared nanocomposites were tested for mechanical/thermal/electrical properties, and the irradiation properties were also determined. The aim of this work is to obtain nanocomposites and improved properties that those materials can display.

A TPU is a multi-phase block copolymer that is created when three basic raw materials are combined together in a specific way; the three raw materials required are a polyol or long-chain diol, chain extender or short-chain diol, and diisocyanate [1]. The soft block, built out of a polyol and isocyanates, is responsible for the flexibility and elastomeric character of a TPU. The hard block, constructed from a chain extender and isocyanates, gives a TPU its toughness (elastomeric property) and physical performance properties. The following structures make clear the difference between a thermoplastic elastomer, thermoset, and a thermoplastic type of polyurethane (Fig. 13.1a–c). The TPU elastomer does not show chemical crosslinks as compared to thermoset polyurethane rubber, where in the case of TPU where physical crosslinks are broken down/ melted when heated and repacked when the material is cooled. Now let us get into some more detail by describing the nanosilica that is used in the preparation of nanocomposite. Fillers in the form of fine particulates have been used in compounding. Particulate fillers are usually divided into two groups: inert fillers and reinforcing fillers. Reinforcing fillers are added in an adequate amount to increase mechanical properties. Inert fillers are added to increase the bulk and reduce costs [2].

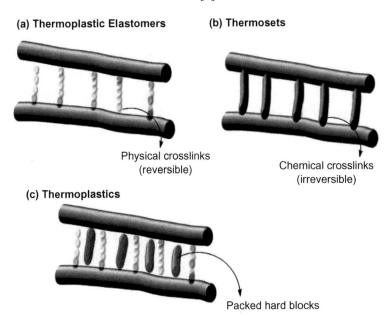

Figure 13.1 Types of polyurethanes: (a) Thermoplastic elastomers, (b) thermosets, (c) thermoplastics.

Silica has an extremely large surface area and smooth non-porous surface, which could promote strong physical contact between the filler and the polymer matrix [3]. For the preparation of silica nanocomposites, fumed silica is commonly used and precipitated silica is seldom used since the precipitated one has more silanol (Si-OH) groups on the surface and consequently it is much easier to agglomerate than the fumed one. The structure of nanosilica shows a three-dimensional network. Silanol and siloxane groups are created on the silica surface, leading to the hydrophilic nature of the particles.

Surfaces of silica are typically terminated with three silanol types: free or isolated silanol, hydrogen-bonded or vicinal silanol, and geminal silanol. The silanol groups residing on adjacent particles, in turn, form hydrogen bonds and lead to the formation of aggregates. These bonds hold individual fumed silica particles together, and the aggregates remain intact even under the best mixing conditions if stronger filler-polymer interaction is not present. The dispersion of nanometer-sized particles in the polymer matrix has a significant impact on the properties of nanocomposites. The unique microphase morphology confers TPUs with a higher tensile strength and toughness when compared with most other elastomers, and the absence of covalent crosslinking allows TPUs to be both melt [4] and solution [5] processed; we have preferred melt blending. However, under continuous and/or cyclic loading, the absence of chemical crosslinking allows the hard domains to restructure, which results in large hysteretic losses and poor creep resistance [6]. The introduction of nanofillers (nanosilica) to this complex TPU morphology showed an improvement in the mechanical properties at an optimum loading of the nanosilica.

A feature of polymer nanocomposites is that the small size of the fillers leads to a dramatic increase in interfacial area as compared with traditional composites [7]. This interfacial area creates a significant volume fraction of interfacial polymer with properties different from the bulk polymer even at low loadings [large (amounts) loading of the nanosilica decreases the properties of the nanocomposites, refer Section 13.3]. In the current research work, nanocomposites based on TPU and nanosilica (with varying amounts) were prepared by melt blending, and the properties obtained by using nanosilica as a reinforcing phase were compared with normal silica (for one batch). Now let us have a look at the steps for experimentation.

13.2 Preparation of Thermoplastic Polyurethane/Nanosilica Composite

The TPU (polyester type) for the study was of Bayer Material Science. The nanosilica was supplied by a retailer, and the formulation of the nanocomposites based on nanosilica is given in Table 13.1, with PU-0, PU-1, PU-3, PU-5, and PU-10. Comparison is made with normal silica S3, in order to find the advances of nanotechnology over conventional technology.

Table 13.1 Formulation of the batches for nanocomposites

Ingredients	PU-0	PU-1	PU-3	PU-5	PU-10	S3*
TPU (phr)	100	100	100	100	100	100
Nanosilica (phr) Normal silica*	0	1	3	5	10	3

13.2.1 Preparation of Nanocomposites

Polyester TPU was incorporated with nanosilica in a laboratory mixer at a temperature just near to the softening temperature, that is, 150°C, maintaining the rotor speed and fill factor, that is, 80 rpm, for a total time of 12 min, for melt intercalation to take place. After melt mixing, the molten mass was taken out from the laboratory mixer and, while hot, passed through a two-roll mixing mill to chill it and sheet it to about 2 mm thick. Plastic molding is carried out in a compression molding machine with water cooling facility, with molding pressure of 50 kg/cm^2. Wax paper was placed between the sheet and the press plates to avoid adhesiveness (as a mold release agent). The sheet was then cooled down to room temperature still under pressure. The test specimens were die-cut from the compression-molded sheet and used for measuring mechanical properties after 24 h of conditioning at room temperature.

13.3 Results and Discussions*

13.3.1 Mechanical Properties

Table 13.2 shows us the mechanical properties of nanocomposites before and after radiating. It showed modulus at 200%, 300%, tensile strength, and elongation at break decreases after 3 phr of nanosilica. It indicates that at 5 and 10 phr loading of filler, agglomeration is more, thereby interaction adhesion between filler and polymer is not good; decrease in tensile strength after radiation is due to the dissociation of bonds between polymers due to high radiation energy and affects the tensile strength of the composite. Increase in tensile strength after radiation may be due to strong adhesion between filler and polymer, thereby effective stress transfer between filler and polymer, which still exists due to strong interfacial interaction between nanosilica and TPUs.

Table 13.2 Mechanical properties of the batches for nanocomposites

Properties	Units	PU-0	PU-1	PU-3	PU-5	PU-10
100% modulus	kg/cm^2	35	56↑	61↑	63↑	70↑
200% modulus	kg/cm^2	64	77↑	83↑	85↑	89↑
300% modulus	kg/cm^2	87	123↑	125↑	124↓	120↓
Tensile strength	kg/cm^2	409	447↑	489↑	408↓	311↓
Elongation at break	%	560	580↑	590↑	540↓	520↓
Hardness	Shore A	72	75↑	79↑	81↑	83↑
Change in properties after radiation resistance (5 MRad for 33.5 h)						
100% modulus	kg/cm^2	50	59↑	66↑	64↓	74↑
200% modulus	kg/cm^2	78	79↑	84↑	86↑	90↑
300% modulus	kg/cm^2	114	125↑	126↑	125↓	122↓
Tensile strength	kg/cm^2	335	358↑	378↑	276↓	267↓
Elongation at break	%	570	580↑	590↑	550↓	510↓
Hardness	Shore A	74	76↑	80↑	82↑	84↑

*Test methods in the development of nanocomposites were taken from Ref. [8].

Properties	Units	PU-0	PU-1	PU-3	PU-5	PU-10
Change in properties after radiation resistance (10 MRad for 67.11 h)						
100% modulus	kg/cm^2	56	65↑	67↑	65↓	75↑
200% modulus	kg/cm^2	82	84↑	86↑	87↑	92↑
300% modulus	kg/cm^2	133	139↑	147↑	126↓	124↓
Tensile strength	kg/cm^2	213	225↑	260↑	180↓	152↓
Elongation at break	%	580	590↑	600↑	560↓	540↓
Hardness	Shore A	75	78↑	81↑	82↑	84↑
Change in properties after radiation resistance (15 MRad for 100.67 h)						
100% modulus	kg/cm^2	63	68↑	69↑	70↑	78↑
200% modulus	kg/cm^2	92	97↑	98↑	90↑	98↑
300% modulus	kg/cm^2	139	140↑	152↑	127↓	125↓
Tensile strength	kg/cm^2	210	213↑	250↑	173↓	147↓
Elongation at break	%	590	600↑	610↑	570↓	550↓
Hardness	Shore A	78	79↑	82↑	83↑	85↑

13.3.2 Electrical Properties

It can be concluded from the electrical properties data that as the nanosilica loading increases till 3 phr, there is an increase in volume resistivity, but in the case of surface resistivity from the above results, it can be concluded that surface resistivity increases when nanosilica is used as a reinforcing phase but in optimum quantity, because surface resistivity decreases to a considerable amount if more loading of nanosilica is done. From the above results, it can be concluded that surface resistivity without adding of nanosilica is much higher than that of surface resistivity obtained after adding 10 phr nanosilica.

From the above experiments, it was concluded that 3 phr of nanosilica was the optimum quantity of the reinforcing filler to be added to polyester TPU, and hence an equal quantity of normal silica was added to polyester TPU and properties were determined. Nanosilica gave excellent properties as compared with normal silica (Table 13.4).

Table 13.3 Electrical properties of the batches for nanocomposites

Properties	Units	PU-0	PU-1	PU-3	PU-5	PU-10
Volume resistivity	ohm-cm	2.60×10^{12}	$2.63 \times 10^{12}\uparrow$	$4.40 \times 10^{12}\uparrow$	$7.85 \times 10^{11}\downarrow$	$8.04 \times 10^{11}\downarrow$
Surface resistivity	ohm	2.15×10^{13}	1.38×10^{13}	2.01×10^{13}	7.33×10^{12}	2.80×10^{12}

Table 13.4 Comparative results of normal silica versus nanosilica for composites

Properties	Units	PU-3	S-3
100% modulus	kg/cm^2	61	43
200% modulus	kg/cm^2	83	65
300% modulus	kg/cm^2	125	122
Tensile strength	kg/cm^2	489	400
Elongation at break	%	590	310
Hardness	Shore A	79	72
Change in properties after radiation resistance (5 MRad for 33.5 h)			
100% modulus	kg/cm^2	66	47
200% modulus	kg/cm^2	84	68
300% modulus	kg/cm^2	126	124
Tensile strength	kg/cm^2	378	246
Elongation at break	%	590	420
Hardness	Shore A	80	73
Change in properties after radiation resistance (10 MRad for 67.11 h)			
100% modulus	kg/cm^2	67	75
200% modulus	kg/cm^2	86	92
300% modulus	kg/cm^2	147	118
Tensile strength	kg/cm^2	260	219
Elongation at break	%	600	460
Hardness	Shore A	81	75

Properties	Units	PU-3	S-3
Change in properties after radiation resistance (15 MRad for 100.67 h)			
100% modulus	kg/cm^2	69	85
200% modulus	kg/cm^2	98	119
300% modulus	kg/cm^2	152	180
Tensile strength	kg/cm^2	250	206
Elongation at break	%	610	470
Hardness	Shore A	82	78

13.3.2.1 Comparison of mechanical properties with normal silica versus nanosilica

From the above data, it can also be made clear that 1 phr of nanosilica gave properties much better than 3 phr normal silica (compare PU-3 and S3). From the above graphs, it can be clearly concluded that the addition of nanosilica was an advantage to increase the mechanical and electrical properties (see Table 13.5) of the prepared nanocomposites.

Table 13.5 Electrical properties of nanocomposites, 3 phr of nanosilica and normal silica

Properties	Units	PU-3	S-3
Volume resistivity	ohm-cm	4.40×10^{12}	8.31×10^{12}
Surface resistivity	ohm	2.01×10^{13}	4.45×10^{13}

13.3.3 Thermal Analysis of Nanosilica Composites

The data generated from thermal analysis via thermal gravimetric analyzer are as mentioned in Table 13.6, which implies that as the filler loading increases, degradation temperature increases when compared to the degradation temperature of the base polyester TPU. However, as the amount (phr) of nanosilica goes on increasing in the composites (above 3 phr), there is a decrease in the degradation temperature. Hence, the optimum loading of 3 phr should be considered (refer Table 13.6).

Table 13.6 Thermogravimetric analysis of nanocomposites

Samples	Polymer content (%)	Low boiling materials (%)	Ash content (%)	Degradation temperature (°C)	Onset temperature (°C)
PU-0	98.919	1.125	Negligible	394.34	331.46
PU-1	97.357	1.549	1.1	411.19↑	325.75
PU-3	93.653	2.575	3.7	412.49↑	321.08
PU-5	90.862	3.845	5.3	389.15↓	315.07
PU-10	82.442	5.663	11.9	383.68↓	315.06

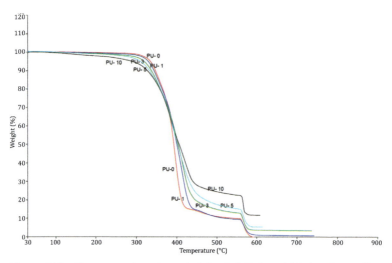

Figure 13.2 Thermogravimetric analysis for 0, 1, 3, 5, and 10 phr of nanosilica in polyester TPU.

13.3.3.1 Comparison of thermal properties with nanosilica versus normal silica

The comparative values signify that there is a slight increase in degradation temperature and results are mentioned in Table 13.7.

Table 13.7 Thermal analysis of nanocomposites, 3 phr of nanosilica and normal silica

Samples	Polymer content (%)	Low boiling materials (%)	Ash content (%)	Degradation temperature (°C)	Onset temperature (°C)
PU-3	93.653	2.575	3.7	412.49	321.08
S-3	95.883	1.254	2.8	421.56	329.82

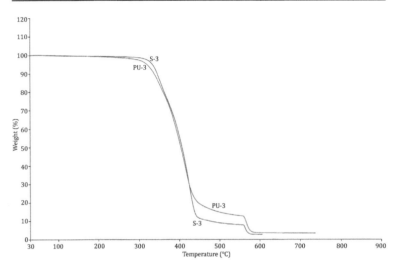

Figure 13.3 Thermogravimetric analysis for 3 phr of normal silica and nanosilica in polyester TPU.

13.4 Conclusion

Polyester TPU nanocomposites were prepared by melt mixing techniques on optimized conditions and various concentrations of nanosilica were added out of which 3 phr was the optimum one which gave excellent properties to nanocomposites. The mechanical, electrical, and thermal properties were improved by adding nanosilica to polyester TPU. Further, the samples were also tested for radiation resistance. Nanosilica-based composites could stand and maintain their properties, at specified dosage and time, but there is a decrease in tensile strength. It can also be concluded that the properties obtained by 3 phr of normal silica could not match the obtained properties of 1 phr nanosilica composites, which means that the use of 1 phr nanosilica can give comparable properties obtained by 3 phr of normal silica.

Acknowledgments

The authors thank Indian Rubber Manufacturers and Research Association, Thane, for carrying out radiation test and Durban University of Technology for RDG grant.

References

1. Brydson, J. A. 1999. *Plastics Materials*. Butterworth-Heinemann.
2. Wypych, G. 1999. *Handbook of Fillers*. ChemTec.
3. Zou, H., Wu, S., and Shen, J. 2008. Polymer/silica nanocomposites: Preparation, characterization, properties, and applications. *Chem. Rev.*, **108**(9), pp. 3893–3957.
4. Alexandre, M. and Dubois, P. 2000. Polymer-layered silicate nanocomposites: Preparation, properties and uses of a new class of materials. *Mater. Sci. Eng. R Rep.*, **28**(1), pp. 1–63.
5. Clemitson, I. R. 2015. *Castable Polyurethane Elastomers*. CRC Press.
6. Pinnavaia, T. J. and Beall, G. W. (Eds.), 2000. *Polymer–Clay Nanocomposites*. John Wiley.
7. Thomas, S. and Stephen, R. 2010. Rubber nanocomposites: Preparation, properties and applications. John Wiley & Sons.
8. Brown, R. 2006. *Physical Testing of Rubber*. Springer Science & Business Media.
9. Rácz, I., Andersen, E., Aranguren, M. I., and Marcovich, N. E. 2009. Wood flour: Recycled polyol based polyurethane lightweight composites. *J. Compos. Mater.*, **43**(24), pp. 2871–2884.

Chapter 14

Removal of Heavy Metals and Textile Dyes in Industrial Wastewater Using Biopolymers and Biocomposites

May Myat Khine, Nang Seng Moe, Kyaw Nyein Aye, and Nitar Nwe

Ecological Laboratory, Advancing Life and Regenerating Motherland, Kan Road, Hlaing Township, Yangon, Myanmar
nitarnwe@gmail.com, mmyatkhine92@gmail.com

High levels of soluble and suspension forms of heavy metals are one of the most toxic materials in soil and water. Adsorption method was used for the removal of heavy metals in wastewater, in which activated carbons and biopolymers were used as common adsorbents. Moreover, most of the wastewater in textile industries composed with discharged from textile dyes. Therefore, many researchers studied the effectiveness of dye removal from wastewaters by different separation techniques such as adsorption, coagulation/flocculation, advanced oxidation technologies, ozonation, membrane filtration, aerobic digestion, and anaerobic digestion. All techniques for separation of dyes have their own limitations in terms of design,

---

Biocomposites: Biomedical and Environmental Applications
Edited by Shakeel Ahmed, Saiqa Ikram, Suvardhan Kanchi, and Krishna Bisetty
Copyright © 2018 Pan Stanford Publishing Pte. Ltd.
ISBN 978-981-4774-38-3 (Hardcover), 978-1-315-11080-6 (eBook)
www.panstanford.com

operation efficiency, and operation cost. This chapter provides extensive information on the removal techniques of dyes and heavy metals using biopolymers and biocomposites.

14.1 Introduction

Naturally, freshwater contains heavy metals such as copper, selenium, and zinc in minute concentrations. These metals are essential for all living organisms in the process of ecosystems [1]. However, high concentration of heavy metals lead to poisoning of the food chain and tend to bioaccumulation (i.e., an increase in the concentration of a chemical in a biological organism over time, compared to the chemical's concentration in the environment).

Pollution of water is the biggest threat in today's world. Most of the wastewaters are discharged directly or indirectly into lakes, rivers, or oceans from industries such as cement, pharmaceutical, food, textile, pulp and paper, rubber, color, photography, leather, cosmetics, plastic, organic compost, metal plating, mining, fertilizer, tanneries, batteries, and pesticides [2, 3]. Most of pollutants from industrial wastewaters sediment in lakes, rivers, and oceans. Each industry discharges different types of wastewater. Most industrial wastewaters contain high amount of heavy metals such as zinc, copper, nickel, mercury, cadmium, lead, chromium, and iron [4, 5]. Biopolymers and biocomposites were applied for the removal of heavy metals under different emerging adsorption methods such as batch experiments, physicochemical method, biosorption and desorption processes, and adsorption process.

During the last few years, an increasing amount of dyes have been used in various industrial processes, including paper and pulp manufacturing, plastics, dyeing of cloth, leather treatment, and printing. Most of the dyes are toxic in nature. The presence of dyes in industrial effluents is a major environmental concern because these dyes are usually recalcitrant to microbial degradation [6]. The removal of various pollutants from the textile industry wastewater at low concentrations used many technologies such as chemical oxidation, precipitation, filtration, aerobic and anaerobic microbial degradation, coagulation, membrane separation, electrochemical treatment, flotation, hydrogen peroxide catalysis, reverse osmosis, ozonation, and biological techniques [7, 8]. Among them, the adsorption process has been found to be more effective, efficient, and economic in removing dyes [8]. The removal of heavy metals and dyes in industrial wastewater using biopolymers and biocomposites is presented in this chapter.

14.2 Removal of Heavy Metals from Industrial Wastewater Using Biopolymers and Biocomposites

Biopolymers (also called renewable polymers) are polymers produced by living organisms, and they are polymeric biomolecules. Biocomposites are composite materials and a reinforcement of natural fibers. Biopolymers and biocomposites are biodegradable and ecofriendly products and have been used for the removal of heavy metals from wastewater. The next section describes the types of heavy metals in industrial wastewaters.

14.2.1 Types of Heavy Metals in Industrial Wastewater

Heavy metals are transported by runoff water and contaminate water sources downstream from the industrial site. Different types of industrial wastewaters contain different types of heavy metals (Table 14.1). Most industrial wastewaters contain Pb, Cr, and Cu. Biopolymers and biocomposites have been used for removing heavy metals from industrial wastewaters.

14.2.2 Removal of Heavy Metals Using Biopolymers

Biopolymers are biorenewable and biodegradable. They have advantages (easy to make complicated items, tailorable physical and mechanical properties, surface modification, immobilize cell, etc.) and disadvantages (leachable compounds, absorb water and proteins, etc., surface contamination, wear and breakdown, and difficult to sterilize). Biopolymers such as alginate, cellulose, and chitosan are the most effective adsorbents and used to remove heavy metals in industrial wastewater [9–12]. Alginate is a natural polymer obtained from abundant natural resources, and it can form salt with metal ions from wastewater [13]. Cellulose is the most abundant polymer in nature and is the main component of plant fibers. It can remove heavy-metal ions from aqueous solution with relatively high adsorption capacity [12]. Chitosan is one of the most important derivatives of chitin, which is obtained from the shells of crustaceans such as crabs and shrimps. Chitosan is used for the removal of heavy metals in industrial wastewater [14]. Table 14.1 summarizes the removal of heavy metals using biopolymers.

Table 14.1 Removal of heavy metals in industrial wastewater using biopolymers

Biopolymers	Metals removed	Source of wastewater	Form of biopolymers	Reference
Alginate	Cr(VI), Pb(II), Cu(II)	Mineral operating industries	Powder	[9]
Cellulose	Pb(II), Cr(III), Ni(II), Zn(II), Cd(II), Cu, Hg	Steel and battery, mining, paper, fertilizer industries	Powder	[2, 3, 12, 15]
Chitosan	Cu(II), Mn, Cd, Zn, Co, Ni, Fe, Pb, Cr	Water pipes, copper water heaters, mining, steel, automobile, batteries and paints industries	Powder	[10, 11]

14.2.3 Removal of Heavy Metals Using Biocomposites

Wastewaters from chemical industries contain cadmium, mercury, lead, chromium, copper, nickel, zinc, iron, and arsenic ions. Discharging these metals in wastewater may cause long-term risk to the ecosystem and humans [16]. Alumina is used as an adsorbent, and its acid–base dissociation leads to positive or negative charges on the surface [16]. Chitosan/ceramic alumina composites have been used as an adsorbent to remove heavy metals such as As(III), As(V), Cr(VI), Cu(II), and Ni(II) [17, 18].

Moreover, chitosan/perlite composites have been applied as adsorbents to remove heavy metals such as cadmium, chromium, copper, and nickel [19]. Magnetite is one of the main iron corrosion products and is used more attractively to remove Pb(II), Cu(II), and Cd(II) from water. Chitosan is used on the surface of magnetic nanoparticles [20].

Cotton, a natural cellulosic fiber, possesses many useful characteristics such as comfort, softness, good absorbency and strength, and color retention. Chitosan/cotton fiber composites have been prepared to remove Pb(II), Ni(II), Cd(II), Cu(II), Hg(II), and Au(III) [21, 22]. Sand has been modified to adsorb heavy metals and dyes in wastewater. Chitosan immobilized on sand has been applied in the adsorption of Cu(II) [23].

Chitosan/montmorillonite nanocomposites have excellent mechanical properties, thermal stability, gas barrier, and flame retardation in comparison to conventional composites. Chitosan-coated montmorillonite has been used for the removal of Cr(VI) [24].

Chitosan/polyvinyl alcohol (PVA) is a highly hydrophilic, non-toxic, biocompatible polymer with excellent mechanical strength, thermal stability, and pH stability and has been used to remove Cu(II) and acted as an emulsifier during the preparation of droplets suspension [25]. Chitosan/polyvinyl chloride (PVC) has high surface area, good physical and chemical stabilities especially in concentrated acidic, basic media and organic solvents for a period of time. Sodium dodecyl sulfate coated PVC beads are used to adsorb copper and nickel ions from aqueous solutions [26]. Alginate is a water-soluble linear polysaccharide extracted from brown seaweed, and it has been used to prepare composite beads [27].

Chitosan/bentonite composites are a good adsorbent for removing mercury ions from wastewater [28]. Table 14.2 summarizes the chitosan composites for removal of various heavy metals from wastewater.

Table 14.2 Removal of heavy metals using biocomposites

Biocomposites	Forms of composites	Types of wastewater	Removing agents	Reference
Chitosan/ ceramic alumina	—	Chemical industrial wastewater	As(II), As(V), Cr(VI), Cu(II), Ni(II)	[17, 18, 29]
Chitosan/perlite	Beads	Chemical industrial wastewater	Cd, Cr, Cu, Ni	[19, 30]
Chitosan/ magnetite	—	Chemical industrial wastewater	Pb(II), Cu(II), Cd(II)	[20]
Chitosan/cotton fiber	Beads	Chemical industrial wastewater	Pb(II), Ni(II), Cd(II), Cu(II), Hg(II)	[21, 22, 31]
Chitosan/sand	Particles	Chemical industrial wastewater	Cu(II)	[23, 32]
Chitosan/ cellulose	Beads	Chemical industrial wastewater	Cu(II), Zn(II), Cr(VI), Ni(II), Pb(II)	[33]
Chitosan/ montmorillonite	Beads	Chemical industrial wastewater	Cr(VI)	[24]
Chitosan/ polyvinyl alcohol (PVA)	Beads	Chemical industrial wastewater	Cu(II), Cd(II)	[25, 34]
Chitosan/ polyvinyl chloride (PVC)	Beads	Chemical industrial wastewater	Cu(II), Ni(II)	[26]

Biocomposites	Forms of composites	Types of wastewater	Removing agents	Reference
Chitosan/ calcium alginate composites	Beads	Chemical industrials wastewater	Pb(II), Cu(II), Cd(II), Fe(II), Ni(II)	[27]
Chitosan/ bentonite		Chemical industrials wastewater	Hg(II)	[28]

14.2.4 Method for Treatment of Heavy Metals in Wastewater

Heavy metals from inorganic effluents have been removed using conventional treatment processes, including chemical precipitation, coagulation, complexation, activated carbon adsorption, ion exchange, solvent extraction, foam flotation, electro-deposition, cementation, membrane operations, and electro-remediation methods. Therefore, numerous novel approaches have been studied to develop cost-effective and more efficient heavy-metal adsorption techniques [29–35]. Among these methods, precipitation is most economical and hence widely used, but many industries still use chemical procedures for treatment of effluents due to economic factors. A summary of heavy metal–removal techniques with their removing agents is presented in Table 14.3.

14.2.5 Adsorption Process

Adsorption is the process of accumulating substances (adsorbate in solution) on as suitable interface and adsorbent (such as solid, liquid, or gas phase). These interaction forces are broadly described as physisorption (physical adsorption) and chemisorption (chemical adsorption) [49].

Physical adsorption (physisorption) is relatively non-specific and is due to the operation of weak forces between molecules. In this process, the adsorbed molecule is not affixed to a particular site on the solid surface; it is free to move over the surface [50].

Table 14.3 Methods for analysis and treatment of heavy metals in wastewater

Types of wastewater	Methods for analysis	Pollutants	Methods for treatments	Reference
Industrial wastewater	—	Cu, Zn	Batch method	[36]
Domestic wastewater	—	Zn	Physicochemical methods • Membrane filtration • Adsorption • Ion exchange • Reverse osmosis • Chemical precipitation or solvent extraction Biological methods	[37]
Industrial wastewater	Atomic absorption spectrometer (AAS)	Fe, Zn, Cu	Biosorption process using sea weed	[2]
Aqueous solutions	-	Cr(VI), Pb(II), Cu(II)	Biosorption and desorption processes Using calcium alginate beads	[38]
Industrial wastewater	Fourier transform infrared spectroscopy (FTIR)	Cu(II)	Adsorption using chitosan	[10]

Types of wastewater	Methods for analysis	Pollutants	Methods for treatments	Reference
Industrial wastewater	—	Pb(II), Cd(II), Zn(II), Cu(II), Ni(II), Co(II), Cr(VI)	• Physicochemical removal processes • Adsorption on new adsorbents	[4]
Industrial wastewater (fertilizer, mining operations, batteries, paper, tanneries, pesticides)	—	Cu(II), Cr(VI), Cr(III), Cd(II), Pb(II), Ni(II), Ag(II), Zn(II)	• Chemical precipitation • Hydroxide sulfide • Adsorption • Biosorption • Membrane filtration • Ultrafiltration • Nanofiltration • Coagulation and flocculation • Flotation • Electrodialysis • Electrochemical treatment	[3]
Aqueous solution	—	Cu(II), Cr(VI)	• Batch processes (using chitosan)	[39]

(Continued)

Table 14.3 (Continued)

Types of wastewater	Methods for analysis	Pollutants	Methods for treatments	Reference
Agricultural wastewater	—	As, Cd, Cr, Cu, Ni, Zn, Pb, Hg	• Adsorption capacities • Binding mechanisms • Operation factors • Pretreatment method	[40]
Industrial wastewater	—	Fe(II), Cu(II), Zn(II), Pb(II)	Batch sorption experiment	[41]
Industrial wastewater	—	Cr(VI), Cr(III)	Biosorption process (using new composite biosorbent prepared by coating chitosan)	[42]
Industrial wastewater	—	Cu(II), Ni(II), Zn(II), Pb(II)	Physical measurements	[43]
Chemical industrial; mining industrial	.	Cd, Pb, Zn, Ni, Cu, Cr, Cr(III)	Batch adsorption studies	[44]
Industrial wastewater	—	Cu(II)	(Using chitosan and sodium alginate)	[13]
Industrial wastewater	—	Hg, Cd, Pb, As, Cr, Tl	Adsorption processes (using egg shell)	[45]

Types of wastewater	Methods for analysis	Pollutants	Methods for treatments	Reference
Industrial wastewater	—	Cu, Ag, Zn, Cd, Hg, Pb, Cr, Fe, Ni, As, Co, Mn, Al	• Physicochemical removal processes • Chemical precipitation • Coagulation and flocculation • Electrochemical treatments • Ion exchange • Membrane filtration • Electrodialysis • Biological method	[46]
Chemical industrial	—	Se, Cr, Pb, Cu, Ni	• Biosorption (using algae) • By bacteria and microorganism • Activated sludge process • Biofilter • Anaerobic digestion • Stabilization ponds	[47]
Aqueous solution	—	Cu(II)	Batch and continuous sorption studies (using marine alga, *Sargassum tenerrimum*)	[48]

Chemical adsorption (chemisorption) is also based on electrostatic forces, but much stronger forces act on this process. In chemisorption, the attraction between adsorbent and adsorbate is a covalent or electrostatic chemical bond between atoms, with shorter bond length and higher bond energy [51].

Adsorption using activated carbon has been considered one of the best alternative treatments for water and wastewater due to its high removal efficiency without the production of harmful byproducts. A summary of properties of physisorption and chemisorption is presented in Table 14.4.

Table 14.4 Properties of physisorption and chemisorption

Characteristics of adsorption	Physisorption	Chemisorption
Adsorption type	Multilayer	Monolayer
Adsorption specificity	Low degree of specificity	High degree of specificity, depends on the number of active sites
Identity of molecule	Desorption is possible (adsorbed molecule keeps its identity)	Desorption is impossible (adsorbed molecule loses its identity)
Thermal properties	Exothermic	Exothermic or endothermic

Source: Ref. [52].

14.2.6 Advantages and Disadvantages of Heavy Metal–Removal Techniques

Heavy metal–removal techniques are precipitation (the most widely used technique for the removal of heavy metals in inorganic effluents from industry; it produces insoluble precipitates of heavy metals as hydroxide, sulfide, carbonate, and phosphate), chemical coagulation (based on zeta potential measurement as the criteria to define the electrostatic interaction between pollutants and coagulant–flocculant agents), ion exchange (a widely used method and can attract soluble ions in water treatment industry that involves effective low-cost materials for removing heavy metals from aqueous solutions), electrochemical (used to remove metals from wastewater streams; uses electricity to pass a current through an aqueous metal-bearing solution containing a cathode plate and an insoluble anode), and adsorption (activated carbon is used for removal of trace heavy metals). Moreover, membrane filtration (ultrafiltration, nanofiltration, and reverse osmosis), biosorption (biological removal of heavy metals in wastewater using biological techniques), and electrodialysis (a membrane separation and passed through an ion exchange membrane by applying an electric potential) are used to remove heavy metals from wastewater [46]. A summary of techniques for removal of heavy metals is presented with their advantages and disadvantages in Table 14.5.

Table 14.5 Advantages and disadvantages of heavy metal–removal techniques

Methods	Advantages	Disadvantages
Chemical precipitation	• Low capital cost • Simple operation • Inexpensive • Can remove most of metals	• Sludge generation • Extra operation cost for sludge disposal • Large amounts of sludge
Chemical coagulation	• Sludge settling dewatering	• High cost • Large consumption of chemicals
Ion exchange	• High regeneration of materials • Metal selective	• High cost • Less number of metal ions removed
Electrochemical	• Metal selective • No consumption of chemicals • Pure metals can be achieved	• High capital and running cost • Initial solution pH and current density
Adsorption using activated carbon	• Most metals can be removed • High efficiency (>99%)	• Cost of activated carbon • No regeneration • Performance depends on adsorbent

(*Continued*)

Table 14.5 (Continued)

Methods	Advantages	Disadvantages
Adsorption with new adsorbents	• Low cost • Easy operation conditions • Having wide pH range • High metal binding capacities	• Low selectivity • Production of waste products
Membrane filtration	• Small space requirement • Low pressure • High separation selectivity	• High operational cost due to membrane fouling
Biosorption	• Low cost • High efficiency • Minimization of sludge • Regeneration of biosorbents • No additional nutrient requirement • Metal recovery	• Early saturation • Limited potential for biological process improvement • No potential for biologically altering the metal valence state
Electrodialysis	• High separation selectivity	• High operational cost due to membrane fouling energy consumption
Photocatalysis	• Removal of metals and organic pollutant simultaneously • Less harmful by products	• Long duration time • Limited applications

Source: Kurniawan et al. (2006), Babel and Kurniawan (2003), Aklil et al. (2004), Kurniawan et al. (2006), Mohammadi et al. (2005), Barakat et al. (2004), and Kajitvichyanukula et al. (2005) cited in Refs. [4] and [40].

14.2.7 Types of Heavy Metals and Their Effect on Human Health

Living organisms require trace amounts of some heavy metals (including cobalt, copper, iron, manganese, and zinc). Most heavy metals are well-known toxic and carcinogenic agents and, even at low concentrations, can cause toxicity to humans and other forms of life. Contaminated water represents a serious threat to human population. The toxicity of metal ions is due to their ability to bind with protein molecules and prevent replication of DNA. To avoid health hazards, it is essential to remove these toxic heavy metals from wastewater before disposal [2]. The effects on human health are quite evident, as shown in Table 14.6.

Table 14.6 Types of heavy metals and their effect on human health

Pollutants	Major sources	Effect on human health	Permissible level (mg/L)
Arsenic	• Pesticides • Fungicides • Metal smelters • As a wood preservative • Tobacco smoke • Production of iron and steel	• Bronchitis • Dermatitis • Poisoning • Carcinogen (lung cancer) • Death • Diarrhea	0.02
Cadmium	• Welding • Electroplating • Pesticides, fertilizers • Cd and Ni batteries • Nuclear fission plant • Cigarette smoke	• Kidney damage • Bronchitis • Gastrointestinal disorder • Bone marrow • Cancer • Severe pain in joints	0.06
Lead	• Paint • Pesticides • Smoking • Automobile emission • Mining • Burning of coal • Pipes • Batteries • Sinkers in fishing	• Liver damage • Kidney disorder • Gastrointestinal damage • Mental retardation in children • Memory loss • Headaches • Tiredness • Transferred postnatally from the mother through breast milk	0.1

(Continued)

Table 14.6 (Continued)

Pollutants	Major sources	Effect on human health	Permissible level (mg/L)
Manganese	• Welding • Fuel addition • Ferromanganese production	• Inhalation or contact causes damage to central nervous system	0.2
Mercury	• Pesticides • Batteries • Paper industry • Electrical switches • Burning of coal	• Damage to nervous system • Protoplasm poisoning • Skin burns • Damage to the kidney • Damage to the brain function • Death • Severe brain damage	0.01
Zinc	• Refineries • Brass manufacture • Metal plating • Plumbing • Batteries	• Zinc fumes have corrosive effect on skin, cause damage to nervous membrane	15
Chromium	• Mining • Mineral sources	• Damage to the nervous system • Fatigue • Lung cancer • Death • Kidney and liver damage	0.05
Copper	• Mining • Pesticide production • Chemical industry • Metal piping	• Anemia • Kidney and liver damage • Stomach and intestinal irritation	0.1

Source: From Refs. [2, 29, 53].

14.3 Removal of Textile Dyes in Industrial Wastewater Using Biopolymers and Biocomposites

Dyes are colored organic compounds used to give color to various substrates, including paper, leather, hair, drugs, foods, cosmetics, plastics, and textile. Dyes consist of two main groups of compounds: chromophores and auxochromes. Chromophores determine the color of the dye, while auxochromes determine the intensity of the color [54]. Textile industry effluents contain various kinds of synthetics dyes, which is the main problem for wastewater treatment [55]. Dye wastes are very harmful to the environment even when they are present in concentrations less than 1 mg/L in wastewater. Dyes are classified into three groups: anionic, cationic, and insoluble. They can also cause allergic dermatitis and skin irritation.

14.3.1 Classification of Dyes Based on Their Applications

Dyes have been classified based on chemical composition and applications. Dyes are widely used to impart color to fabrics, plastics, food, print, and leather [6]. Azo dyes are immensely used as commercial dyes in industries such as textiles, cosmetics, pulp and paper, paint, pharmaceutical, carpet and printing, leather, and food. In humans, contact with colored wastewater may cause serious health problems and hazards-induced diseases such as allergy, skin diseases, mutation, and cancer [56]. It can also be harmful for kidneys, liver, brain, and the central nervous system. A summary of classification of dyes is presented with their applications in Table 14.7.

Table 14.7 Classification of dyes based on their applications

Types of dye	Examples	Application
Acid dyes	Methyl orange, methyl red, orange I, orange II, and Congo red acid (blue, black, violet, yellow)	Wool, silk, polyurethane fibers nylon

(Continued)

Table 14.7 (Continued)

Types of dye	Examples	Application
Basic dyes	Aniline yellow, butter yellow, methylene blue, malachite green, basic red, basic brown, basic blue, crystal violet, brilliant green	Reinforced nylon, polyesters, wool, silk, mod-acrylic
Direct dyes	Martius yellow and Congo red, direct black, direct orange, direct blue, direct violet, direct red	Cotton, rayon, wool, silk and nylon, flax, leather in (alkaline or neutral bath)
Disperse dyes	Celliton fast pink B, celliton fast blue B, disperse blue, disperse red, disperse orange, disperse yellow, disperse brown	Synthetic polyamide fibers, polyesters, nylon and polyacrylonitriles
Fiber reactive dye	Procion dye (2,4,6-trichloro 1,3,5-triazine), reactive red, reactive blue, reactive yellow, reactive black, remazol (blue, yellow, red, etc.)	Cotton, wool, and silk, cellulosic fibers, polyamide
Ingrain azo dye	Para red	Cotton (cellulose), silk, nylon, polyester, polyester and leather, coloring agent in food
Vat dyes	Indigo, tyrian purple, benzanthrone indigo, vat blue, vat green	Wool, coloring agent in food, flax, rayon fibers
Mordant	Alizarin	Cotton and wools

Source: From Refs. [6, 56].

14.3.2 Types of Textile Dyes in Industrial Wastewater

Textile dyes are found in wastewater from various industries. Table 14.8 summarizes the dyes removed from some industrial wastewater.

Table 14.8 Dyes in some industrial wastewaters

Types of industrial wastewater	Dyes
Plastics industry	Disperse blue, disperse red, disperse orange, disperse yellow, disperse brown
Dyeing of cloth	Congo red, methyl (orange and red), orange (I, II), acid (blue, black, violet, yellow)
Leather	Martius yellow, direct black, direct orange, direct blue, direct violet, direct red

Source: From Refs. [6, 57].

14.3.3 Removal of Textile Dyes in Industrial Wastewater Using Biopolymers

Textile dyes are removed from industrial wastewaters using biopolymers such as poly(propyleneimine), chitin, and chitosan. Chitin and chitosan efficiently remove many different dyes and are widely used for the removal of dyes as biosorbents. Table 14.9 summarizes the removal of dyes from industrial wastewater using some biopolymers.

Table 14.9 Removal of textile dyes in industrial wastewater using biopolymers

Biopolymers	Removing agents
Chitosan-polypropyleneimine (CS-PPI)	Reactive black 5 (RB 5), reactive red 198 (RR 198)
Chitin	Anionic dyes
Chitosan	Anionic and cationic dyes

Source: From Refs. [58–60].

14.3.4 Removal of Textile Dyes in Industrial Wastewater Using Biocomposites

Montmorillonite-forming chitosan composites are used to remove Congo red. The molar ratio of chitosan to montmorillonite could influence the chemical environment of composites. It was found that the adsorption capacity of Congo red increased till the molar ratio of chitosan and montmorillonite exceeded 1:1, after which the adsorption remained almost constant. There are two possible reasons for this scenario. First, this could be due to the balancing of initial negative charge of montmorillonite by chitosan, which would enhance the adsorption capacity of Congo red. Second, it may be caused by the montmorillonite being saturated with the amount of intercalated chitosan [61].

Polyurethane has various applications such as insulator in walls and roofs, flexible foam in upholster furniture, medical devices, and foot wears [62]. Polyurethane used to form chitosan composites in adsorbing Acid Violet 48. Clay has a wide variety of uses due to its chemical and physical properties, and modified clays are used to adsorb dyes and heavy metals [63]. Montmorillonite is mainly composed of SiO_2, Al_2O_3, CaO, MgO, Fe_2O_3, Na_2O, and K_2O. Bentonites have been used to remove aromatic organics from oily liquid wastes and chitosan/bentonite composites to adsorb tartrazine, a dye containing azo group, which is harmful to living things [64].

In addition, chitosan/oil palm composite beads remove reactive blue 19 [65]. Kaolinite is a 1:1 aluminosilicate, consisting of SiO_2, Al_2O_3, and H_2O. A new chitosan bead was prepared, which was blended with maghemite and kaolin [66]. Perlite is a glassy volcanic rock varying in color from grey to black and used in the adsorption of dyes such as methyl violet. The list of chitosan biocomposites used to remove dyes in wastewater is summarized in Table 14.10.

Table 14.10 Removal of textile dyes in industrial wastewater using biocomposites

Biocomposites	Forms of composites	Types of wastewater	Dye	Reference
Chitosan/ montmorillonite		Textile industrial wastewater	Congo red	[61]

Biocomposites	Forms of composites	Types of wastewater	Dye	Reference
Chitosan/ polyurethane		Textile industrial wastewater	Acid violet	[62]
Chitosan/ activated clay	Beads	Textile industrial wastewater	Methylene blue, reactive dye RR22	[63]
Chitosan/ bentonite	Beads	Textile industrial wastewater	Tartrazine malachite green	[64]
Chitosan/oil palm ash	Beads	Textile industrial wastewater	Reactive blue 19	[65]
Chitosan/ kaolin-γ-Fe$_2$SO$_3$	Beads	Textile industrial wastewater	Methyl orange	[66]
Chitosan/perlite		Textile industrial wastewater	Methyl violet	[66]

14.3.5 Method for Treatment of Textile Dye in Wastewater

Most of the dyes are stable to photodegradation and biodegradation. Colored wastewater poses a challenge to conventional wastewater treatment techniques such as coagulation, flocculation, membrane separation, oxidation, or ozonation. Adsorption is an effective, cheap, and potential technique for removing dyes. In recent years, natural polymeric materials have drawn considerable attention because they are renewable, biodegradable, non-toxic, and has potential as an environment friendly material [60]. A summary of dye-removal techniques is presented with their removing agents in Table 14.11.

Table 14.11 Method for treatment of textile dye in wastewater

Types of wastewater	Methods	Removing agents	Reference
Textile wastewater	Physical and chemical methods • Oxidation • Adsorption • Membrane technologies • Coagulation/ flocculation	Color	[7]
Industrial wastewater (plastics, dyeing of cloth, leather)	• Bioflocculation (using bacteria, *Sphingomonas*, gram-negative, rod-shaped, aerobic)	Dyes	[57]
Industrial wastewater	• Batch adsorption experiments (using ferric oxide as an adsorbent)	Color	[8]
Textile industrial	• Biosorption processes (using chitosan microcapsules)	Cd(II), Zn(II)	[67]
Synthetic dye house effluents	• Physical and chemical methods (using activated carbon)	Dyes	[68]

14.3.6 Advantages and Disadvantages of Various Dye-Removal Techniques

Dyes in wastewater effluents have been treated using different separation techniques such as physiochemical, chemical, and biological methods. The advantages and disadvantages of techniques to remove dyes in wastewaters are given in Table 14.12.

Table 14.12 Advantages and disadvantages of various dye-removal techniques

Separation techniques	Advantages	Disadvantages
Adsorption	Most effective adsorbent	Ineffective against disperse and vat dyes
Ion exchange	No loss of sorbents, effective	Economic constraints, not effective for disperse dyes

Separation techniques	Advantages	Disadvantages
Membrane filtration	Effective for all dyes with high-quality effluent	High pressures, expensive, incapable of treating large volumes
Electrokinetic coagulation	Simple, economically feasible	Needs further treatments by flocculation and filtration and production of sludge
Fenton reagent	Effective process and cheap reagent	Sludge production and disposal problems
Ozonation	No production of sludge	Half-life is very short (20 min) and high operational cost
Photocatalyst	Economically feasible and low operational cost	Degradation of some photocatalyst into toxic byproducts
Aerobic degradation	Efficient in the removal of azo dyes and low operational cost	Very slow process and provide suitable environment for growth of microorganisms
Anaerobic degradation	Byproducts can be used as energy sources	Need further treatment under aerobic conditions and yield of methane and hydrogen sulfide

Source: Refs. [6, 69, 70].

14.4 Conclusion

Many investigators have tried various methods for the removal of heavy metals and textile dyes from industrial wastewater. In recent years, a wide range of technologies, such as chemical precipitation, adsorption, membrane filtration, electrodialysis, and photocatalysis, have been developed for removing heavy metals from wastewater. It is important to note that the selection of the most suitable technology depends on some basic parameters such as pH, initial metal concentration, the overall treatment performance, environmental impacts, and economic parameters such as the capital investment and operational costs. Finally, technical applicability, plant simplicity, and cost-effectiveness are the key factors that play major roles in the selection of the most suitable treatment system for inorganic effluents. All the factors mentioned above should be taken into consideration in selecting the most effective and inexpensive treatment in order to protect the environment.

Acknowledgment

The authors thank the European Union for financial support, Mr. Win MyoThu, President, Advancing Life and Regenerating Morther land (ALARM), Yangon, Myanmar for his encouragement and members of Ecological Laboratory, Advancing Life and Regenerating Morther land (ALARM), Yangon, Myanmar for their support.

References

1. Bagul, V. R., Shinde, D. N., Chavan, R. P., Patil, C. L., and Pawar, R. K. (2015). New perspective on heavy metal pollution of water, *J. Chem. Pharm. Res.*, **7**(12), pp. 700–705.
2. Abdullah, S. B. (2010). Heavy metals removal from industries wastewater by using sea weed through biosorption process, Dissertation thesis, Faculty of Civil Engineering and Earth Resources, University Malaysia Pahang.
3. Fenglian, F. and Wang, Q. (2011). Removal of heavy metal ions from wastewater: A review, *J. Environ. Manag.*, **92**, pp. 407–418.
4. Barakat, M. A. (2011). New trends in removing heavy metals from industrial wastewater. *Arabian J. Chem.*, **4**, pp. 361–377.
5. Jaros, K., Kaminski, W., Albinska, J., and Nowak, U. (2005). Removal of heavy metal ions: Copper, zinc and chromium from water on chitosan beads, *Environ. Protection Eng.*, **31**, pp. 1–10.
6. Gonawala, K. H. and Mehta, M. J. (2014). Removal of color from different dye wastewater by using ferric oxide as an adsorbent, *J. Eng. Res. Appl.*, **4**, pp. 102–109.
7. Dawood, S. and Sen, T. K. (2014). Review on dye removal from its aqueous solution into alternative cost effective and non-conventional adsorbents, *J. Chem. Process Eng.*, **1**, pp. 1–11.
8. Pearce, C. I., Lioyd, J. R., and Guthrie, J. T. (2003). The removal of colour from textile waste water using whole bacterial cell: A review, *Dyes Pigment.*, **58**, pp. 179–196.

9. Gotoh, T., Matsushima, K., and Kikuchi, K. I. (2004). Preparation of alginate-chitosan hybrid gel beads and adsorption of divalent metal ions, *Chemosphere*, **55**, pp. 135–140.

10. Hadi, A. G. (2013). Synthesis of chitosan and its use in metal removal, *Chem. Mater. Res.*, **3**(3), pp. 2224–3224.

11. Rana, M. S., Halim, M. A., Safiullah, S., and MamunMollah, M. (2009). Removal of heavy metal from contaminated water by biopolymer crab shell chitosan, *J. Appl. Sci.*, **9**(15), pp. 2762–2769.

12. Sungur, S. and Babaoglu, S. (2005). Synthesis of a new cellulose ion exchanger and use for the separation of heavy metals in aqueous solutions, *Sep. Sci. Technol.*, **40**, pp. 2067–2078.

13. Qin, Y., Shi, B., and Liu, J. (2006). Application of chitosan and alginate in treating wastewater containing heavy metal ions, *Indian J. Chem. Technol.*, **13**, pp. 464–469.

14. Knorr, D. (1984). Use of chitinous polymers in food: A challenge for food research and development, *Food Technol.*, **38**(1), pp. 85–97.

15. Aziz, H. A., Adlan, M. N., and Ariffin, K. S. (2008). Heavy metals [Cd, Pb, Zn, Ni, Cu, Cr (III)] removal from water in Malaysia: Post treatment by high quality limestone, *Bioresour. Technol.*, **99**, pp. 1578–1583.

16. Wan Ngah, W. S., Teong, L. C., and Hanafiah, M. A. K. M. (2011). Adsorption of dyes and heavy metal ions by chitosan composites: A review, *Carbohydr. Polym.*, **83**, pp. 1446–1456.

17. Veera, M. B., Krishnaiah, A., Ann, J. R., and Edgar, D. S. (2008). Removal of copper (II) and nickel (II) ions from aqueous solutions by a composite chitosan biosorbent, *Sep. Sci. Technol.*, **43**, pp. 1365–1381.

18. Veera, M. B., Krishnaiah, A., Jonathan, L. T., Edgar, D. S., and Richard, H. (2008). Removal of arsenic (III) and arsenic (V) from aqueous medium using chitosan-coated biosorbent, *Water Res.*, **42**, pp. 633–642.

19. Shameem, H., Abburi, K., Tushar, K. G., Dabir, S. V., Veera, M. B., and Edgar, D. S. (2006). Adsorption of divalent cadmium [Cd(II)] from aqueous solutions onto chitosan coated perlite beads, *Ind. Eng. Chem. Res.*, **45**, pp. 5066–5077.

20. Tran, H. V., Tran, L. D., and Nguyen, T. N. (2010). Preparation of chitosan/magnetite composite beads and their application for removal of Pb(II) and Ni(II) from aqueous solution, *Mater. Sci. Eng.*, **30**, pp. 304–310.

21. Qu, R. J., Sun, C. M., Fang, M., Zhang, Y., Ji, C. N., and Xu, Q. (2009). Removal and recovery of Hg(II) from aqueous solution using chitosan-coated cotton fibers, *J. Hazard. Mater.*, **167**, pp. 717–727.

22. Qu, R. J., Sun, C. M., Wang, M. H., Ji, C. N., Xu, Q., and Zhang, Y. (2009). Adsorption of Au(III) from aqueous solution using cotton fiber/ chitosan composite adsorbents, *Hydrometallurgy*, **100**, pp. 65–71.

23. Wan, M. W., Kan, C. C., Lin, C. H., Buenda, D. R., and Wu, C. H. (2007). Adsorption of copper (II) by chitosan immobilized on sand, *Chia-Nan Annu. Bull.*, **33**, pp. 96–106.

24. Fan, D. H., Zhu, X. M., Xu, M. R., and Yan, J. L. (2006). Adsorption properties of chromium (VI) by chitosan coated montmorillonite, *J. Biol Sci.*, **6**, pp. 941–945.

25. Kumar, M., Bijay, P. T., and Vinod, K. S. (2009). Crosslinked chitosan/ polyvinyl alcohol blend beads for removal and recovery of Cd(II) from wastewater, *J. Hazard. Mater.*, **172**, pp. 1041–1048.

26. Srinivasa, R. P., Vijaya, Y., Veera, M. B., and Krishnaiah, A. (2009). Adsorptive removal of copper and nickel ions from water using chitosan coated PVC beads, *Bioresour. Technol.*, **100**, pp. 194–199.

27. Vijaya, Y., Srinivasa, R. P., Veera, M. B., and Krishnaiah, A. (2008). Modified chitosan and calcium alginate biopolymer sorbents for removal of nickel (II) through adsorption, *Carbohydr. Polym.*, **72**, pp. 261–271.

28. Yang, Y. Q. and Chen, H. J. (2007). Study on the intercalation organic bentonite and its adsorption, *J. Xinyang Normal University*, **20**, pp. 338–340.

29. Krishnamurthy, S. (1992). Biomethylation and environmental transport of metals, *J. Chem. Educ.*, **69**(5), pp. 347.

30. Kalyani, S., Ajitha, P. J., Srinivasa, R. P., and Krishnaiah, A. (2005). Removal of copper and nickel from aqueous solutions using chitosan coated on perlite as biosorbent, *Sep. Sci. Technol.*, **40**, pp. 1483–1495.

31. Zhang, G. Y., Qu, R. J., Sun, C. M., Ji, C. N., Chen, H., and Wang, C. H. (2008). Adsorption metal ions of chitosan coated cotton fiber, *J. Appl. Polym. Sci.*, **110**, pp. 2321–2327.

32. Wan, M. W., Kan, C. C., Buenda, D. R., and Maria, L. P. D. (2010). Adsorption of copper (II) and lead (II) ions from aqueous solution on chitosan-coated sand, *Carbohydr. Polym.*, **80**, pp. 891–899.

33. Sun, X. Q., Peng, B., Jing, Y., Chen, J., and Li, D. Q. (2009). Chitosan (chitin)/cellulose composite biosorbents prepared using ionic liquid for heavy metal ions adsorption, *Separations*, **55**, pp. 2062–2069.

34. Wan Ngah, W. S., Kamari, A., and Koay, Y. J. (2004). Equilibrium kinetics studies of adsorption of copper (II) on chitosan and chitosan/PVA beads, *J. Biol. Macromol.*, **34**, pp. 155–161.

35. Gunatilake, S. K. (2015). Methods of removing heavy metals from industrials wastewater, *J. Multidiscip. Eng. Sci. Studies*, **1**, pp. 12–18.
36. Jo, Y. H., Do, S. H., Jang, Y. S., and Kong, S. H. (2010). The removal of metal ions (Cu^{2+}, Zn^{2+}) using waste reclaimed adsorbent for plating wastewater treatment process, *Proc. World Congr. Eng. Comput. Sci.*, **2**, pp. 1–5.
37. Gakwisiri, C., Raut, N., Al Saadi, A., Al Aisri, S., and Al Ajmi, A. (2012). A critical review of removal of zinc from wastewater, *Proc. World Congr. Eng. Comput. Sci.*, **1**, pp. 1–5.
38. Pandey, A., Bera, D., Shukla, A., and Ray, L. (2007). Studies on Cr(VI), Pb(II) and Cd(II) adsorption–desorption using calcium alginate as biopolymer, *Chem. Speciat. Bioavailab.*, **18**(1), pp. 17–24.
39. Schmuhl, R., Krieg, H. M., and Keizer, K. (2001). Adsorption of Cu(II) and Cr(VI) ions by chitosan: Kinetics and equilibrium studies, *Water SA*, **27**, pp. 1–7.
40. Nguyen, T. A. H., Ngo, H. H., Guo, W. S., Zhang, J., Liang, S., Yue, Q. Y., Li, Q., and Nguyen, T. V. (2013). Applicability of agricultural waste and by-products for adsorptive removal of heavy metal from wastewater, *Bioresour. Technol.*, **148**, pp. 574–585.
41. Dhabab, J. M. (2011). Removal of Fe(II), Cu(II), Zn(II) and Pb(II) ions from aqueous solution by duckweed, *J. Oceanogr. Marine Sci.*, **2**(1), pp. 17–22.
42. Nomanbbay, S. M. and Palanisamy, K. (2005). Removal of heavy metal from industrial wastewater using chitosan coated oil palm shell charcoal, *Electron. J. Biotechnol.*, **8**(1), DOI: 10.2225/vol8-issue1-fulltext-7.
43. Ahmad Bhat, M., Mukhtar, F., Chisti, H., and Ahmad Shah, S. (2014). Removal of heavy metal ions from wastewater by using oxalic acid: An alternative method, *J. Latest Res. Sci. Technol.*, **3**, pp. 61–64.
44. Aziz, H. A., Adlan, M. N., and Ariffin, K. S. (2008). Heavy metals [Cd, Pb, Zn, Ni, Cu, Cr (III)] removal from water in Malaysia: Post treatment by high quality limestone, *Bioresour. Technol.*, **99**, pp. 1578–1583.
45. Devi, R. (2015). Removal of heavy metals from wastewater using low cost adsorbents: A review, *Int. J. Recent Res. Aspects*, **2**, pp. 5–7.
46. Gunatilake, S. K. (2015). Methods of removing heavy metals from industrials wastewater, *J. Multidiscip. Eng. Sci. Studies*, **1**, pp. 12–18.
47. Dhokpande, S. R. and Jayant, P. K. (2013). Biological methods for heavy metals removal: A review, *J. Eng. Sci. Innovative Technol.*, **2**, pp. 304–309.

48. Sivaprakash, B., Rajamohan, N., and Mohamed Sadhik, A. (2010). Batch and column sorption of heavy metal from aqueous solution using a marine alga *Sargassum tenerrimum, J. Chem. Tech. Res.*, **2**, pp. 155–162.
49. Rouquerol, F. (1999). *Adsorption by Powders and Porous Solids* (Academic Press, London), pp. 1–21, 355–361, 378–382.
50. Sawyer, N. C., Mc Carty, P. L., and Parkin, G. F. (1994). *Chemistry for Environmental Engineering* (McGraw Hill International Edition, Singapore), pp. 1–19.
51. Montgomery, J. M. (1985). *Water Treatment Principles and Design* (Consulting Engineers Inc., USA), pp. 312–326.
52. Atkins, P. V. (1994). *Physical Chemistry*, 5th ed. (Oxford University Press, Oxford), pp. 324–326.
53. Baird, C. (2000). *Environmental Chemistry*, 3rd ed. (W. H. Freeman and Company, New York), pp. 1–17.
54. Moussavi, G. and Mahmoudi, M. (2009). Removal of azo and anthraquinone reactive dyes by using MgO nanoparticles, *J. Hazard. Mater.*, **168**, pp. 806–812.
55. Crini, G. (2006). Low-cost adsorbents for dye removal: A review, *Bioresour. Technol.*, **97**, pp. 1061–1085.
56. Sarkheil, H., Noormohammadi, F., Rezaei, A. R., and Borujeni, M. K. (2014). Dye pollution removal from mining and industrial wastewaters using chitson nanoparticles, *Int. Conf. Agriculture Environ Biol Sci.*, June 4–5, 2014, Antalya, Turkey, pp. 37–43.
57. Buthelezi, S. P., Olaniran, A. O., and Pillay, B. (2012). Textile dye removal from wastewater effluents using bioflocculants produced by indigenous bacterial isolates, *Molecules*, **17**, pp. 14260–14274.
58. Kiakhani, M. S., Arami, M., and Gharanjig, K. (2013). Dye removal from colored textile waste water using chitosan-PPI dendrimer hybrid as a biopolymer: Optimization, *Kinetic Isotherm Studies*, **127**, pp. 2607–2619.
59. Longhinotti, E. and Pozza, F. (1998). Adsorption of anionic dyes on the biopolymer chitin, *J. Braz. Chem. Soc.*, **9**(5), http://dx.doi.org/10.1590/S0103-50531998000500005.
60. Saraswathi, P., Nirmala Devi, V., and Makeswari, M. (2016). Removal of dyes from aqueous solution by using modified chitosan as an adsorbent, *J. Chem. Pharm. Res.*, **8**(6), pp. 468–471.
61. Wang, L. and Wang, A. (2007). Adsorption characteristics of Congo Red onto the chitosan/montmorillonite nanocomposite, *J. Hazard. Mater.*, **147**, pp. 979–985.

62. Won, S. L., Lee, H. C., Jeong, Y. G., Min, B. G., and Lee, S. C. (2009). Preparation and acid dye adsorption behavior of polyurethane/chitosan composite foams, *Fibers Polym.*, **10**, pp. 636–642.

63. Chang, M. Y. and Juang, R. S. (2004). Adsorption of tannic acid, humic acid and dyes from water using the composite of chitosan and activated clay, *J. Colloid Interface Sci.*, **278**, pp. 18–25.

64. Wan Ngah, W. S., Ariff, N. F. M., and Hanafiah, M. A. K. M. (2010). Preparation, characterization, and environmental application of crosslinked chitosan-coated bentonite for tartrazine adsorption from aqueous solutions, *Water, Air, Soil Pollut.*, **206**, pp. 225–236.

65. Hameed, B. H., Hasan, M., and Ahmad, A. L. (2008). Adsorption of reactive dye onto cross-linked chitosan/oil palm ash composite beads, *J. Chem. Eng.*, **136**, pp. 164–172.

66. Zhu, H. Y., Jiang, R., and Xiao, L. (2010). Adsorption of an anionic dye bychitosan/kaolin/γ-Fe$_2$O$_3$ composites, *Appl. Clay Sci.*, **48**, pp. 522–526.

67. Sargin, I. and Arslan, G. (2015). Chitosan/sporopollenin microcapsules: Preparation, characterization and application in heavy metal removal, *J. Biol. Macromol.*, **75**, pp. 230–238.

68. Sivamani, S. and Grace, B. L. (2009). Removal of dyes from wastewater using adsorption: A review, *J. Biosci. Technol.*, **2**, pp. 47–51.

69. Kharub, M. (2012). Use of various technologies, methods and adsorbents for the removal of dye: A review, *J. Environmental Research and Development.*, **6**, pp. 879–883.

70. Sharma, S., Saxena, R., and Gaur, G. (2014). Study of removal techniques for Azo dyes by biosorption: A review, *J. Applied Chemistry.*, **7**(10), pp. 6–21.

Chapter 15

Bio-based Material Protein and Its Novel Applications

Tanvir Arfin and Pooja R. Mogarkar
*Environmental Materials Division, CSIR-NEERI, Nehru Marg,
Nagpur 440020, India*
tanvirarfin@gmail.com

Proteins are one of the vital ecofriendly macromolecules consisting long chains of amino acid residues known as polypeptide. They have unique structural, chemical, mechanical, and biological properties. Due to the variant properties of proteins, there are abundant innovative protein applications. This chapter mainly attempts a brief description of classification, structure, properties, and applications of proteins in various fields such as food, biomedicine, agriculture, packaging, tissue engineering, textiles, biosensors, and electronics. The nutritional importance of protein is also highlighted in the present chapter. Special attention is given toward the biocomposite of protein in order to grow ecofriendly materials such as films, gels, particles, hydrogels, tubes, fibers, as well as electrical and optical devices having excellent physical and chemical properties that are

Biocomposites: Biomedical and Environmental Applications
Edited by Shakeel Ahmed, Saiqa Ikram, Suvardhan Kanchi, and Krishna Bisetty
Copyright © 2018 Pan Stanford Publishing Pte. Ltd.
ISBN 978-981-4774-38-3 (Hardcover), 978-1-315-11080-6 (eBook)
www.panstanford.com

environmental friendly and cost effective. Extensive research is being carried out for enhancing the characteristics of protein and its composites to produce a variety of promising products in packaging, biomedicine, agriculture, and tissue engineering.

15.1 Introduction

The name protein was introduced from the Greek word "Proteios," meaning primary or first. The name itself indicates the importance of proteins and is suitable since they are concerned with almost all physiological processes, playing a multiple role in biological processes. One can define proteins as naturally occurring nitrogenous polypeptide compounds, which give a mixture of various α-amino acids upon hydrolysis. Macro-biomolecular proteins are complex nitrogenous organic compounds present in plants and animals (i.e., in all living cells, muscles, blood, hairs, nails, leathers, skin, silk, wool). They are molecules of large size, complexity, and variety. Proteins are composed of carbon, hydrogen, oxygen, nitrogen, and usually sulfur. Proteins may also contain trace elements (e.g., phosphorus, iron). The molecular weight of protein ranges from a few thousand to a million or more. The polymeric compounds of α-amino acids, having molecular weight up to 10,000, are called polypeptides, and those having molecular weight more than 10,000 are regarded as proteins. Proteins perform numerous functions other than those molecules concerned with the compounds of food. Enzymes, hormones, and antibodies are also proteinaceous in nature. Enzymes play the role of biocatalysts; hormones are used to regulate chemical reactions in the body. Enzymes and hormones act as vital molecules for controlling various life processes such as metabolic activities in the form of digestion and execration and also for converting chemical energy to mechanical function. Antibodies act as a natural defense agent against attack of foreign substances or microorganisms responsible for different diseases. Nourishment sensitivities result when certain ingested proteins cause an obvious alteration in the protection components. Proteins are excellent transport agents. In order to modulate the osmotic pressure and pH of body fluids, blood plasma proteins and hemoglobin play a vital role in transporting nutrients, oxygen, etc. to different parts of the body. Insulin regulates the amount of sugar present in the blood. Proteins such as actin and myosin present in the body fluids function as carriers of inorganic and organic compounds. Plants have the ability to synthesize proteins from inorganic nitrogen sources, such as ammonia, nitrate, and nitrite. Animals, unlike plants, cannot synthesize proteins in this manner. Thus, all animals, either directly or indirectly, depend on plants to satisfy their protein needs.

15.2 Amino Acids

Though all proteins are built up of similar building blocks, the amino acids, they have different biological functions and properties as we have seen above. Proteins consist of 20 amino acids. Amino acids are mainly composed of a basic amino group and an acidic carboxyl group attached to the same carbon atom, the α-carbon atom. Additionally, they also have a third group referred to as the side chain denoted by the letter R [1]. The general structural formula of an α-amino acid in the unionized and ionized condition is shown in Fig. 15.1.

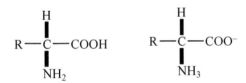

Figure 15.1 α-amino acid in the unionized and ionized condition.

15.2.1 Classification of Amino Acids

As we have seen above, amino and carboxyl groups are common to all amino acids. Hence, we differentiate one amino acid from the other with respect to the R group. On the basis of side chains, amino acids are distinguished into four groups as follows:

- **Non-polar R groups**: Alanine, valine, leucine, isoleucine, proline, phenylalanine, tryptophan, methionine
- **Polar uncharged R group**: Glycine, serine, threonine, cysteine, tyrosine, asparagine, glutamine
- **Negatively charged R groups**: Aspartic acid, glutamic acid
- **Positively charged R groups**: Lysine, arginine, histidine

15.3 Classification of Proteins

Twenty odd natural amino acids could have produced an infinite number of proteins. There are a number of ways of classification of proteins as they carry out a wide variety of biological functions. As per the functions of proteins, they are classified as catalytic proteins, contractile proteins, and structural proteins. According to the products of hydrolysis or compositional basis, proteins are mainly classified into three categories: simple proteins, conjugated proteins, and derived proteins. Classification of proteins is shown in Fig. 15.2.

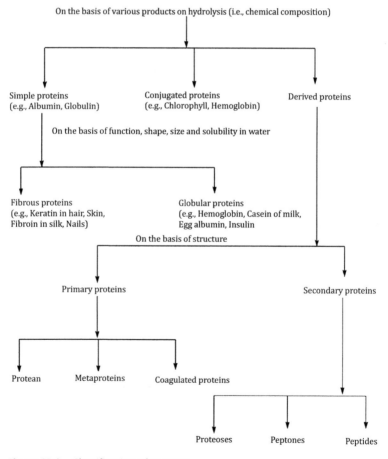

Figure 15.2 Classification of proteins.

15.3.1 Simple Proteins

Simple proteins, on hydrolysis, simply yield α-amino acids. These proteins are also known as holoproteins. The holoproteins are subdivided according to solubility in different solvents (water, salt solution, acid, alkali, alcohol 80%). It is shown in Table 15.1. On the basis of solubility, simple proteins are classified as albumins, globulins, scleroproteins, histones, prolamines, and protamines. For example, egg albumin, serum albumin, lactalbumin, serum (blood) globulin, keratin in hair, oryzenin from rice, zein from corn, salmine from salmon, collagens, glutenins. Many enzyme and hormone proteins fit into either the albumin or globulin category. Plant seed proteins are mostly glutelins.

Table 15.1 Classification of simple proteins on the basis of solubility in different solvents

Name	Solubility in				Food source
	Water	Salt solution	Acid/ Alkali	Alcohol 80%	
Albumins	Soluble	Soluble	—	—	Milk, egg, plant and animal cells
Globulins	—	Soluble	—	—	Milk, egg, meat, plant cells, particularly in seed proteins
Glutelins	—	—	Soluble	—	Cereal grains and related plant materials
Prolamines	—	—	—	Soluble	Cereal grains and related plant materials
Histones	Soluble	—	Soluble	—	Glandular tissues, pancreas, thymus, fish
Protamines	Soluble	—	Soluble	—	Fish sperm
Scleroproteins (albuminoids)	—	—	—	—	Meat

Simple proteins are also classified into two groups according to shape and molecular structure.

15.3.1.1 Fibrous proteins

Fibrous proteins are long, thread-like proteins having very elongated or asymmetric shape, like that of thread. Intramolecular hydrogen bond is comparatively strong. These proteins have helical or sheet structure. They are insoluble in water but soluble in concentrated acid and alkali. Examples of these proteins are fibroin (silk protein), keratin (protein of hair, nails), feathers, skin, horn, silk, cartilage, and wool and collagen (in bone marrow).

15.3.1.2 Globular proteins

Globular proteins are found in spherical, oval, or elliptical shape. The peptide chains in globular proteins are also held by intramolecular hydrogen bonds, but these forces are comparatively weak. Because of highly ordered pattern of folding, these proteins have compact structures. Globular proteins are insoluble in water. Examples of globular proteins are egg albumin (egg white), insulin (hormone), myoglobin, cytochromes, casein of milk, pepsin, enzymes, antibodies, and venom of snake, scorpion, and bees.

15.3.2 Conjugated Proteins

Conjugated proteins, on hydrolysis, yield α-amino acids and a non-proteinous part known as prosthetic group or cofactor. The classification of conjugated proteins on the basis of prosthetic group is provided in Table 15.2. Prosthetic group is a simple or complex non-peptide organic molecule or an inorganic ion or organometallic complex that is loosely or firmly bound to the polypeptide chain of conjugated protein. The prosthetic groups of conjugated proteins are carbohydrates, lipids, nucleic acids, metal ions, or phosphates. The prosthetic group governs the biological functions of proteins. These groups play a vital role in conjugated protein; without it, the protein will lose its function. The prosthetic group is bound to the protein by linkages other than salt linkages. The protein component of a conjugated protein is stabilized by combination with the prosthetic group. Depending on the prosthetic group, proteins are further classified as follows:

Table 15.2 Classification of conjugated proteins on the basis of prosthetic group

Conjugated protein	Prosthetic group	Example
Glyco-proteins	Carbohydrate	Egg white
Lipo-proteins	Fat (lipid)	Cell membrane
Nucleo-proteins	Nucleic acid	Chromosomes
Phospho-proteins	Phosphoric acid	Casein of milk
Chromo-proteins	Metals (Fe, Mg, Cu, Co)	Chlorophyll

15.3.2.1 Glycoproteins or mucoproteins

These proteins contain carbohydrate as the prosthetic group. Glycoproteins are proteins whose prosthetic groups are heterosaccharides containing hexosamine, galactose, mannose, fucose, and sialic acid. A covalent bond joins the protein to the heteropolysaccharide by either *O*-glycosidic (with serine or threonine) or *N*-glycosidic bonds (with asparagines). Glycoproteins are found in mucous secretions of mammals, and they function as lubricating agents. Egg white contains ovomucoid, which cannot be coagulated by heat and is a glycoprotein. Certain fractions of pulse proteins are glycoproteins, for example, egg white yolk (ovomucoid of egg white), mucin in mucous (saliva), jellyfish, tendomucoid (tendon), etc.

15.3.2.2 Lipoproteins

These proteins contain lipid (fat) as prosthetic group. Lipoproteins are proteins complexed with lipids and are found in cells and the blood stream. The lipids are very firmly held to the proteins and cannot be easily removed. The lipids in lipoproteins are triglycerides, phospholipids, cholesterol, or derivatives of cholesterol. Lipoproteins serve as transporters of lipids in blood. Based on density, lipoproteins are grouped into three groups: high-density, low-density, and very low-density lipoproteins. Some commonly observed lipoproteins include cell membrane, cholesterol, cephalin, lecithin, nerve tissue lipovitellin and lipovitellenin from egg yolk, lipoproteins of blood containing about 75% of lipid.

15.3.2.3 Nucleoproteins

There are mainly the proteins that have nucleic acids in the form of prosthetic groups containing the nucleus of the cell, chromosomes, ribose, protamines, and histones. They are accompanied by the DNA and are known as nucleoproteins and nucleohistones. Nucleoproteins are complexes of proteins and nucleic acids. Nucleic acids readily combine with proteins to form the complexes. Phosphoproteins are proteins conjugated with inorganic phosphate. The most widely known phosphoproteins are the milk protein casein and the enzyme pepsin.

15.3.2.4 Phosphoproteins

These proteins contain phosphoric acid as the prosthetic group (e.g., casein in milk, ovovitellin of egg yellow yolk).

15.3.2.5 Chromoproteins or metalloproteins

These are proteins carrying metal ions such as Fe, Mg, Cu, and Co or a colored compound as the prosthetic group due to which the protein appears colored. Examples include chlorophyll in plant, hemoglobin in blood, myoglobin, cytochromes (red colored), flavoproteins (yellow colored), and hemocyanin (blue colored). Metalloproteins are complexes of proteins and heavy metals. In most metalloproteins, the metal is loosely bound and can be easily removed. However, in some proteins such as hemoglobin and myoglobin, the metal iron is firmly bound to the prosthetic group. Liver and spleen contain the metalloproteins ferritin and hemosiderin with about 20% iron content. These are storage forms of iron in animals, which release iron from the proteins when required. Conalbumin from egg can form complex with iron, and it also combines with copper and zinc.

15.3.3 Derived Proteins

These are degradation products obtained with the help of acids, alkalis, or enzymes acting on natural proteins. They undergo some structural changes due to the action of heat chemical reagent. Thus, before final degradation into α-amino acids, partial hydrolysis of proteins yields such intermediate products as proteoses, peptones, and polypeptides, which are often described as derived proteins. The nature of product formed depends on the extent of hydrolysis. Denatured proteins are formed due to the coagulation of natural colloidal proteins.

15.4 Structure of Protein

The miscellaneous biological functions of proteins result from their structure. The structure of a protein is explained under four stages: primary structure, secondary structure, tertiary structure, and quaternary structure.

15.4.1 Primary Structure

The nature of amino acids and their linear sequence in the polypeptide chain is referred to as the primary structure, as shown in Fig. 15.3. The determination of the primary structure, which was once a formidable job, has now become easy due to the modern analytical tools available for amino acid analysis. The exclusive sequences of amino acids are responsive for several essential properties of the proteins. For example, the replacement of one amino acid residue in the β-chains of hemoglobin, which contains 574 amino acid residues, can bring about profound changes in its biological properties. The sequence of amino acids also determines, to a large extent, the secondary and tertiary structures of proteins [2].

— Ala — Glu — Val — Thr — Asp — Pro — Gly —

Figure 15.3 Primary structure of protein.

15.4.2 Secondary Structure

An extended peptide chain is not stable, and it folds into itself. The secondary structure is referred to as three-dimensional structure where the particles of proteins are arranged in a chain. The common structure of protein shows minimal possible free energy. Hence, the structure of a protein is not arbitrary but, to some degree, ordered. The secondary structure of a protein depends on the structural characteristics of peptide bond repeating in the chain. X-ray studies indicate that the peptide bond is, to some degree, shorter than other single C–N bonds. Single C–N bonds indicate the features of double bond as well. Thus, groups contiguous to the peptide bond pivot uninhibitedly. The unbending nature of the peptide bond holds the six atoms shown in the diagram in a single plane. The amino group (–NH–) do not show any ionization between pH 0 and 14 because of the double bond features of the peptide bond. In addition, the R groups of amino acid deposits, on account of stearic hindrance, force oxygen and hydrogen bond to obtain in *trans* configuration. Therefore, the hydrogen of the peptide bonds helps in the formation of *trans* configuration in the backbone of peptides. Hence, it is noticed that the backbone of peptides as well as protein shows free rotation in the two bonds between amino acids and not in the third bond, which is indicated in Fig. 15.4. A right-handed coil along with α-helix is found in the stable feasible structure as the restriction of peptide bond as imposed on the poly amino acid chain. The α-helix consists of 3.6 amino acid deposits for every turn of the protein backbone, with the R groups of the amino acids, which is moving outside along the pivot of the helical structure. Hydrogen bonding occurs among the nitrogen of one peptide bond and the oxygen of another peptide bond in the four residues through the backbone structure of protein [3]. This arrangement enhances the stability of the structure.

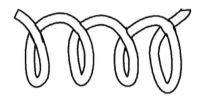

Figure 15.4 Secondary structure of protein.

Another secondary structure observed in various fibrous proteins is the β-pleated sheet setup. In this setup, the peptide backbone makes a crisscross example, with the R groups of the amino acids lengthening above and underneath the peptide chain. Since all peptide bonds are accessible for hydrogen bonding, this setup permits highest crosslinking between the adjacent polypeptide chains and thus ensures superior solidness. When the polypeptide chains run in the same direction, parallel-pleated sheets, and when they run in the opposite directions, antiparallel pleated sheets, are possible. Silk and insects fibers are best examples of the β-sheet structure. Most proteins do not have the regular secondary structure due to some factors that prevent the formation of long uninterrupted regions of α-helix or β-pleated sheets. For example, if a proline residue is present in the polypeptide chain, the α-helix is interrupted because the amide nitrogen of proline, when involved in peptide bond formation, does not possess an attached hydrogen bond. In addition, hydrogen bonding in both the pleated sheet and α-helix is interrupted because the amide nitrogen of proline, when involved in peptide bond formation, does not possess an attached hydrogen bond. In addition, hydrogen bonding in both the pleated sheet and α-helical structures may be disturbed by unfavorable side-chain interactions, such as the presence of two bulky side chains next to each other or the electrostatic repulsion produced by two similar groups.

Another kind of secondary structure of fibrous proteins is the collagen helix. Collagen, found in skin, tendons, and numerous other parts of the body, frames the 33% of the aggregate body protein. Collagen contains 33% glycine and one-fourth proline or hydroxyproline residues. The rigid R groups and the inadequate amount of hydrogen bonds by peptide linkages including proline and hydroxyproline force the collagen polypeptide chain into an odd wrinkle sort helix. The peptide bonds comprising glycine lead to the formation of interchain hydrogen bonds with two collagen polypeptide chains which results in a stable triple helix structure known as "tropocollagen."

15.4.3 Tertiary Structure

The tertiary structure of proteins defines a specific three-dimensional configuration, as shown in Fig. 15.5. The tertiary structure comprises the specific units of secondary structure folded with each other which has a pattern of the peptide chain. The folded fractions are attached together by means of hydrogen bonds produced among R groups, by electrostatic interaction between chains possessing oppositely charged groups such as those of lysine, arginine, glutamic, and aspartic acids, hydrophobic interactions between non-polar regions and covalent disulfide linkages [4]. In the formation of the tertiary structure, all the polar groups are on the surface of the molecule and the interior consists almost entirely of non-polar hydrophobic residues, such as those of leucine, valine, methionine, and phenylalanine. The presence of polar R groups on the surface of proteins usually accounts for their solubility in aqueous solutions.

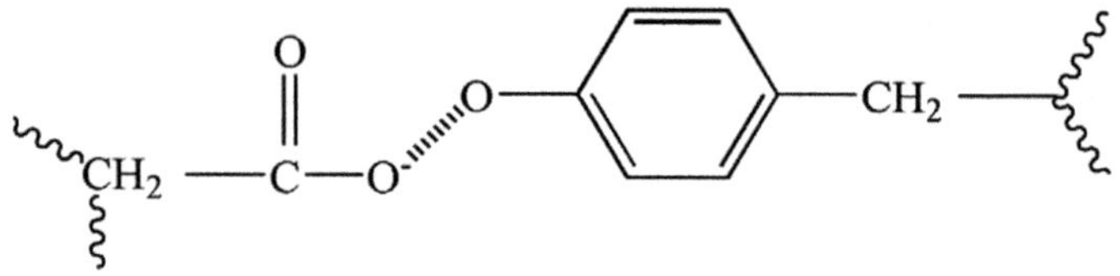

Figure 15.5 Tertiary structure of protein.

15.4.4 Quaternary Structure

The primary, secondary, and tertiary structural organization discussed above applies to all proteins with a single polypeptide chain. The quaternary structure is formed when protein with two or more polypeptide chains interacts, forming a native protein molecule, as shown in Fig. 15.6. The bonding mechanisms holding protein chains collectively are usually similar to those included in the tertiary structure, apart from the fact that disulfide bonds do not support in maintaining the quaternary structure of proteins [2].

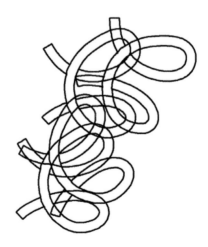

Figure 15.6 Quaternary structure of protein.

15.5 Properties of Proteins

On the exterior of protein molecule, hydrophilic R groups are present, while hydrophobic non-polar R groups are positioned in the interior of the protein molecule. The behavior of protein is similar to amino acids due to the presence of hydrophilic R groups on the surface of proteins. The multiplicity of hydrophilic R groups makes the behavior of proteins much more complex [5].

15.5.1 Electrolytic Properties of Protein

Proteins act as electrolyte. A protein obeys similar physical and chemical principles of an electrolyte. The amino acid composition of individual proteins greatly varies, and thus their net charge varies. Proteins with high content of acidic groups such as aspartic and glutamic acids have low isoelectric pH; on the other hand, proteins with maximum basic amino acids such as arginine and lysine have a high isoelectric point.

15.5.2 Ionic Characteristics

Many methods of fractionation of proteins from biological systems are a result of the variation in the ionic properties of proteins. Methodologies such as electrophoresis (particularly zone electrophoresis on polyacrylamide gel) and ion-exchange chromatography have been successfully employed in the isolation and purification of proteins on the basis of their ionic properties.

15.5.3 Solubility

Solubility of protein is also influenced by electrical charges. The protein present in the solution represents the change in solubility by the action of pH, ionic strength, temperature, and dielectric properties of the solvent. Using these variables, protein mixtures can be resolved.

15.5.4 Hydrolytic Characteristic

Proteins get easily hydrolyzed with acid, alkali, and enzymes. Heating of proteins with 6 M HCl for 8–10 h at 120°C leads to complete hydrolysis. Acid hydrolysis avoids racemization of amino acids, but it may destroy tryptophan. The amino acids asparagines and glutamine are hydrolyzed to aspartic and glutamine acids during acid hydrolysis. Proteins undergo alkaline hydrolysis with 2 M sodium or barium hydroxide, resulting in substantial racemization of amino acids. During alkaline hydrolysis of protein, the amino acids arginine and cysteine, and a portion of lysine, are destroyed, although tryptophan is retained. Proteins are completely hydrolyzed by enzymes without any destruction of amino acids. This kind of hydrolysis takes place in the body during digestion of proteins.

15.5.5 Putrefaction

Protein food gets deteriorated by microorganisms. Under unsatisfactory conditions when the food is not properly processed, spoilage organisms grow. Microbial proteases bring about decarboxylation and determination ensuing in undesirable changes in flavor and texture, and production of offensive odors and toxins, a process referred to as putrefaction.

15.6 Native Proteins and Their Denaturation

Native proteins are proteins that are naturally available in living tissues or cells.

15.6.1 Denaturation

As discussed earlier, proteins are very delicate, ordered three-dimensional structural molecules. This structure undergoes changes with the help of mild agents and results in breakdown of peptide bonds. The drastic slowdown of the conformation structure leads to alterations in typical characteristics of proteins, and this is called denaturation. Many changes occur during denaturation in protein. Denaturation allows peptide bonds to be available for the process of hydrolysis by proteolytic enzyme. Denaturation results in decreased solubility, and also biological properties such as catalysis are nowhere to be found. Hence, crystallization of protein could be carried out, leading to an increase in viscosity and optical rotation.

The rise in viscosity suggests the unfolding of the molecule, resulting in more asymmetry. This would expose more hydrophobic residues, leading to the decreasing solubility of proteins. Denaturation is irreversible, but under specific conditions, reversible denaturation occurs. Denaturing agents include acids, alkalies, alkylids, heavy metals, salts, urea, ethanol, ions (bromide, chloride, iodide), and synthetic detergents at low concentration. Sometimes denaturation can be produced by mechanical processes. Denaturation is the result of the alteration of the secondary, tertiary, or quaternary structure of the protein molecule, barring the breakage of covalent bonds. Denaturation is, accordingly, a procedure by which hydrogen bonds, hydrophobic interactions, and salt linkages are broken and the protein completely unfolds and assumes a random coil structure, in which state the protein molecules readily form aggregates (coagulation). Denaturation is generally reversible phenomenon if the methodology followed for the denaturation is not strong. Reversible denaturation may also occur if the molecular weight of the native protein is extremely larger. Many a times, in spite of using milder methods for denaturation, reversible denaturation is not observed in some smaller proteins.

Both physical and chemical agents bring about denaturation. Heat plays a vital role as a physical agent. At each 10°C increment in temperature, the denaturation rate raises up by 600 fold. The effect of denaturation can be minimized by working at a lower temperature. The speed of heat denaturation is influenced by factors such as water content of a protein, ionic strength, pH, and types of ions existing in the solution. Layering of proteins at an interface can result in denaturation. Therefore, the creation of interfaces, such as those of foams, should be avoided to preserve the native properties of proteins. Stirring, shaking, high pressure, and ultraviolet radiations lead to protein denaturation. Among the chemical agents, the pH of the medium has a profound effect on the denaturation of proteins. Most proteins are stable within a fairly narrow pH range, and exposure to pH values outside this range causes denaturation. A 6–8 M concentration of urea, and guanidine hydrochloride, which tends to break hydrogen bonds, also causes denaturation of proteins. Synthetic detergents such as sodium dodecyl sulfate (SDS) are the most effective among the denaturing agents known. In food processing, the denaturation phenomenon has great importance.

When most foods are prepared, they are heat coagulated as in the processing of milk by pasteurization, evaporation, and spray drying, where it is desirable to retain the natural properties of proteins. It is believed that during denaturation, the chain unfolds and unfills. The denatured protein is more radically attacked by proteolytic enzyme.

The general effects of denaturation are as follows:

- The peptide bonds of proteins become readily available for hydrolysis by proteolytic enzymes.
- The solubility of protein decreases and textural changes are observed.
- Enzyme activity, if originally present, decreases or vanishes.
- Crystallization of protein cannot be carried out any more.
- Intrinsic viscosity increases.
- Optical rotation of protein solution increases.

15.7 Protein Gels

Dry proteins have the ability to absorb water. A few proteins can form gels capable of immobilizing water, equaling to nearly 10 times the weight of hydrated proteins. Gel formation of protein occurs at low concentrations. For example, gelatin dispersion in water with concentration as low as 1% forms a gel and fibrinogen concentration of 0.04% in plasma forms a gel. When colloidal dispersion of some relatively large molecules is cooled then its viscosity increases to the point at which some rigidity is attained and this point is called gel point. Through hydration, proteins are able to bind approximately 1 g of water per 5 g of dry protein. However, few proteins are capable of immobilizing water 10 times more than that through hydration. This immobilized water is not tightly bound to the protein and can be physically removed. On standing for some time, many gels lose solvents and eventually shrink. This phenomenon is known as syneresis or weeping.

There are three theories on gel formation.

15.7.1 Adsorption

On cooling the adsorption of solvent molecules by the solute results in the formation of large particles. These enlarged particles touch or overlap, enclosing more solvent and immobilizing the system, causing the rigidity. Adsorption increases with reduction in temperature.

15.7.2 Three-Dimensional Network Theories

It is postulated that a compound capable of gelation is either fibrous in structure or can react with itself to form fibers. On cooling, the fibers form a three-dimensional network by reacting at relatively small distances. The bonds that tie the network are either primary or secondary or attractive forces. This theory can explain gel formation and system, which depends on concentration, pH, temperature, and salt concentration.

15.7.3 Particle Orientation Theory

This theory postulates that some systems have a tendency to orientate themselves in a definite configuration. Proteins that form gels have structures with a high degree of asymmetry. These long proteinaceous fibers form a three-dimensional matrix, primarily by the establishment of inter-protein hydrogen bonds, and this crosslinked structure is sufficiently well developed to hold water in an immobilized state. Ionized functional groups on proteins also aid in immobilizing water. If the attractive forces on proteins are increased, for example, by changing the pH to a value closer to the isoelectric point of the proteins, the gel tends to shrink. The shrinkage would expel some of the immobilized water (syneresis). Gelatin and casein are good examples of gel-forming proteins, which coagulate with the help of the enzyme rennin.

15.8 Food Proteins

Both plants and animals require protein for growth, survival, and propagation of species. Proteins are present in many foods in varying amounts. Most proteins have to be processed or modified prior to use by human beings. Some major food proteins are considered briefly in this section.

15.8.1 Animal Proteins

Meat is an important source of protein from animal sources. It is the edible muscle of cattle, sheep, and swine. It is designated as red meat because the color of beef, lamb mutton, and pork is light or dark red due to the presence of respiratory pigments myoglobin in them. Muscle from adult mammalian sources, stripped of all external fat, contains about 18–20% protein on wet basis. Muscle proteins are categorized on the basis of their origin and solubility as myofibrillar, sarcoplasmic, and stroma (connective tissue) proteins, which amount to 49–55%, 30–34%, and 10–17%, respectively, of the total amount of protein. Milk is an excellent source of protein in our diet. Cow milk contains about 3.5% protein. Milk proteins are generally divided into two classes: casein and whey proteins. Casein, which is insoluble in water, is a heterogeneous group of phosphoproteins and accounts for 80% of the total milk protein. Whey proteins, making up the other 20%, are the soluble proteins of milk. Egg contains 13–14% protein, about two-thirds of which is present in egg white and rest in egg yolk. Egg white consists of a number of proteins that are readily denatured and coagulated. Yolk is a mixture of lipoproteins and phosphoproteins. Fish contains 40–60% edible flesh. The protein content of fish varies from 10% to 21%. Fish muscles are similar to mammalian skeletal muscles with respect to structure and function, but are easily damaged. The pigmented reddish-brown muscles of fish contain enzymes that, following harvest, cause changes responsible for much of the instability of fish proteins.

15.8.2 Vegetable Proteins

Fresh vegetables are not good sources of proteins. Many contain 1% of proteins. Potatoes and green beans contain about 2% and fresh peas about 6.5% protein. Proteins from potatoes are considered to be of good quality because they are relatively high in the levels of lysine and tryptophan. Cereal grains contain proteins in the range of 6–20%. The protein content of rice is 7–9%, while that of wheat is 12–15%. Proteins are found in various morphological tissues of the grains such as embryo, germ, bran or seed coat, and the endosperm. The germ proteins are mainly globulins or albumins and several enzymes are present in them. Bran is poorly digested by humans, and bran proteins are difficult to separate. Bran is mostly used as animal feed. The endosperm proteins act as structural components and also as a food reserve for the growing seedling. The endosperm proteins of wheat are mostly prolamines, gliadins, and glutelins. Rice contains high levels of glutelins and low prolamine. Cereal proteins are generally of relatively poor nutritional quality. Seeds contain protein in excess of 15%. Pulses (legumes) contain, on an average, more than 20% proteins. Proteins of seeds are mostly concentrated in aleurone grains, which are subcellular granules of the cotyledon cells. Seed proteins function as structural elements of cell walls and various membranes and also as food reserves. The proteins of most seeds are globular. Owing to a decrease in the availability of meat proteins, seed proteins are gaining importance. Newer techniques have been developed to produce textured or shaped proteins from seeds. Nutritionally, seed proteins contain less lysine and are also deficient in methionine and threonine. Seed proteins contain some anti-nutritional factors. They should be subjected to proper heat treatment to destroy or inactivate the anti-nutritional quality.

15.9 Non-traditional Proteins

People in many parts of the world are experiencing varying degrees of protein malnutrition largely because of rapid increase in population. Therefore, there is a need to increase the production of proteins from traditional sources and to develop proteins from non-traditional sources. Some success has been achieved in the production of proteins from some unconventional sources. Microorganisms grow rapidly, their yields are high, and their growing conditions can be controlled. Therefore, microbes have been used to obtain food proteins (single-cell proteins). Two species of yeasts, *Candida utilis* (torula yeast) and *Saccharomyces carlsbergensis* (brewer's yeast), have been used for human food. Torula yeast grows well on sulfite waste liquor (waste product from paper industry) and wood hydrolysates, by utilizing pentoses as the carbon source. Brewer's yeast can be collected after beer fermentation. These yeasts contain approximately 50% of proteins on dry-weight basis. They are, however, deficient in methionine, but by adding 0.3% methionine, their biological value can be increased to more than 90%.

One disadvantage of food yeasts is their nucleic acid content. Nucleic acid metabolic products are relatively insoluble and may lead to the formation of kidney stones or aggravate arthritic or gouty conditions. Strains of the yeast *Candida lipolytica* can grow on petroleum. The carbon and energy for the growth of organisms are provided by alkanes (straight-chain hydrocarbon molecules of petroleum). A commercial product named Toprina has been prepared by this method. Toprina is toxicologically safe. However, the product has not been a success due to the rising cost of petroleum. The bacterium *Methylophilus methylotrophus* can oxidize and use methane (or methanol) as a source of carbon and energy. A product named "Pruteen" is being produced using this method. Two genera of algae—*Chlorella* (green algae) and *Spirulina* (blue-green algae, now classified as blue-green bacteria)—when grown under controlled conditions, contain 50–60% protein on dry-weight basis. Algal proteins contain all essential amino acids (methionine content is low). But high algal protein in the diet results in nausea, vomiting, and abdominal pain. Poor digestibility and other undesirable characteristics can be eliminated by proper processing.

Fungi are used as a source of food. Mushroom, a filamentous fungus containing 27% protein (dry-weight basis), is commercially grown and used as food. Attempts are being made to produce large amounts of food protein by culturing fungi in liquid media containing carbohydrates and inorganic nitrogen salts. However, there is a danger of formation of microbial toxins (mycotoxins) in proteins produced by this method. Leaf proteins extracted from green plant leaves can be used as food protein. The dried product contains 50–70% protein. The nutritional value of leaf proteins is greater than that of proteins of other plants. Their lysine content is high (5–7%). The cost, yield, and the palatability of leaf proteins come in the way of their use to alleviate the world's shortage of food proteins. However, attempts are being made to resolve these difficulties in using leaf proteins as food.

15.10 Nutritional Importance of Proteins

Proteins play some functional roles in food because they can form gels, sols, and emulsions and can contribute color and flavor. Their most important role, however, is their nutritional value. The primary function of dietary proteins is to supply nitrogen and amino acids for the synthesis of body proteins and other nitrogen-containing substances. Human body tissues contain 20 amino acids. Of these, nine cannot be produced in the body and have to be supplied through food. These nine amino acids are histidine, isoleucine leucine, lysine, methionine, phenylalanine, threonine, tryptophan, and valine. These amino acids are designated as essential. The other amino acids, which are regarded as non-essential and can be created in the inner body from a utilizable source of nitrogen, usually protein. The diet should provide all the essential amino acids in amounts required by the body, together with a sufficient amount of utilizable nitrogen for the synthesis of body proteins. If any single amino acid is deficient, protein synthesis ceases or is greatly slowed. The quality or balance of a protein depends on the types and quantities of amino acids it contains. A balanced or superior class protein consists of all the essential amino acids required for the human body.

Proteins of animal origin are generally of higher quality than those of plant origin. Cereal proteins are low in lysine and deficient in methionine, tryptophan, and, occasionally, threonine. Pulse proteins are deficient in methionine, and oil seed and nut proteins in lysine, methionine, and sometimes in threonine. The amino acids not contained in a protein are designated as limiting amino acids. While proteins deficient in some essential amino acids are fed in amounts sufficient to provide adequate amounts of limiting amino acids, some amino acids that are in excess for body growth and maintenance are utilized as source of energy. When the dietary pattern of amino acids differs from the ideal pattern, it results in amino acid imbalance, leading to depressed growth and impairment of mental capabilities in children. Except mental impairment, other defects can be overcome by supplementing the diet with the limiting amino acids. The level of protein intake required for adequate maintenance has been worked out by an expert group from the Food and Agriculture Organization (FAO) and the World Health Organization (WHO). According to them, the recommended everyday intake is 0.59 g of protein per kilogram of body mass for an average individual. The daily requirement for protein remains constant during the lifetime of most adults. FAO and WHO suggest that kids in the age group of 1–10 years should intake 0.88 g of protein per kilogram of body weight every day. During pregnancy and lactation, women require some 20–30 g of additional protein per day. During disease and injury, which cause breakdown of tissue proteins and increased excretion of nitrogen, more protein is required to compensate for losses [6].

15.11 Applications of Protein-Based Biocomposites

Since many decades, it is observed that protein-based biomaterials are exclusively applied to generate various physical features as border line spectrum to fulfil the needs leading to elastic nature which yields for supporting the tissues. By optimizing the molecular interfaces of the protein structure, composite materials are fabricated in the form of films and gel. The affinity to synthesize the polymer is exclusively elaborated due to the characteristics such as tenability of material, and biosensor.

15.11.1 Protein-Based Biocomposites as Biodegradable Packaging Materials

One of the commonly used protein, wheat gluten, is an advanced bio-based polymer appropriate for manufacturing plastics due to its excellent functional properties (mechanical and gas barrier, viscoelasticity, film formation, foam formation, biocompatibility) [7, 8]. Kuktaite et al. [9] state the possible use of nanoclay-based wheat gluten films for food packaging applications due to their attractive gas barrier properties. Wheat gluten protein is a mixture of gliadins and glutenins [9]. Both gliadins and glutenins have individual importance for their use as thermoplastic films since both have variant properties; for instance, gliadins have higher elongation, while glutenins possess higher strength and stiffness, hence can be used separately for making films [10]. Biocomposites made from wheat gluten and soy protein, reinforced with natural fibers (such as hemp, jute, and bamboo fibers), display enhanced mechanical properties. Likewise, biocomposites made from egg albumin and potato starch as well as extruded composites made from wheat gluten and modified potato starch are eligible for packaging applications due their superior mechanical properties and excellent gas barrier characteristics [8].

15.11.2 Protein-Based Thermoplastics in Biomedical Applications

Protein-based biocomposites are promising materials for biomedical applications because of their characteristics such as non-hazardous along with their native properties (e.g., mechanical, optical, electrical, chemical, and thermal). Several protein-based composite materials, for example, protein–inorganic ceramic materials, protein-synthetic polymer materials, play vital roles in the recent growth of biomaterials. Collagens and elastins are frequently found collectively in the body to give a mix of quality and adaptability required for particular tissue properties. Vaz et al. have developed and characterized novel meltable polymers and composites based on casein and soybean proteins [11]. They confirm biomaterials. The above studies reveal that thermoplastics based on casein and soybean protein possess adequate mechanical and degradation properties and also bioactive character. Nanoparticles produced using proteins have been proposed as option carriers and have benefits particular to remedial protein conveyance [12]. Elastin-like polypeptides (ELPs) fit under the category of thermal-responsive biopolymer class. These are processed to yield a broad range of nanoparticles for protein and peptide delivery applications. ELPs are composed of a sequence of repeated pentapeptides of Val–Pro–Gly–Xaa–Gly, where Xaa is amino acid other than proline. Skopinska-Wisniewska et al. have developed collagen–elastin thin films with variant mixing ratios [13]. Both the components, collagen and elastin, have their own importance in making composites: Collagen provides tensile strength for regenerated tissues, while elastin gives resilience. Hu et al. investigated a novel category of biomedical materials where they blended semi-crystalline silk protein with tropoelastin in different proportions [14]. Outcomes of the study reveal that for controlling the bulk material features, the hydrophobic and hydrophilic interactions between silk and tropoelastin protein serve as a significant factor. Several scientists have come to the point that domesticated silk fibroin does not have specific cell attachment sites such as the arginine–glycine–aspartic acid (RGD) sequence; on the other hand, it was present in other wild-type silkworm silks. Because of this, wild silk-based composite materials are framed for in vivo control of cell differentiation process.

Nowadays, biocomposites formed by combining fibroin with cellulose or starch are one of the best options to customize cell adhesion and proliferation characteristics. As per an earlier discussion, protein–polysaccharide composites can be used as coating materials for porous membranes, which enhanced fibroblast adhesion and proliferation, and consequently raised the scaffold strength and hydrophilicity [15]. Sionkowska et al. have crosslinked silk fibroin with chitosan and developed three-dimensional silk fibroin–chitosan composite sponges [16]. The sponges with enough mechanical integrity are required for implantation. Physical properties of sponges further improved by using variant ratio of silk and chitosan. When silk and gelatin are intermixed with methanol, it forms a silk–gelatin hydrogel. Disulfide bonds are responsible for grouping fibrous protein keratin. The connective tissue is in protective function with β-sheet structure. It is possible to incorporate ultra-fine inorganic nanosilica particles in protein films, and such silk–silica and collagen–silica composite films have found their application in osteogenesis for bone repair due to their better stability and reinforcement performance in the coming years [15].

15.11.3 Agriculture

Protein-based composites find their application in agricultural sciences. Sartore et al. have proposed the use of recyclable polymeric materials in view of hydrolyzed proteins, synthesized from waste products of the leather industry, and they make use of such bio-based materials in the agricultural routine of mulching [17]. The biocompatible mulching films exhibited excellent mechanical and agronomical exhibitions in the field. Their mulching impact remains for no less than 12 months. The ecofriendly mulches based on hydrolyzed proteins can be projected as substitutes to low-density polyethylene plastic films utilized for soil mulching, which are constructed with non-renewable oil-based crude materials and create a lot of plastic waste.

15.11.4 Tissue Engineering

Tissue engineering is the branch of science involving combination of cells, tissues, or organs to generate functional organs for implantation. It also has applications related to repair and replacement of tissues such as bone, cartilage, muscle, and blood vessel. Protein-based materials are used in tissue engineering in terms of meeting with enhanced clinical demand for technologies to advance the regeneration of functional organs and living tissues. Hu discussed the impact on stem cells in knitted silk collagen scaffolds for tendon tissue engineering [14]. Xiao et al. manufactured gelatin methacrylate (GelMA)–silk fibroin (SF) interpenetrating polymer network (IPN) hydrogels [18]. They mixed gelatin methacrylate with SF solution and photo-crosslinked with the use of UV irradiation to produce the GelMA–SF IPN hydrogel, followed by methanol treatment to induce silk fibroin crystallization. These mechanically robust and tunable IPN hydrogels could be of use for a range of microscale tissue engineering applications. Buttafoco et al. determined electrospun collagen–elastin nanofiber meshes from aqueous solutions for artificial blood vessels [19]. Haslik et al. proposed clinically evaluated collagen–elastin three-dimensional matrices (Matriderm®) as a dermal alternative for the treatment of severe burns [20]. In 2010, Serban et al. proposed that chemical crosslinkage of soluble elastin, hyaluronic acid, and silk fibroin can be effectively used to control properties of modular elastic patches [21].

15.11.5 Textile Industry

In the textile industry, natural protein fibers have been used extensively in the past decades because besides having attributes such as toughness, slow degradability, strength, elongation, moisture absorbance, and vast biological compatibility, they are ecofriendly, cost-effective, renewable, and non-hazardous.

15.11.6 Other Applications

A lot of protein-based composite materials are investigated for various applications, according to their need in different fields. Ecofriendly, biocompatible crosslinked hydrogels have been made from poly(γ-glutamic acid) and gelatin composites [15]. Characteristic properties of protein composites are improved with the use of inorganic materials (CdTe, magnetite, gold) due to their intrinsic properties [22]. Inoue et al. proposed the use of protein–inorganic materials as biomimetic muscle having enhanced density [23]. Steven et al. (2013) determined that silk and carbon nanotubes (CNT–silk) composites can be formed with excellent features like high toughness, flexible shape, and better strain-humidity sensitivity, which qualify them for electronic applications in near future [24]. Biofoams made from wheat gluten and silica are highly porous and flame retardant. They find application in house insulation, sound and thermal insulations, and also useful when light weightiness and porosity are necessary [25].

15.12 Conclusion and Future Perspectives

To conclude, protein is regarded as an important bio-based macromolecule with divergent physicochemical characteristics. Proteins and their composites have been innovatively generated and serve useful applications in packaging, biomedicine, agriculture, tissue engineering, biosensors, and electronics. To meet the targets and demands of different biomedical, tissue engineering, and packaging applications, the configuration and functions of proteins are further designed and modified. In the near future, research in the development of efficient protein composites will definitely pave the way for possibilities in many fields due to their good characteristic properties.

References

1. Greenstein, J. P. and Winitz, M. (1961). *Chemistry of Amino Acids* (John Wiley & Sons, New York).
2. Dockerson, R. F. and Geiss, I. (1983). *Proteins: Structure, Function and Evolution* (Benjamin Cummings, Menlo Park, California).
3. Chakraverty, A. and Singh, R. P. (2014). *Postharvest Technology and Food Process Engineering* (CRC Press).
4. Schultz, G. E. and Schirmer, R. H. (1985). *Principles of Protein Structure* (Springer-Verlag, New York).
5. Cherry, J. P. (1981). *Protein Functionality in Foods*, Vol. 147 (American Chemical Society).

6. Chawanje, C. M., Barbeau, W. E., and Grun, I. (2001). Nutrient and antinutrient content of an underexploited Malawian water tuber *Nymphaea petersiana* (Nyika), *Ecol. Food Nutr.*, **40**(4), 347–366.
7. Blomfeldt, T. O. J., Kuktaite, R., Johansson, E., and Hedenqvist, M. S. (2011). Mechanical properties and network structure of wheat gluten foams, *Biomacromolecules*, **12**(5), 1707–1715.
8. Muneer, F. (2014). Biocomposites from natural polymers and fibers. Introductory paper at the Faculty of Landscape Architecture, Horticulture and Crop Production Science, Swedish University of Agricultural Sciences.
9. Kuktaite, R., Türe, H., Hedenqvist, M. S., Gällstedt, M., and Plivelic, T. S. (2014). Gluten biopolymer and nanoclay-derived structures in wheat gluten–urea–clay composites: Relation to barrier and mechanical properties. *ACS Sustain. Chem. Eng.*, **2**(6), 1439–1445.
10. Chen, L., Reddy, N., Wu, X., and Yang, Y. (2012). Thermoplastic films from wheat proteins, *Ind. Crops Products*, **35**(1), 70–76.
11. Vaz, C. M., Fossen, R. F., van Tuil, L. A., de Graaf, R. L., and Cunha, A. M. (2003). Casein and soybean protein-based thermoplastics and composites as alternative biodegradable polymers for biomedical applications, *J. Biomed. Mater. Res.*, **65A**(1), 60–70.
12. Herrera Estrada, L. P. and Champion, J. A. (2015). Protein nanoparticles for therapeutic protein delivery, *Biomater. Sci.*, **3**, 787–799.
13. Skopinska-Wisniewska, J., Sionkowska, A., Kaminska, A., Kaznica, A., Jachimiak, R., and Drewa, T. (2009). Surface characterization of collagen/elastin based biomaterials for tissue regeneration, *Appl. Surf. Sci.*, **255**(19), 8286–8292.
14. Hu, X., Cebea, P., Weissb, A. S., Omenettoa, F., and Kaplana, D. L. (2012). Protein-based composite materials, *Mater. Today*, **15**(5), 208–215.
15. Wang, F., Yang, C., and Hu, X. (2014). Advanced Protein Composite Materials (American Chemical Society, Washington, DC).
16. Sionkowska, A. and Płanecka, A. J. (2013). Preparation and characterization of silk fibroin/chitosan composite sponges for tissue engineering, *J. Mol. Liq.*, **178**, 5–14.
17. Sartore, L., Vox, G., and Schettini, E. (2013). Preparation and performance of novel biodegradable polymeric materials based on hydrolyzed proteins for agricultural application, *J. Polym. Environ.*, **21**(3), 718–725.
18. Xiao, W., He, J., Nichol, J. W., Wang, L., Hutson, C. B., Wang, B., Du, Y., Fan, H., and Khademhosseini, A. (2011). Synthesis and characterization of

photo-crosslinkable gelatin and silk fibroin interpenetrating polymer networks hydrogels, *Acta Biomater*, **7**(6), 2384–2393.

19. Buttafoco, L., Kolkman, N. G., Engbers-Buijtenhuijs, P., Poot, A. A., Dijkstra, P. J., Vermes, I., and Feijen, J. (2006). Electrospinning of collagen and elastin for tissue engineering applications, *Biomaterials*, **27**(5), 724–734.

20. Haslik, W., Kamolz, L. P., Nathschlager, G., Andel, H., Meissi, G., and Frey, M. (2007). First experience with the collagen-elastin matrix matriderm as a dermal substitute in severe burn injuries of the hand, *Burns*, **33**(3), 364.

21. Serban, M. A., Kluge, J. A., Laha, M. M., and Kaplan, D. L. (2010). Modular elastic patches: Mechanical and biological effects, *Biomacromolecules*, **11**(9), 2230–2237.

22. Jin, H.-J. and Kaplan, D. L. (2003). Mechanism of silk processing in insects and spiders, *Nature*, **424**, 1057–1061.

23. Inoue, S., Tanaka, K., Arisaka, F., Kimura, S., Ohtomo, K., and Mizuno, S. J. (2000). Silk fibroin of *Bombyx mori* is secreted assembling a high molecular mass elementary unit consisting of H-chain, L-chain, and P 25, with a 6:6:1 molar ratio, *Biol. Chem.*, **275**, 40517–40528.

24. Steven, E., Saleh, W. R., Lebedev, V., Acquah, S. F. A., Laukhin, V., Alamo, R. G., and Brooks, J. S. (2013). Carbon nanotubes on a spider silk scaffold, *Nat. Commun.*, **4**, 2435–2440.

25. Wu, Q., Andersson, R. L., Holgate, T., Johansson, E., Gedde, U. W., Olsson, R. T., and Hedenqvist, M. S. (2014). Highly porous flame-retardant and sustainable biofoams based on wheat gluten and in situ polymerized silica, *J. Mater. Chem. A*, **2**(48), 20996–21009.

Chapter 16

Biopolyesters: Novel Candidates to Develop Multifunctional Biocomposites

Hafiz M. N. Iqbal[a] and Tajalli Keshavarz[b]

[a]*Tecnologico de Monterrey, School of Engineering and Sciences,*
Campus Monterrey, Ave. Eugenio Garza Sada 2501 Sur Col. Tecnológico C.P. 64849,
Monterrey, Nuevo León, Mexico
[b]*Applied Biotechnology Research Group, Department of Life Sciences,*
Faculty of Science and Technology, University of Westminster,
London W1W 6UW, United Kingdom
hafiz.iqbal@my.westminster.ac.uk, hafiz.iqbal@itesm.mx

This chapter focuses on biopolyesters as potential candidates with novel and multifunctional characteristics to engineer new types of biocomposites. For the past several years, research is under way around the globe in biomaterials-based biotechnology at large and composites in particular. Among the biopolyesters, polyhydroxyalkanoates (PHAs) and more specifically poly(3-hydroxybutyrate) [P(3HB)] are interesting candidates for the preparation of PHA-based composites and other products for a variety of bio- and non-bio-sectors. Owing to the unique chemical structure, bioactivity, non-toxicity, and effectiveness as a biopolymer,

---

Biocomposites: Biomedical and Environmental Applications
Edited by Shakeel Ahmed, Saiqa Ikram, Suvardhan Kanchi, and Krishna Bisetty
Copyright © 2018 Pan Stanford Publishing Pte. Ltd.
ISBN 978-981-4774-38-3 (Hardcover), 978-1-315-11080-6 (eBook)
www.panstanford.com

PHAs possess several complementary properties that position them well in the materials sector in the modern world. In this context, the utilization of biopolyesters provides extensive opportunities for experimentation, interdisciplinary and multidisciplinary scientific research. Among these, PHA-based composites/blends, thin films, nano- and microparticles, and 3D scaffolds are of supreme importance. Researchers have redirected their interests to the engineering of bio-based materials for targeted applications in different industries, including cosmetics, pharmaceuticals, and other biotechnological/biomedical applications.

16.1 Introduction

Bio-based natural materials are moving into the mainstream applications, changing the dynamics of 21st century materials and their utilization in various research strategies. Owing to the increasing consciousness and elevated demands in healthcare facilities, the engineering aspects of novel materials are considered a potential solution to such a problematic issue [1]. These materials have not only been a motivating factor for the materials scientists, but also they provide potential opportunities for improving living standards [1, 2]. In the past years, several authors reported several types of novel materials, including PHAs [3–8]. In the recent decades, there have been an ever-increasing research interest for multipurpose applications in biotechnology at large and biomedical, pharmaceutical, and cosmeceutical applications in particular [9]. Words such as renewability, recyclability, and sustainability are emphasized in growing scientific and ecological awareness. The green agenda principles have directed this search toward ecofriendly materials with multifunctional features [10]. The legislation authorities are the driving force behind the development of these new types of materials, which are antimicrobial and green in nature [1].

16.2 Biopolyesters

PHAs, along with others, are among the most representative bio-based polyesters from microbial origin. PHAs belong to a family of biopolyesters produced by microbes under limited nutritional conditions (e.g., nitrogen or phosphate) [11, 12], or excess carbon source [13–16]. The unbalanced nutritional supply causes the bacteria to accumulate PHAs in the form of granules as an internal energy storage, as shown in Fig. 16.1. In 1888, Beijerinck first observed these intracellular granules within bacterial cells. During the 1920s, a French microbiologist Maurice Lemoigne was the first who discovered polyester, P(3HB), as an intracellular granule in the gram-positive bacterium *Bacillus megaterium* [14, 17]. A wide spectrum of gram-positive and gram-negative bacteria (approximately over 300 species, examples of which include *Pseudomonas* spp., *Bacillus* spp., and *Methylobacterium* spp.) has been identified with the capability to biosynthesize PHAs. However, some bacterial species, including *Azotobacter vinelandii* UWD, *Alcaligenes eutrophus*, *Alcaligenes latus*, and a mutant *Azotobacter vinelandii*, are also able to accumulate PHAs under non-limiting conditions [15, 16, 18]. Figure 16.2 shows the generic structural formula for PHAs, where x is 1 or higher, and R can be either hydrogen or hydrocarbon chains of up to C16 in length. Based on Fig. 16.2, the main members of the PHA family are presented in Table 16.1.

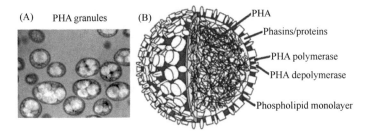

Figure 16.1 PHA granules (A) and schematic of a PHA granule (B). The core consists of PHA polymer, which is enwrapped by a phospholipid monolayer and proteins on the outside. The proteins consist of PHA polymerase, PHA depolymerase, structural proteins, and proteins of unknown function [1].

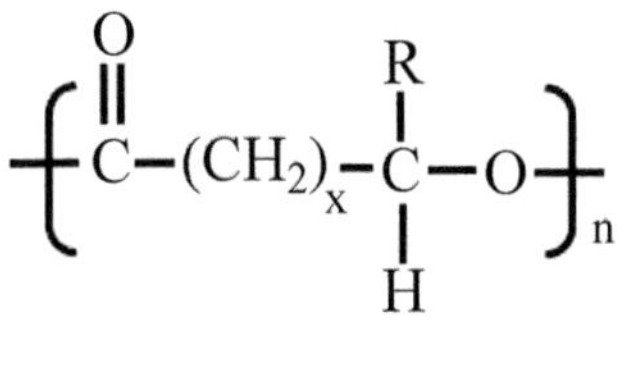

$$\left\{ \begin{matrix} O \\ \| \\ C-(CH_2)_x \end{matrix} - \begin{matrix} R \\ | \\ C-O \\ | \\ H \end{matrix} \right\}_n$$

Figure 16.2 Generic chemical structure of polyhydroxyalkanoates (PHAs) [1].

Table 16.1 Main PHA structures based on Fig. 16.2

Name	Abbreviation	x value	R group
Poly(3-hydroxypropionate)	P(3HP)	1	Hydrogen
Poly(3-hydroxybutyrate)	P(3HB)	1	Methyl
Poly(3-hydroxyvalerate)	P(3HV)	1	Ethyl
Poly(3-hydroxyhexanoate)	P(3HHx)	1	Propyl
Poly(3-hydroxyheptanoate)	P(3HHp)	1	Butyl
Poly(3-hydroxyoctanoate)	P(3HO)	1	Pentyl
Poly(3-hydroxynonanoate)	P(3HN)	-	Hexyl
Poly(3-hydroxydecanoate)	P(3HD)	1	Heptyl
Poly(3-hydroxyundecanoate)	P(3HUD) or P(3HUd)	1	Octyl
Poly(3-hydroxydodecanoate)	P(3HDD) or P(3HDd)	1	Nonyl
Poly(3-hydroxyoctadecanoate)	P(3HOD) or P(3HOd)	1	Pentadecanoyl
Poly(4-hydroxybutyrate)	P(4HB)	2	Hydrogen
Poly(5-hydroxybutyrate)	P(5HB)	2	Methyl
Poly(5-hydroxyvalerate)	P(5HV)	3	Hydrogen

Source: Ref. [1].

The types of monomer being synthesized by the bacterium are determined by the carbon source used in the fermentation medium [1]. It has now been well established that the major monomer has the same chain length as the carbon source. Monomers containing odd numbers of carbon atoms are synthesized when a carbon source with odd numbers of carbon atoms is utilized, while monomers containing even numbers of carbon atoms are synthesized from carbon sources with even numbers of carbon atoms. For example, when a bacterium is cultivated with octane (eight carbon atoms) as the only carbon source, the produced PHAs consist mainly of 3-hydroxyoctanoate units (eight carbon atoms), with small amounts of 3-hydroxyhexanoate units (six carbon atoms) [19]. More than 100 different monomers can be combined within this family to give materials with different properties; they can be either thermoplastic or elastomeric material. PHAs have attracted great scientific and technological interest due to their good biocompatibility, biodegradability, and thermoplastic properties [20, 21] and are expected to contribute to the construction of environmentally sustainable products.

16.3 Physiochemical Characteristics of Biopolyesters

Polymers from the aforementioned polyester family exhibit a wider range of structural, physicochemical, and thermomechanical properties. Depending on the length of the alkyl group, R, PHAs can be categorized into short-chain-length PHAs (scl-PHAs) and medium-chain-length PHAs (mcl-PHAs). The scl-PHAs, which contain 3–5 carbon atoms, are thermoplastic, exhibiting a high degree of crystallinity. The mcl-PHAs, which contain 6–14 carbon atoms, are elastomers with a low degree of crystallinity. With variations in the length of R, PHAs change their properties [1]. Grafting/blending of different PHA monomers allows optimizing their properties for various applications and, in particular, for a biomedical sector where biocompatibility, biodegradability, and thermomechanical properties are considered critically. To date, approximately 150 different types of biosynthetic PHAs have been reported, making them the largest group of natural polyesters [16, 22–24]. PHA nomenclature and classification may still evolve as new structures continue to be discovered. So far several PHAs, including P(3HB), copolymers of 3-hydroxybutyrate and 3-hydroxyvalerate, P(3HB-co-3HV), poly(4-hydroxybutyrate) [P(4HB)], copolymers of 3-hydroxybutyrate and 3-hydroxyhexanoate P(3HB-co-3HHx), and poly(3-hydroxyoctanoate) [P(3HO)] are available in sufficient quantity for research purposes [12, 21].

16.4 Poly(3-hydroxybutyrate)

P(3HB) belongs to scl-PHA type and is the most often used PHA since its discovery in 1926 by Lemoigne. It represents the simplest member of the PHA family, with its chemical structure shown in Fig. 16.3. Mechanical properties of P(3HB) are comparable to that of the synthetic polymers such as polypropylene [25]. P(3HB) is an amorphous to highly crystalline material with a degree of crystallinity of 30–90% [26], due to the presence of a short methyl side chain within its structure [27]. In spite of its relatively brittle and stiff properties, with a strain at break typically less than 5%, P(3HB) can be fabricated with other suitable natural and synthetic polymers to achieve satisfactory flexibility [28]. The properties of P(3HB) strongly depend on various factors, including the type of microbial culture, production, and extraction protocols. Due to its high crystallinity, P(3HB) exhibits a very slow degradation rate of 3.6 wt% per week in activated sludge, 1.9 wt% per week in soil, 1.5 wt% per week in lake water, and 0.8 wt% per week in Indian Ocean sea water [29, 30]. Besides the processing conditions, the microstructure and properties of PHA materials themselves can significantly affect the degradation rates [31, 32]. Thus, it has been investigated for tissue engineering applications that require a longer retention time or a high stability in the surrounding environment [12, 33], for example, bone repair [34, 35], nerve conduits [36, 37], and pericardial substitutes [38, 39]. In vitro tests have shown that P(3HB) is biocompatible with various cell lines, including osteoblasts, epithelial cells, and rabbit chondrocytes [34, 40].

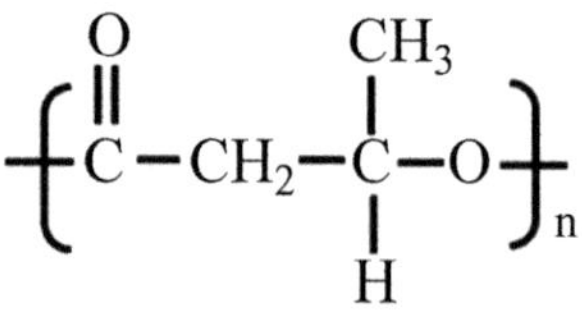

$$\left\{ \begin{matrix} O & CH_3 \\ \parallel & | \\ C-CH_2-C-O \\ & | \\ & H \end{matrix} \right\}_n$$

Figure 16.3 Chemical structure of P(3HB) [1].

The material properties of P(3HB) can be fine-tuned for specific applications by incorporating it with a second monomer unit. There are two approaches: (i) co-synthesis of P(3HB) with hydroxyalkanoate monomeric units of higher chain length, by co-feeding of the culture with different carbon sources. Some common examples are poly(3-hydroxybutyrate-co-3-hydroxyvalerate) [P(3HB-co-3HV)], which are also available commercially as Biopol [41–43]), poly(3-hydroxybutyrate-co-3-hydroxyhexanoate) [P(3HB-co-3HHx)] [44, 45], and poly(3-hydroxybutyrate-co-4-hydroxybutyrate) [P(3HB-co-4HB)] [46]; (ii) physical blending of P(3HB) with higher-chain-length PHAs, e.g., P(3HV) [47, 48], P(3HHx) [49–52], and P(3HO) [53, 54].

The physical and thermal properties of microbial copolyesters can be regulated by varying their molecular weights and compositions. In general, the resulting copolyesters are more flexible and elastic than P(3HB) [55]. The blending approach has several advantages in comparison to synthesizing new copolyesters, including the ease of preparation and optimization of its final properties [56]. Blending reduces the crystallinity of P(3HB) and, as a result of macrophase separation and the effective surface area of the blended material, increases the surface erosion rate [56, 57].

16.5 Biocomposites

A composite consists of two or more distinct materials/polymers to obtain tailor-made characteristics or to improve or impart ideal properties. Such characteristics include, but not limited to, specific strength, thermal properties, surface properties, biocompatibility, and biodegradability. The individual counterparts from a biocomposite fail to demonstrate the features mentioned above on their own. There are several means to modify polymers to make them useful for a wider range of applications [58]. These techniques include alkaline hydrolysis, chemical, gamma radiation, photochemical, UV, plasma-induced techniques, and enzymatic grafting [1, 5–7, 59–65].

Recently, bio-based composite materials have been engineered for target applications in different sectors such as bio-based packaging, biomedical, pharmaceutical, textiles, paper, and others [66–70], to address the growing environmental concerns of a globally unsustainable dependence on non-renewable petroleum-based resources [71, 72]. Owing to the ever-increasing environmental consciousness, the manufacture, use, and removal of traditional synthetically produced polymers or composite structures are considered more critically [73]. The "green biocomposites" consist of biocompatible and biodegradable biopolymers [74]. Biopolymers generated from renewable natural sources by microorganisms are often biodegradable, biocompatible, and non-toxic in nature. Therefore, manufacturing of green composites using one or more individual biopolymers is very desirable. Sustainability requirement is changing the dynamics of the materials industry, offering new opportunities and prospects. The sustainability concept is shown in Fig. 16.4.

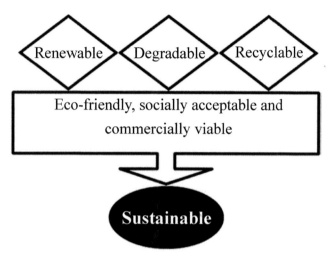

Figure 16.4 Concept of "sustainability" [1].

16.6 Properties of Biocomposites for Biomedical Applications

16.6.1 Biocompatibility and Biodegradability

The unique capability of a material to perform with an appropriate host response in a specific application is termed biocompatibility. Such interpretation of biocompatibility may seem futuristic but is, in fact, much closer than one would expect. It is recognized that cell interaction with a test surface is a simplification of physiological conditions, which usually involves full immersion of the cell in a culture environment [1].

The versatility of in vitro cell studies is affirmed by the vast amount of well-established techniques. Apart from the typical biochemical quantification methods, new microscopic techniques are emerging steadily owing to their wider coverage and depiction of cell morphology about biomolecules. It is often considered necessary to match, as much as possible, the physicochemical and mechanical characteristics of the support biomaterials surrounding tissues. Before the design and development of biocomposite biomaterials, their physicochemical, mechanical, morphological, and toxicological characteristics must be evaluated carefully, and critically about the biomedical applications. Over the last decade, substantial efforts have been made to develop biocomposites with novel characteristics to optimize both in vitro and in vivo performances, while retaining the anticipated bulk properties. As far as the use of tools and materials in medicine are concerned, owing to the emergence of novel green technologies, the benefits of carefully selected and crafted materials have been well established [1]. Over the last 50 years, innovative devices such as joint replacements, pacemakers, lenses, cochlear implants, artificial heart valves, and blood vessels have significantly extended the lifetime and life quality of patients [75]. These devices are termed "implantable medical devices," and the materials suitable for producing them are termed "biomaterials." Although highly successful in several clinical applications, the design of such materials is far from optimum [76]. Consequently, the anticipation and inspiration for further research in biomaterials with novel characteristics intensify. The interdisciplinary research area is more active and innovative than ever and ranges from physics and chemistry to molecular and cell biology and medicine.

As regards biodegradability, "a potential of a target material undergoing decomposition into carbon dioxide, new biomass, and water (in the presence of oxygen, i.e., aerobic conditions) and methane (in the absence of oxygen, i.e., anaerobic conditions)." The predominant mechanism is the enzymatic action of microorganisms. However, different media (liquid, inert, or compost medium) are also considered for the analysis of biodegradability. Biodegradation involves living microorganisms, promoted by their enzymes, and can occur under aerobic and anaerobic conditions leading to complete or partial removal of the target material from the environment. Linear polymers are more biodegradable than branched polymers. Several researchers have examined the biodegradability of aliphatic homo- and co-polyester-based materials in various environments such as soil, freshwater, and seawater [1, 7, 77–82]. As described earlier, in practice, most of the synthetic polymers are petroleum based and are not biodegradable. Therefore, in this context, biodegradable biopolymers or bio-based polymers contribute significantly to the sustainable development of a wider range of disposal polymers with minor adverse environmental impact. Biodegradation is an important factor that should be considered during the design, and the products must be engineered from "conception to reincarnation," the so-called "cradle-to-cradle" approach [1]. Moreover, the choice of the designed materials relates to the intended biotechnological and biomedical applications. In recent years, with increasing scientific knowledge and consciousness, people are more aware that efforts have to be made to rebalance the carbon cycle by reducing the amount of carbon dioxide. Part of the "going green" concept is based on the development of products based on renewable and biodegradable resources [1, 7]. In this background, Fig. 16.5 illustrates some possible degradation steps of phenol-grafted keratin-EC based biocomposite [7].

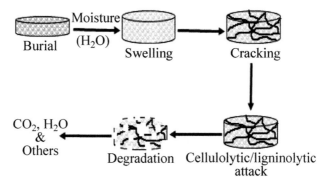

Figure 16.5 A schematic representation of proposed mechanism of soil burial degradation cycle. Reproduced from Ref. [7], with permission of The Royal Society of Chemistry.

16.7 Biomedical and Biotechnological Applications

The use of biopolymers such as PHA-based biocomposites for biomedical and biotechnological applications has many intrinsic advantages such as biocompatibility, biodegradability, renewability, sustainability, and non-toxicity. In the recent years, from a biological point of view, a wide spectrum of (bio)-polymers-based biocomposites have been engineered for target applications. All of the biopolymers above are characterized and well organized/developed into value-added structures, thus can provide a proper route to emulate biosystems—a biomimetic approach. Herein, Fig. 16.6 illustrates an overview of the recent uses of biopolymers for biomedical and biotechnological applications.

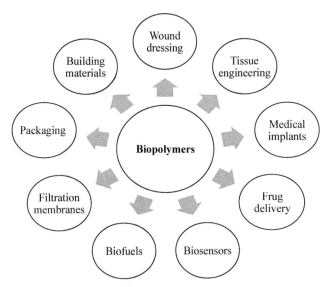

Figure 16.6 Use of biopolymers for various biomedical and biotechnological applications [1].

16.7.1 Biomedical Applications

Owing to the aforementioned properties, that is, biocompatibility and biodegradability, PHAs and PHA-based co-materials have now been considered tailor-made constructs for applications in the medical sector of the modern era. Furthermore, the abovementioned biocompatibility characteristics are underlined because of the natural occurrence of P(3HB) in the human blood and tissue. Therefore, in this context, PHAs and/or PHA-based constructs have been successfully investigated for potent in vivo applications such as implantable constructs, surgical materials, meshes, and sutures (various 2D and 3D shapes), and as a novel carrier constructs at micro- and nanolevel for controlled drug release [83, 84]. Moreover, thanks to the key technical advances in the functional tissue engineering, the highly sophisticated constructs with novel characteristics for artificial blood vessels, bone marrow scaffolds, vascularized tissue constructs, spinal fusion cages, implantable joints, and regeneration devices are among the big achievements [12, 85, 86].

However, before considering the above-mentioned medical applications, it is very critical to consider/distinguish the hydrolytic sensitivity/stability. The hydrolytic sensitivity/stability ratio of the material-based constructs solely depends on the type of application as some required fast degradation whereas other demanding withstand features. In this context, the unique structural composition of PHAs allows the engineering of novel constructs with a fine-tuned thermos-mechanical and tailor-made in vivo degradability properties. For example, P(3HB)- and P(HBHV)-based materials and co-materials normally take a longer degradation under in vitro conditions. On the other hand, some P(3HB)-based co-materials such as P(3HB4HB) possess highly accelerated bio-based degradation rate [1].

Owing to the increasing consciousness and demands to reduce bacterial contaminations in healthcare facilities and possibly to cut pathogenic infections, the engineering aspects of novel active antimicrobial materials are considered a potential solution to such a problematic issue [1]. In the past years, several authors have already reported antibacterial features of several materials, including silver nanoparticles [3, 4, 7, 8]. However, excess release of silver nanoparticles inhibits osteoblasts growth and can also cause many severe side effects such as cytotoxicity [4]. Among natural materials, keratinous proteins are attractive candidates to prepare keratin-based composites, which in turn may find potential applications in biomedical, pharmaceutical, tissue engineering, and cosmetic industries [87]. By this evidence, we hypothesized that natural phenols are among the practical choice for inhibiting bacterial infections and investigated the antibacterial features of these compounds, incorporated materials. Figure 16.7 illustrates the development and antibacterial behavior of phenol-g-keratin-EC based materials [7]. Based on an earlier published data, most of the phenolic compounds, including gallic acid, p-4-hydroxybenzoic acid, and thymol, have the ability to disrupt the lipid structure of the bacterial cell wall, further leading to destruction of the cell membrane, cytoplasmic leakage, and cell lysis, which ultimately leads toward cell death [88, 89]. Furthermore, the delocalization of the electrons on their structure has also been reported to contribute to their antibacterial activity as well [90, 91].

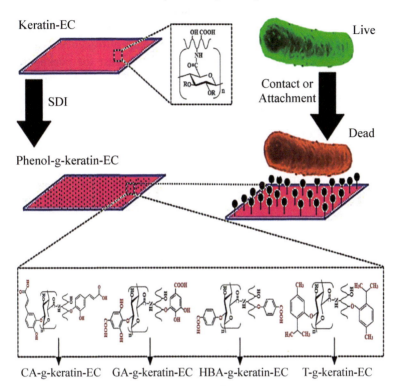

Figure 16.7 The design and antibacterial behavior of phenol-g-keratin-EC–based materials. Reproduced from Ref. [7], with permission of The Royal Society of Chemistry.

16.7.2 Biotechnological Applications

Since the last few decades, there has been a continuously increasing interest in the development of stronger, stiffer, lightweight, and multifunctional engineering material for a variety of industrial and biotechnological applications. To compensate the demand for better performance, extensive research has been devoted to biopolymers and different polymer-based green composites [1]. So far, the most well-known and structured application of P(3HB) and P(3HB)-based co-material such as P(3HB-co-3HV) is a potential alternative to the above-mentioned conventional and non-biodegradable plastics for packaging and other biotechnological purposes. Some of the successful examples include, but not limited to, the development of bio-based plastic bottles for shampoos and other household commodities, using biopolyesters [16]. Likewise, plastic containers and cups have also been well prepared for nutraceutical food products. Moreover, PHAs are of supreme interest for packaging applications, owing to their oxygen permeability barrier potential. Such novel features, in turn, avoid/prevent oxidative spoilage of various food products and ultimately enhance the shelf life period. Here, the pretensions for substrate purity, on the one hand, and for isolation and refining, on the other hand, are lower than for higher sophisticated applications. Interestingly, other potent applications of the various PHAs are in agriculture for a controlled release of growth factors, that is, a wider spectrum of essential nutrients and fertilizers, etc. or pesticidal and herbicidal agents.

16.8 Concluding Remarks and Future Considerations

In summary, the present chapter aimed to critically overview the literature to establish the stability and infective capacity of naturally occurring materials. The chapter also aimed at judicious design, novel characteristics of the developed material that can be modified to achieve an optimal infective capability. Such materials include, but not limited to, biodegradable and biocompatible films and highly porous 3D constructs. Moreover, a novel type of potent materials could be designed for the management and skin regeneration/repair from injury, particularly burns and ulcers, where the risk of bacterial infection is high. Material structure and performance integrity need to be accessed using a range of analytical and imaging techniques.

To date, several efforts have been made to develop novel biomaterials using pristine PHAs extracted from various resources. However, there is still much left to address the concerns of global dependence on petroleum-based materials by degradable and ecofriendly biomaterials. Therefore, in the recent years, much attention has been directed to the engineering of bio-based biocomposite materials for targeted applications in different industries. The development of hybrid biomaterials by in situ modifications, through effective exploitation of biotechnology, can lead to the development of green products with enhanced material properties for applications in cosmetics, pharmaceuticals, and other biotechnological and biomedical sectors of the modern world.

Green chemistry needs to overcome many challenges for successful implementation of innovative technologies to accomplish pollution prevention, reduction and elimination of harmful waste materials during the entire production process. In this regard, ever-increasing environmental awareness and the demand for sustainable technology have gained substantial consideration by the academia and industry to develop ecofriendly processing designs. Moreover, to address the challenges of green chemistry, laccase-assisted grafting processes are simple, ecofriendly, and provide energy-saving reactions. In addition to the non-toxic nature and other benefits of laccase, its use as a biocatalyst, for grafting purposes, offers a possibility to replace the hazardous solvent-based techniques.

Acknowledgments

Authors are thankful to the Tecnologico de Monterrey, Mexico, and the University of Westminster, London, UK, for providing literature facilities.

References

1. Iqbal, H. M. N. (2015). *Development of Bio-composites with Novel Characteristics through Enzymatic Grafting*. Doctoral dissertation, University of Westminster, London, UK.
2. Nair, L. S. and Laurencin, C. T. (2007). Biodegradable polymers as biomaterials. *Progress in Polymer Science*, **32**(8), 762–798.
3. Michl, T. D., Locock, K. E., Stevens, N. E., Hayball, J. D., Vasilev, K., Postma, A., and Griesser, H. J. (2014). RAFT-derived antimicrobial polymethacrylates: Elucidating the impact of end-groups on activity and cytotoxicity. *Polymer Chemistry*, **5**(19), 5813–5822.
4. Wang, L., He, S., Wu, X., Liang, S., Mu, Z., Wei, J., and Wei, S. (2014). Polyetheretherketone/nano-fluorohydroxyapatite composite with antimicrobial activity and osseointegration properties. *Biomaterials*, **35**(25), 6758–6775.

5. Iqbal, H. M., Kyazze, G., Tron, T., and Keshavarz, T. (2014). "One-pot" synthesis and characterisation of novel P(3HB)–ethyl cellulose based graft composites through lipase catalysed esterification. *Polymer Chemistry*, **5**(24), 7004–7012.

6. Iqbal H. M. N., Kyazze, G., Locke, I. C., Tron, T., and Keshavarz, T. (2015). Development of bio-composites with novel characteristics: Evaluation of phenol-induced antibacterial, biocompatible and biodegradable behaviours. *Carbohydrate Polymers*, **131**, 197–207.

7. Iqbal, H. M. N., Kyazze, G., Locke, I. C., Tron, T., and Keshavarz, T. (2015). In situ development of self-defensive antibacterial biomaterials: Phenol-g-keratin-EC based bio-composites with characteristics for biomedical applications. *Green Chemistry*, **17**(7), 3858–3869.

8. Lu, Z., Zhang, X., Li, Z., Wu, Z., Song, J., and Li, C. (2015). Composite copolymer hybrid silver nanoparticles: Preparation and characterization of antibacterial activity and cytotoxicity. *Polymer Chemistry*, **6**(5), 772–779.

9. Ruiz-Ruiz, F., Mancera-Andrade, E. I., and Iqbal H. M. N. (2016). Marine-derived bioactive peptides for biomedical sectors: A review. *Protein and Peptide Letters.* In Press. http://www.ncbi.nlm.nih.gov/pubmed/27491381.

10. Iqbal, H. M. N., Kyazze, G., Tron, T., and Keshavarz, T. (2015). Laccase-assisted approach to graft multifunctional materials of interest: Keratin-EC based novel composites and their characterisation. *Macromolecular Materials and Engineering*, **300**(7), 712–720.

11. Sudesh, K., Abe, H., and Doi, Y. 2000. Synthesis, structure and properties of polyhydroxyalkanoates: Biological polyesters. *Progress in Polymer Science,* **25**, 1503–1555.

12. Chen, G. Q. and Wu, Q. (2005). The application of polyhydroxyalkanoates as tissue engineering materials. *Biomaterials*, **26**(33), 6565–6578.

13. Dawes, E. A. and Senior, P. J. (1973). The role and regulation of energy reserve polymers in micro-organisms. *Advances in Microbial Physiology,* **10**, 135–266.

14. Lee, S. Y. (1996). Bacterial polyhydroxyalkanoates. *Biotechnology and Bioengineering*, **49**(1), 1–14.

15. Ojumu, T. V., Yu, J., and Solomon, B. O. (2004). Production of polyhydroxyalkanoates, a bacterial biodegradable polymers. *African Journal of Biotechnology*, **3**(1), 18–24.

16. Keshavarz, T. and Roy, I. (2010). Polyhydroxyalkanoates: Bioplastics with a green agenda. *Current Opinion in Microbiology*, **13**(3), 321–326.

17. Lemoigne, M. (1926). Products of dehydration and of polymerization of ß-hydroxybutyric acid. *Bull Soc Chem Biol*, **8**, 770–782.

18. Chou, K. S., Chang-Ho, H. W. R., and Goodrich, P. R. (1997). Poly(hydroxybutyrate-co-hydroxy-valerate) from swine waste liquor by *Azotobacter vinelandii* UWD. *Biotechnology Letters*, **19**(1), 7–10.

19. De Smet, M. J., Eggink, G., Witholt, B., Kingma, J., and Wynberg, H. (1983). Characterization of intracellular inclusions formed by *Pseudomonas oleovorans* during growth on octane. *Journal of Bacteriology*, **154**(2), 870–878.

20. Stevens, M. M. (2008). Biomaterials for bone tissue engineering. *Materials Today*, **11**(5), 18–25.

21. Bettinger, C. J. (2011). Biodegradable elastomers for tissue engineering and cell-biomaterial interactions. *Macromolecular Bioscience*, **11**, 467–482.

22. Zhang, B., Carlson, R., and Srienc, F. (2006). Engineering the monomer composition of polyhydroxyalkanoates synthesized in *Saccharomyces cerevisiae*. *Applied and Environmental Microbiology*, **72**(1), 536–543.

23. Li, Z. and Loh, X. J. (2015). Water soluble polyhydroxyalkanoates: Future materials for therapeutic applications. *Chemical Society Reviews*, **44**(10), 2865–2879.

24. Rehm, B. H. A. (2015). Microbial synthesis of biodegradable polyesters: Processes, products, applications, in *Biodegradable Polyesters* (Fakirov, S., Ed.), pp. 47–72, Wiley-VCH Verlag GmbH & Co. KGaA, Weinheim, Germany.

25. Engelberg, I. and Kohn, J. (1991). Physico-mechanical properties of degradable polymers used in medical applications: A comparative study. *Biomaterials*, **12**, 292–304.

26. Sudesh, K., Abe, H., and Doi, Y. (2000). Synthesis, structure and properties of polyhydroxyalkanoates: Biological polyesters. *Progress in Polymer Science*, **25**, 1503–1555.

27. Kawaguchi, Y. and Doi, Y. (1992). Kinetics and mechanism of synthesis and degradation of poly(3-hydroxybutyrate) in *Alcaligenes eutrophus*. *Macromolecules*, **25**, 2324–2329.

28. Misra, S. K., Valappil, S. P., Roy, I., and Boccaccini, A. R. (2006). Polyhydroxyalkanoate (PHA)/inorganic phase composites for tissue engineering applications. *Biomacromolecules*, **7**, 2249–2258.

29. Akmal, D., Azizan, M. N., and Majid, M. I. A. (2003). Biodegradation of microbial polyesters P(3HB) and P(3HB-co-3HV) under the tropical

climate environment. *Polymer Degradation and Stability*, **80**(3), 513–518.

30. Liu, Q., Zhang, H., Deng, B., and Zhao, X. (2014). Poly(3-hydroxybutyrate) and poly(3-hydroxybutyrate-co-3-hydroxyvalerate): Structure, property, and fiber. *International Journal of Polymer Science*, Article ID 374368, 11 pages.

31. Abe, H. and Doi, Y. (1999). Structural effects on enzymatic degradabilities for poly[(R)-3-hydroxybutyric acid] and its copolymers. *International Journal of Biological Macromolecules*, **25**(1), 185–192.

32. Plackett, D. (Ed.) (2011). Front matter, in *Biopolymers: New Materials for Sustainable Films and Coatings*, John Wiley & Sons, Ltd, Chichester, UK. doi: 10.1002/9781119994312.fmatter.

33. Chen, Q., Liang, S., and Thouas, G. A. (2013). Elastomeric biomaterials for tissue engineering. *Progress in Polymer Science*, **38**(3), 584–671.

34. Doyle, C., Tanner, E. T., and Bonfield, W. (1991). In vitro and in vivo evaluation of polyhydroxybutyrate and of polyhydroxybutyrate reinforced with hydroxyapatite. *Biomaterials*, **12**, 841–847.

35. Luklinska, Z. B. and Bonfield, W. (1997). Morphology and ultrastructure of the interface between hydroxyapatite-polyhydroxybutyrate composite implant and bone. *Journal of Materials Science: Materials in Medicine*, **8**(6), 379–383.

36. Hazari, A., Wiberg, M., Johansson-Ruden, G., Green, C., and Terenghi, G. (1999). A resorbable nerve conduit as an alternative to nerve autograft in nerve gap repair. *British Journal of Plastic Surgery*, **52**(8), 653–657.

37. Young, R. C., Terenghi, G., and Wiberg, M. (2002). Poly-3-hydroxybutyrate (PHB): A resorbable conduit for long-gap repair in peripheral nerves. *British Journal of Plastic Surgery*, **55**(3), 235–240.

38. Duvernoy, O., Malm, T., Ramström, J., and Bowald, S. (1995). A biodegradable patch used as a pericardial substitute after cardiac surgery: 6- and 24-month evaluation with CT. *The Thoracic and Cardiovascular Surgeon*, **43**(5), 271–274.

39. Kalangos, A. and Faidutti, B. (1996). Preliminary clinical results of implantation of biodegradable pericardial substitute in pediatric open heart operations. *The Journal of Thoracic and Cardiovascular Surgery*, **112**(5), 1401–1402.

40. Zheng, Z., Bei, F. F., Tian, H. L., and Chen, G. Q. (2005). Effects of crystallization of polyhydroxyalkanoate blend on surface physicochemical properties and interactions with rabbit articular cartilage chondrocytes. *Biomaterials*, **26**(17), 3537–3548.

41. Köse, G. T., Korkusuz, F., Özkul, A., Soysal, Y., Özdemir, T., Yildiz, C., and Hasirci, V. (2005). Tissue engineered cartilage on collagen and PHBV matrices. *Biomaterials*, **26**(25), 5187–5197.

42. Sun, J., Wu, J., Li, H., and Chang, J. (2005). Macroporous poly(3-hydroxybutyrate-co-3-hydroxyvalerate) matrices for cartilage tissue engineering. *European Polymer Journal*, **41**(10), 2443–2449.

43. Weng, Y. X., Wang, X. L., and Wang, Y. Z. (2011). Biodegradation behavior of PHAs with different chemical structures under controlled composting conditions. *Polymer Testing*, **30**(4), 372–380.

44. Doi, Y., Kitamura, S., and Abe, H. (1995). Microbial synthesis and characterization of poly(3-hydroxybutyrate-co-3-hydroxyhexanoate). *Macromolecules*, **28**(14), 4822–4828.

45. Wang, Y. W., Yang, F., Wu, Q., Cheng, Y. C., Peter, H. F., Chen, J., and Chen, G. Q. (2005). Effect of composition of poly(3-hydroxybutyrate-co-3-hydroxyhexanoate) on growth of fibroblast and osteoblast. *Biomaterials*, **26**(7), 755–761.

46. Ying, T. H., Ishii, D., Mahara, A., Murakami, S., Yamaoka, T., Sudesh, K., and Iwata, T. (2008). Scaffolds from electrospun polyhydroxyalkanoate copolymers: Fabrication, characterization, bioabsorption and tissue response. *Biomaterials*, **29**(10), 1307–1317.

47. Satoh, H., Yoshie, N., and Inoue, Y. (1994). Hydrolytic degradation of blends of poly(3-hydroxybutyrate) with poly(3-hydroxybutyrate-co-3-hydroxyvalerate). *Polymer*, **35**(2), 286–290.

48. Gassner, F. and Owen, A. J. (1996). Some properties of poly(3-hydroxybutyrate)–poly(3-hydroxyvalerate) blends. *Polymer International*, **39**(3), 215–219.

49. Deng, Y., Zhao, K., Zhang, X. F., Hu, P., and Chen, G. Q. (2002). Study on the three-dimensional proliferation of rabbit articular cartilage-derived chondrocytes on polyhydroxyalkanoate scaffolds. *Biomaterials*, **23**(20), 4049–4056.

50. Deng, Y., Lin, X. S., Zheng, Z., Deng, J. G., Chen, J. C., Ma, H., and Chen, G. Q. (2003). Poly(hydroxybutyrate-co-hydroxyhexanoate) promoted production of extracellular matrix of articular cartilage chondrocytes in vitro. *Biomaterials*, **24**(23), 4273–4281.

51. Kai, Z., Ying, D., and Guo-Qiang, C. (2003). Effects of surface morphology on the biocompatibility of polyhydroxyalkanoates. *Biochemical Engineering Journal*, **16**(2), 115–123.

52. Zheng, Z., Bei, F. F., Tian, H. L., and Chen, G. Q. (2005). Effects of crystallization of polyhydroxyalkanoate blend on surface

physicochemical properties and interactions with rabbit articular cartilage chondrocytes. *Biomaterials,* **26**(17), 3537–3548.

53. Dufresne, A. and Vincendon, M. (2000). Poly(3-hydroxybutyrate) and poly(3-hydroxyoctanoate) blends: Morphology and mechanical behavior. *Macromolecules,* **33**(8), 2998–3008.

54. Basnett, P., Ching, K. Y., Stolz, M., Knowles, J. C., Boccaccini, A. R., Smith, C., and Roy, I. (2013). Novel poly(3-hydroxyoctanoate)/poly(3-hydroxybutyrate) blends for medical applications. *Reactive and Functional Polymers,* **73**(10), 1340–1348.

55. Barker, P. A., Mason, F., and Barham, P. J. (1990). Density and crystallinity of poly(3-hydroxybutyrate/3-hydroxyvalerate) copolymers. *Journal of Materials Science,* **25**(4), 1952–1956.

56. Ha, C. S. and Cho, W. J. (2002). Miscibility, properties, and biodegradability of microbial polyester containing blends. *Progress in Polymer Science,* **27**(4), 759–809.

57. Satoh, H., Yoshie, N., and Inoue, Y. (1994). Hydrolytic degradation of blends of poly(3-hydroxybutyrate) with poly(3-hydroxybutyrate-co-3-hydroxyvalerate). *Polymer,* **35**(2), 286–290.

58. Akaraonye, E., Keshavarz, T., and Roy, I. (2010). Production of polyhydroxyalkanoates: The future green materials of choice. *Journal of Chemical Technology and Biotechnology,* **85**(6), 732–743.

59. Mitomo, H., Watanabe, Y., Yoshii, F., and Makuuchi, K. (1995). Radiation effect on polyesters. *Radiation Physics and Chemistry,* **46**(2), 233–238.

60. Grøndahl, L., Chandler-Temple, A., and Trau, M. (2005). Polymeric grafting of acrylic acid onto poly(3-hydroxybutyrate-co-3-hydroxyvalerate): Surface functionalization for tissue engineering applications. *Biomacromolecules,* **6**(4), 2197–2203.

61. Lao, H. K., Renard, E., Linossier, I., Langlois, V., and Vallée-Rehel, K. (2007). Modification of poly(3-hydroxybutyrate-co-3-hydroxyvalerate) film by chemical graft copolymerization. *Biomacromolecules,* **8**(2), 416–423.

62. Lao, H. K., Renard, E., Langlois, V., Vallée-Rehel, K., and Linossier, I. (2010). Surface functionalization of PHBV by HEMA grafting via UV treatment: Comparison with thermal free radical polymerization. *Journal of Applied Polymer Science,* **116**(1), 288–297.

63. Iqbal, H. M. N., Kyazze, G., Locke, I. C., Tron, T., and Keshavarz, T. (2015). Development of novel antibacterial active, HaCaT biocompatible and biodegradable CA-g-P(3HB)-EC biocomposites with caffeic acid as a functional entity. *eXPRESS Polymer Letters,* **9**, 764–772.

64. Iqbal, H. M. N., Kyazze, G., Locke, I. C., Tron, T., and Keshavarz, T. (2015). Poly(3-hydroxybutyrate)-ethyl cellulose based bio-composites with novel characteristics for infection free wound healing application. *International Journal of Biological Macromolecules*, **81**, 552–559.

65. Iqbal, H. M. N., Kyazze, G., Tron, T., and Keshavarz, T. (2016). Laccase from *Aspergillus niger*: A novel tool to graft multifunctional materials of interests and their characterization. *Saudi Journal of Biological Sciences*, In-Press, DOI: 10.1016/j.sjbs.2016.01.027.

66. Klemm, D., Schumann, D., Udhardt, U., and Marsch, S. (2001). Bacterial synthesized cellulose—artificial blood vessels for microsurgery. *Progress in Polymer Science*, **26**(9), 1561–1603.

67. Grunert, M. and Winter, W. T. (2002). Nanocomposite of cellulose acetate butyrate reinforced with cellulose nanocrystals. *Journal of Polymers and the Environment*, **10**, 28–30.

68. Gindl, W. and Keckes, J. (2004). Tensile properties of cellulose acetate butyrate composites reinforced with bacterial cellulose. *Composites Science and Technology*, **64**(15), 2407–2413.

69. Svensson, A., Nicklasson, E., Harrah, T., Panilaitis, B., Kaplan, D. L., Brittberg, M., and Gatenholm, P. (2005). Bacterial cellulose as a potential scaffold for tissue engineering of cartilage. *Biomaterials*, **26**(4), 419–431.

70. Czaja, W., Krystynowicz, A., Bielecki, S., and Brown Jr, R. M. (2006). Microbial cellulose: The natural power to heal wounds. *Biomaterials*, **27**(2), 145–151.

71. Srubar, W. V., Pilla, S., Wright, Z. C., Ryan, C. A., Greene, J. P., Frank, C. W., and Billington, S. L. (2012). Mechanisms and impact of fiber–matrix compatibilization techniques on the material characterization of PHBV/oak wood flour engineered biobased composites. *Composites Science and Technology*, **72**(6), 708–715.

72. Iqbal, H. M. N., Kyazze, G., and Keshavarz, T. (2013). Advances in the valorization of lignocellulosic materials by biotechnology: An overview. *BioResources*, **8**(2), 3157–3176.

73. Herrmann, A. S., Nickel, J., and Riedel, U. (1998). Construction materials based upon biologically renewable resources: From components to finished parts. *Polymer Degradation and Stability*, **59**(1), 251–261.

74. Mohanty, A. K., Misra, M., and Drzal, L. T. (2002). Sustainable bio-composites from renewable resources: Opportunities and challenges in the green materials world. *Journal of Polymers and the Environment*, **10**(1–2), 19–26.

75. Ratner, B. D., Hoffman, A. S., Schoen, F. J., and Lemons, J. E. (2004). *Biomaterials Science: An Introduction to Materials in Medicine*, Academic Press.
76. Whitesides, G. M. (2005). Nanoscience, nanotechnology, and chemistry. *Small*, **1**(2), 172–179.
77. Rizzarelli, P., Puglisi, C., and Montaudo, G. (2004). Soil burial and enzymatic degradation in solution of aliphatic co-polyesters. *Polymer Degradation and Stability*, **85**(2), 855–863.
78. Tokiwa, Y. and Calabia, B. P. (2004). Review degradation of microbial polyesters. *Biotechnology Letters*, **26**(15), 1181–1189.
79. Lenz, R. W. and Marchessault, R. H. (2005). Bacterial polyesters: Biosynthesis, biodegradable plastics and biotechnology. *Biomacromolecules*, **6**(1), 1–8.
80. Volova, T. G., Boyandin, A. N., Vasiliev, A. D., Karpov, V. A., Prudnikova, S. V., Mishukova, O. V., and Gitelson, I. I. (2010). Biodegradation of polyhydroxyalkanoates (PHAs) in tropical coastal waters and identification of PHA-degrading bacteria. *Polymer Degradation and Stability*, **95**(12), 2350–2359.
81. Boyandin, A. N., Prudnikova, S. V., Filipenko, M. L., Khrapov, E. A., Vasil'ev, A. D., and Volova, T. G. (2012). Biodegradation of polyhydroxyalkanoates by soil microbial communities of different structures and detection of PHA degrading microorganisms. *Applied Biochemistry and Microbiology*, **48**(1), 28–36.
82. Burlein, G. A. and Rocha, M. C. (2014). LDPE/PHB blends filled with castor oil pressed cake. *Materials Research*, **17**(1), 203–212.
83. Doi, Y. and Steinbüchel, A. (Eds.), (2002). *Biopolymers, Polyesters III: Applications and Commercial Products* (Vol. 4), Wiley-Blackwell.
84. Williams, S. F. and Martin, D. P. (2005). Applications of polyhydroxyalkanoates (PHA) in medicine and pharmacy. *Biopolymers Online*.
85. Zinn, M., Witholt, B., and Egli, T. (2001). Occurrence, synthesis and medical application of bacterial polyhydroxyalkanoate. *Advanced Drug Delivery Reviews*, **53**(1), 5–21.
86. Valappil, S. P., Misra, S. K., Boccaccini, A. R., and Roy, I. (2006). Biomedical applications of polyhydroxyalkanoates: An overview of animal testing and in vivo responses. *Expert Review of Medical Devices*, **3**(6), 853–868.
87. Khosa, M. A. and Ullah, A. (2013). A sustainable role of keratin biopolymer in green chemistry: A review. *Journal of Food Processing and Beverages*, **1**(1), 1–8.

88. Veras, H. N., Rodrigues, F. F., Colares, A. V., Menezes, I. R., Coutinho, H. D., Botelho, M. A., and Costa, J. G. (2012). Synergistic antibiotic activity of volatile compounds from the essential oil of *Lippia sidoides* and thymol. *Fitoterapia*, **83**(3), 508–512.
89. Shahidi, S., Aslan, N., Ghoranneviss, M., and Korachi, M. (2014). Effect of thymol on the antibacterial efficiency of plasma-treated cotton fabric. *Cellulose*, **21**(3), 1933–1943.
90. Ultee, A., Bennik, M. H. J., and Moezelaar, R. (2002). The phenolic hydroxyl group of carvacrol is essential for action against the food-borne pathogen *Bacillus cereus*. *Applied and Environmental Microbiology*, **68**(4), 1561–1568.
91. Elegir, G., Kindl, A., Sadocco, P., and Orlandi, M. (2008). Development of antimicrobial cellulose packaging through laccase-mediated grafting of phenolic compounds. *Enzyme and Microbial Technology*, **43**(2), 84–92.

Chapter 17

Treatment of Industrial Wastewater Using Biopolymers and Biocomposites

Nang Seng Moe,[a] May Myat Khine,[a] Kyaw Nyein Aye,[a] Hiroshi Tamura,[b] Hideki Yamamoto,[c] and Nitar Nwe[a]

[a]*Ecological Laboratory, Advancing Life and Regenerating Motherland, Kan Road, Hlaing Township, Yangon, Myanmar*
[b]*Faculty of Chemistry, Materials and Bioengineering, Kansai University, Suita, Osaka 564-8680, Japan*
[c]*Faculty of Environmental and Urban Engineering, Department of Chemical, Energy and Environmental Engineering, Kansai University, Osaka, 564-8680, Japan*
nangsengmoe@gmail.com, nitarnwe@gmail.com

Most industrial wastewaters contain various amounts and different types of pollutants. Organic matters (such as proteins, pigments, oils, and sugars) and inorganic constituents (such as heavy metals) are the most common constituents in industrial wastewaters. Biological and chemical treatments are applied to remove organic and inorganic matters from industrial wastewaters. For these treatments, reactors such as anaerobic fluidized bed (AFB) reactors for removal of organic materials and mixed reactor for removal of high solid concentrations have been designed and applied to treat industrial wastewaters. Moreover, membrane technologies such as ultrafiltration for the removal of proteins, pigments, oils, sugar, and

Biocomposites: Biomedical and Environmental Applications
Edited by Shakeel Ahmed, Saiqa Ikram, Suvardhan Kanchi, and Krishna Bisetty
Copyright © 2018 Pan Stanford Publishing Pte. Ltd.
ISBN 978-981-4774-38-3 (Hardcover), 978-1-315-11080-6 (eBook)
www.panstanford.com

organic microparticles; nanofiltration for the removal of pigments, sulfates, divalent cations, divalent anions, lactose, sucrose, and sodium chloride have also been applied for wastewater treatments. The easiest, cost-effective, and ecofriendly method for the treatment of wastewater is using biopolymers and biocomposites such as sodium alginate, poly-aluminum ferric chloride, and cationic polyacrylamide. These materials are used as flocculants for the removal of turbid materials. For example, chitosan is used to remove heavy metals and turbid materials. Therefore, this chapter presents innovative processes for the treatment of industrial wastewaters using biopolymer and biocomposite materials and different types of reactors for the reduction of toxicity and for technology-based treatment standards.

17.1 Introduction

Nowadays, human population is increasing day by day. As a consequence, there are industrial and technological expansion, increase in energy utilization and high amount of waste generation from domestic and industrial sources. A high amount of wastewaters from these processes is also disposed in rivers, seas, land, etc. Depending on the discharged types of wastewaters, these are generally divided into domestic wastewaters, wastewaters from institutions, industrial wastewaters, infiltration into sewers, storm water, leachate, and septic tank wastewaters. These wastewaters are hazardous to humans and other living resources [1, 2]. Industrial wastewaters come from two sources: food-producing industries and other human accessories manufacturing. Food industries such as distillery and slaughterhouse release high concentration of organic matters in wastewaters. However, other human accessories production industries, such as metal plating facilities, mining operations, nuclear powerhouse, fertilizer industries, paints and pigments, municipal and storm water run-off, battery and tannery industries release a huge amount of heavy metals in wastewaters [1, 3]. Various physical (screening and filtration), biological (aerobic and anaerobic), and chemical methods are used to treat wastewaters up to an acceptable level of quality for discharge [4]. Moreover, mixed flow reactors, plug flow reactors, fluidization and membrane filtration have been used in these treatments [5, 6]. Nowadays, some reactors are fixed filters, which are made more useful by upgrading with microfiltration (MF), ultrafiltration (UF), nanofiltration (NF), and reverse osmosis (RO) [7]. In the recent years, researchers have been investigating low-cost adsorbents of organic or biological origin, zeolites, industrial byproducts, agricultural wastes, biomass, and polymeric materials [8, 9]. For actual wastewater treatment, the method should be not only efficient but also cost-effective and green. Due to these facts, biopolymers and biocomposites are used because they have different functional groups of hydroxyls and amines for biosorption and physisorption [10]. This chapter describes the types of wastewaters from food industries and human accessories industries, various types of treatments, common types of reactors used in wastewater treatment, and applications of biopolymer and biocomposite materials. Some low-cost biosorbents such as chitosan, alginate, biocomposites, and byproducts from agriculture used in wastewater treatment are also described.

17.2 Wastewater from Various Industries

17.2.1 Wastewater from Food Industries

Nowadays, food-processing industries are behind one of the major environmental problems due to the production of wastewaters from processing plants. According to industries and products, concentrations of constituents contained in wastewaters are different. Most wastewaters contain high concentrations of organic matter and other corresponding materials.

17.2.2 Wastewater from Distillery Plants

Distillery wastewater, stillage obtained from the processing of distillery pot ale, slops, spent wash, dunder, mosto, vinasse and thin stillage, and the volume and concentration of wastewaters depend on feedstock and the process of ethanol production [11]. Some characteristics of distillery wastewaters are given in Table 17.1. According to this table, the amount of chemical oxygen demand (COD) (i.e., the amount of oxygen required to degrade matter by chemical interactions) and the amount of biological oxygen demand (BOD) (i.e., the amount of oxygen required to degrade organic matter biologically) in wastewater released from feedstock based on sugarcane and molasses is higher than that based on wheat crop. However, the main problem in most distillery plants is high concentration of BOD and COD in wastewater.

Table 17.1 Compositions in distillery effluent

Parameters	Compositions [1, 12]
pH	7–3.8
BOD	43,000–60,000 (mg/L)
COD	70,000–98,000 (mg/L)
Cl^-	5,000–10,650 (mg/L)
NO_3^-	-
SO_4^-	2,000–5,000 (mg/L)
Tot P	500–1,500 (mg/L)
Zn	-
Tot N	1,000–1,200 (mg/L)
Tot K	5,000–12,000 (mg/L)
Tot Na	150–356 (mg/L)
Tot Ca	6,800–16,000 (mg/L)
TDS	58,000–91,700 (mg/L)
TSS	2,000–26,560 (mg/L)
Total solids	60,000–118,260 (mg/L)
Color	Dark brown

17.2.3 Wastewater from Coffee Processing

Coffee-processing industries discharge highly polluted wastewater [13]. These industries produce a large amount of wastewater that contain high concentrations of organic matter, nutrients, suspended matter, and acidic compounds (Table 17.2).

Table 17.2 Characteristics of coffee wet wastewater

Characteristics	Compositions [13, 14]
Total COD (mg/L)	2,545–7,903
Total BOD (mg/L)	4,820
pH	3
ST (mg/L)	8,638–1,228.5
TVS (mg/L)	4,452–1,141.6
SST (mg/L)	11–315.7
SSV (mg/L)	1,415– 271.2

17.2.4 Wastewater from Milk Industries

Milk plays a vital role in human life. Dairy industries produce various products such as raw milk, pasteurized milk, butter, and cheese. The required amount of water in milk processing depends on the plant size, and then it is also disposed as wastewater. Wastewater from milk-processing units contain soluble organics, suspended solids, trance organics which causes odor, color, and turbidity of wastewater. All these components could promote eutrophication [15]. These wastewaters contain high BOD and COD and a high amount of oil and grease than the permissible limits. Characteristics of effluents from milk processing are given in Table 17.3.

Table 17.3 Compositions of wastewaters from dairy industry

Parameters	Compositions
pH	3–8
Total dissolved solids	1060–5000 mg/L
Suspended solids	760–1500 mg/L
BOD	1240–3600 mg/L
COD	3000–6000 mg/L
Total nitrogen	84–200 mg/L
Phosphorus	11–50 mg/L
Oil and grease	15–290 mg/L
Chloride	105 mg/L

Source: Adapted from Refs. [16, 17].

17.2.5 Wastewater from Slaughterhouses

Wastewaters from slaughterhouses contain blood from slaughtered animals, suspended solids due to rumen contents, undigested food, feathers, flesh, bone, and highly proteinaceous materials, leading to environmental pollution. Wastewaters from slaughterhouses have a BOD/COD ratio of 0.6, indicating that these waters are highly biodegradable. The blood of slaughtered animals contribute a COD of about 375,000 mg/L (Trittand and Schuehard, 1992, cited in Ref. [11]). Moreover, microorganisms in these wastewaters can cause many diseases, such as tuberculosis, salmonellosis, and helminthosis. Therefore, proper treatment is necessary before the disposal of these wastewaters [11]. The physicochemical characteristics of slaughterhouse wastewaters are given in Table 17.4.

Table 17.4 Physicochemical characteristics of slaughterhouse wastewaters

Parameters	Range
pH	6–7
Alkalinity as $CaCO_3$	3,000–4,000 mg/L
Total solids	9,000–10,000 mg/L
Total volatile solids	5,000–6,000 mg/L
Suspended solids	2,000–3,000 mg/L
Chemical oxygen demand (COD)	20,000–30,000 mg/L
Biochemical oxygen demand (BOD)	10,000–20,000 mg/L
Sulfate as SO_4	90–100 mg/L
Phosphate as PO_4	70–80 mg/L
Chloride (Cl)	400–500 mg/L
Sodium (Na)	200–300 mg/L
Potassium (K)	250–350 mg/L
Total ammonia as NH_3–N	250–325 mg/L
Total nitrogen as N	900–1,000 mg/L
Oil and grease	200–300 mg/L

Source: Reprinted from Ref. [11], Copyright © 2015 IJCPS Journal. All rights reserved.

17.2.6 Wastewater from Other Industries

Nowadays, the number of tannery factories has increased due to the growth of population. These factories discharge wastewater containing toxic organic compounds and heavy metal ions such as lead and chromium [18]. Table 17.5 shows the effluents of the tannery industry.

Table 17.5 Initial effluents of the tannery industry

Parameters	Concentration
Color	Blackish color
Odor	Unacceptable smell
pH	7–7.5
BOD (mg/L)	1,000–1,500
COD (mg/L)	4,000–4,500
Total dissolved solids (TDS) (mg/L)	10,000–17,000
Total solids (TS) (mg/L)	30,000–35,000
Total hardness (TH) (mg/L)	900–950
Turbidity (NTU)	400–500
Sodium (mg/L)	4,500–5,500
Chromium (Cr) (mg/L)	1,000–1,500
Lead (Pb) (mg/L)	0.5–0.35

Source: Reprinted from Ref. [18], with permission from Springer Nature.

Synthetic dyes are now commercially used in the society due to low production cost, brighter colors, better resistance toward environmental factors, and ease of application [19]. Because of these properties, synthetic dyes are used more than natural dyes in most industrial applications. Synthetic dyes are often highly toxic and carcinogenic; they consist of two main groups of compounds: chromophores and auxochromes [19].

Dyes are one of the main sources of severe water pollutions as these are used more in textile industries. So the colored effluents from textile industries have triggered a major concern for human health and marine lives [19].

Moreover, arsenic-containing wastes are produced from chromated copper arsenate wood treatment [8]. Chromium compounds and cadmium sulfide are released from inorganic pigment manufacturing. Nickel, vanadium, and chromium are released from wastes of petroleum refining. Touching, inhaling, and accidental discharge of these heavy metals cause serious health effects, including reduced growth and development, cancer, organ damage, nervous system damage, and death, in extreme cases [8].

Heavy metals such as chromium (Cr), lead (Pb), arsenic (As), copper (Cu), iron (Fe), manganese (Mn), vanadium (V), nickel (Ni), mercury (Hg), cobalt (Co), molybdenum (Md), and bismuth (Bi) discharged by industries are listed in Table 17.6.

Table 17.6 Heavy metals found in wastewaters from major industries

Industry	A	As	Cd	Cr	C	Hg	Pb	Ni	Zn
Pulp and paper mills				X	X	X	X	X	X
Organic chemicals	X	X	X	X		X	X		X
Alkalis, chlorine			X	X	X		X	X	X
Fertilizers	X	X	X	X	X	X	X	X	X
Petroleum refining	X	X	X	X	X		X	X	X
Steel works			X	X	X	X	X	X	X
Aircraft plating, finishing	X		X	X	X	X		X	
Flat glass, cement				X					
Textile mills				X					
Tanning				X					
Power plants				X					
Pharmaceutical									X
Mining industries									X
Paint and dynes				X					
Pesticides				X					X

Source: From Refs. [8, 20].

Metal ions from these industries might harm aquatic lives and humans. Hazard levels of heavy metals are given in Table 17.7.

Table 17.7 Standard maximum contaminant level (MCL) for the most hazardous heavy metals

Metal names	Side infection	Limiting range of MCL (mg/L)
Arsenic	Skin manifestations, visceral cancers, vascular disease	0.01–0.05
Cadmium	Kidney damage, renal disorder, human carcinogen	0.005–0.01
Chromium	Headache, diarrhea, nausea, vomiting, carcinogenic	0.05–0.1
Copper	Damaging liver, Wilson disease, sleeplessness	0.25–0.3
Nickel	Dermatitis, nausea, chronic asthma, coughing, human carcinogen	0.20
Zinc	Depression in mind, fatigue, nervous signs, and increased dehydration	0.8–5
Lead	Damage the fetal brain, diseases of the kidneys, circulatory system, and nervous system	0.006–0.015
Mercury	Rheumatoid arthritis, and diseases of the kidneys, circulatory system, and nervous system	0.00003–0.002

Source: Data adapted from Ref. [8];
http://www.pollutionissues.com/Fo-Hi/Heavy-Metals.html; and
http://www.jmess.org/wpcontent/uploads/2015/11/JMESSP13420004.pdf.

17.3 Methods of Wastewater Treatment

There are various methods of wastewater treatment, basically physical treatment, biological treatment, and chemical treatment.

17.3.1 Physical Treatment

Physical treatments such as screening, filtration, and sedimentation are also known as primary treatments, which are the earliest methods used to remove debris and solids from wastewater. Screening process involves coarse screens and fine screens. Debris and solids are cleaned mechanically using bar screen or manually using trash racks. Size limits for coarse screens are 6 mm (0.25 inch) or larger and those for fine screens are 1.5–6 mm (0.06–0.25 inch) and 0.2–1.5 mm (0.01–0.06 inch). Screening is classified according to type, as given in Table 17.8 [21]. Moreover, solids that are heavier than water settle at the bottom from the wastewater by gravity. Particles entrapped in air float to the top of water and are removed [22].

Table 17.8 Classification of screening devices

Screening types	Classification
Bar screen	It can be cleaned both manually and mechanically.
Fine bar or perforated coarse screen	It has a fine bar, a perforated plate, and a rotary drum.
Fine screen	It has a fixed parabolic and rotary drum and a rotary disk.

Source: Adapted from Ref. [21] and https://www3.epa.gov/npdes/pubs/final_sgrit_removal.pdf

The oldest method is sand filtration, which uses clay and hardpan as natural filters. These are the finest filter media with slow flow rate. If the treatment location is sloped, a pump is not required for flow. Although sand filtration reduces a number of waterborne diseases, it is not adequate for all kinds of microorganisms [23]. A disinfection process might be needed, such as chlorination using hyphochlorite powder or liquid bleach [23].

17.3.2 Biological Treatment

Biological treatment (also called secondary treatment) applies microorganisms that mainly rely on metabolism and growth rate, such as bacteria, algae, and fungi. There are two types of biological treatments: aerobic and anaerobic digestion. Microorganisms use both aerobic and anaerobic digestion to digest organic matter. Anaerobic digestion is more suitable than aerobic digestion for high concentrations of organic matter contained in wastewaters from different industries such as distillery, pulp and paper, slaughterhouse, and dairy [24].

Depending on microbes, it could be used not only in aerobic but also in anaerobic digestion. Microbes are used in various forms such as membrane types, cyclic activated sludge system, media trickling filter known as packed bed biotower, fluidized media bioreactor, and sequencing media. A comparison of the efficiencies of aerobic and anaerobic digestion is given in Table 17.9. Anaerobic is more efficient for using low down organic concentration and generate more biogas. The emission amount of biogas and methane mainly relies on macronutrients (such as carbohydrate, protein, lipid, and cellulose) in food wastes. Nowadays, modifications in the existing reactor designs to a plug flow reactor design improved the efficiency of digestion and low concentration of volatile fatty acids (VFAs) in the effluent. Sometime, it is also used as bacterial sludge immobilization form. Anaerobic sludge blanket reactor and anaerobic baffled reactor could be used to get sludge aggregates that can be easily settled with gas separation. Fluidized bed reactors and anaerobic expanded bed reactors are better applied in bacterial attachment of density and particulate materials. Entrapment of sludge aggregates as packing materials is suitable in downflow and upflow anaerobic filters [2, 25].

Table 17.9 Comparison conditions of anaerobic and aerobic digestion

	Aerobic digestion	Anaerobic digestion
Energy requirement	High	Low
Effluent quality	Excellent	Moderate to poor
Organic loading rate	Moderate	High
Sludge production	High	Low
Nutrient requirement	High	Low
Temperature sensitivity	Low	High
Retention time	Short	Long
Odor	Fewer problems	Bad odor problems

Source: Adapted from Leslie Grady (1999) and Yeoh (1995) cited in Ref. [26] and http://www.ijsrp.org/research-paper-0614/ijsrp-p3007.pdf.

17.3.3 Chemical Treatment

When physical and biological treatments fail to purify water, chemical treatment or tertiary treatment is considered. Tertiary treatments such as chemical precipitation, neutralization, adsorption, ion exchange, and disinfection involve chlorination, ozone, and ultraviolet light [23].

Coagulation and flocculation are processes of chemical precipitation and used for sedimentation of colloidal materials and impurities as sludge. It is flexible in the case of dyeing wastewaters, but it faces some problems as dyes are of different types. Based on the type of treatment, coagulants are separated into three types: organic, inorganic, and biological. In most cases, aluminum is used for coagulation. This coagulation process forms small flocs through a stable and slow method. Ferric coagulants are readily used for precipitation and large flocs [27].

17.4 Types of Reactors Used in Wastewater Treatment

The most common types of reactors used in wastewater treatment are complete mixed reactors (CMRs), mixed plug flow reactors (MPFRs), covered lagoon (CL), plug flow reactors (PFRs), upflow anaerobic sludge blanket (UASB), fixed film anaerobic digester, and sequential reactors (SBRs) [27].

Moreover, membrane bioreactors (MBRs) are also used in pretreatment and conventional activated sludge basin (CAS). First, wastewater passes through a gravity channel to a small basin (around 1 m^3) and then flows to a manual screen (1 cm bars space). This is used as the pretreatment system. For CAS, active sludge is taken from a small municipal wastewater treatment plant and used to feed a MBR (Kubota flat membrane (203 type) with 0.4 μm pore size and 0.11 m^2 filtering surface) [28].

17.4.1 Membrane Filtration

Membranes are roughly classified according to the material from which they are prepared and are considered to be organic or inorganic. Ceramic is the typical inorganic material for microfiltration (MF), ultrafiltration (UF), and nanofiltration (NF) membranes; metals are also used to develop membranes [29]. The organic materials used for MF and UF membranes include polysulfone (PSF), polyethylene

(PE), cellulose acetate (CA), polyacrylonitrile (PAN), polypropylene (PP), polyvinylidene fluoride (PVDF), and polytetrafluoroethylene (PTFE). Polyamides are largely used for NF/RO membranes [6]. Materials and their characteristics are roughly classified according to the material from which they are prepared, and are considered to be organic or inorganic.

The most useful membrane separation processes are MF, UF, NF, RO, electrodialysis (ED), and electrodeionization (EDI) [29]. Among them, the first four processes produce permeate and concentrate. Each membrane has various ranges of pore size: 100–1000 nm for MF, 5–100 nm for UF, 1–5 nm for NF, and 0.1–1 nm for RO [6]. Membranes can be configured in either cylindrical or planar form. The most commonly used membrane designs are hollow fiber (HF), spiral wound, plate and frame, pleated filter cartridge, and tubular [6].

NF is widely used not only in membrane processes for water and wastewater treatment but also in desalination. It has been replaced with RO membranes in many applications because of lower energy consumption and higher flux rates [6]. UF, NF, and RO are used for industries such as dairy, cereal, oil, tomato puree, beer, wine, fish, meat, pickled vegetables, and retained solutes are proteins, pigments, oils, sugar, organics microparticles, sulfates, heavy metals, and salts [30].

A ceramic ultrafiltration membrane bioreactor (CUFMB) includes a capacity volume of 30 L, effluent control system, electromagnetic valve, temperature control system, cooling device, membrane system, TECH-SEP tubular ceramic membrane with seven channels each having a 4.5 mm diameter, and a pore size of about 20 nm and filtration area of 0.04 m^2 [31].

17.4.2 Fluidization

In fluidization, the gas flows upward from the bottom of a bed of solid particles to empty spaces between particles. At this stage, if the velocity of gas is low, the aerodynamic strain on each particle also becomes less and the bed remains in a fixed state. If velocity is high, aerodynamics will begin to counteract the gravitational forces and, therefore, the bed will expand in volume as the particles move away from each other (Krishna, 1993, cited in Refs. [32, 33]).

Anaerobic fluidized bed (AFB) reactors possess sand or granular activated carbon as small media to track bacteria. The conditions of the reactor mainly depend on the pore size and flow velocity of the reactor. If the reactor has large pore spaces and high flow rate, the bed will have less clogging and short circuiting. For high efficiency, bed expansion must be of specific area and small pore size. An upgraded system of AFB had an attached biofilm that contained a correct blend of methanogens to avoid the risk of microorganisms. Some drawbacks were the initial time needed and dilution inlet to reactor, high recycle rate, and high energy cost. A modification of AFB was an expanded granular sludge bed (EGSB) reactor with different upflow velocity [34].

Fluidized bed can be used for various objectives such as strict emission regulation of fuels such as high-sulfur coal, lignite, peat, oil, sludge, petroleum coke, gas, and wastes [34]. Fluidized bed can apply more useful with high technology such as fluidization of combustion, gasification, catalytic cracking, heat treatment furnaces, and solids transport and also effective using in drying or cooling moist substances. Municipal solid wastes are effectively used by fluidized technology [4]. Fluidized bed can be used in the treatment of wastewaters from the production of synthetic starch, real textile, diesel fuel, and brew [34].

17.4.3 Complete Mixed Reactor

A complete mixed reactor consists of insulated materials, driven mixer, and feedstock and can be maintained under mesophilic or thermophilic temperature. The reactor vessel is insulated with reinforced concrete, steel, and heating coils. Circulating hot water can be placed inside the digester or depending on the consistency of the feedstock [33]. The driven mixer is circulated by a recirculation pump and biogas is trapped by a gas tight cover. These reactors need a retention time 10–15 days and are better for 3–10% total solids. Anaerobic complete mixed reactor in treatment system it is mainly depend on hydraulic retention time (HRT) and solids retention time (SRT) and they have nearly same range of 15–40 days to perform provide sufficient retention. It is more suitable for using in high solid concentrations. Disadvantages of this reactor are as follows: (1) It cannot maintain high volumetric loading rate and (2) it has a limited rate of COD content, between 8000 and 50,000 mg/L. So the typical organic loading rate (OLR) is between 1 and 5 kg COD/m^3 per day [34]. Completely mixed reactors are usually used in palm oil mill effluent (POME: condensation wastewater, two-phase olive pomace and olive mill solid residue) treatment by continuous flow and mesophilic temperature, which is the best to run [36].

17.4.4 Anaerobic Filters

Anaerobic filters can be used as upflow and downflow packed bed processes and are widely used in beverage, food-processing, pharmaceutical, and chemical industries due to their high capability of biosolids retention [33]. Various types of support materials in the filter media are sand, plastics, reticulated foam polymers, stone, granite, granular activated carbon (GAC), and quartz [33]. But they have faced the problem of clogging by biosolids and other precipitated minerals and influent suspended solids. Methanogens process has been processed at lower levels of the reactor. Toxicity of hydrogen sulfide is removed by stripping sulfide in the upper section of the reactor and then solid is removed by gas recirculation. Although this method is simple and easy in downflow, upflow cannot occur readily. But there is a higher risk of losing biosolids to the effluent in the downflow systems [34].

Upflow anaerobic sludge blanket (UASB) reactor is widely used in many types of industries, municipal wastewater treatment, food processing, paper, and chemical industries. Inlet flow was set up at the bottom of the reactor and was passed through sludge blanket. The flow was then brought out between the upper part of the reactor and the lower edges of a funnel. By reduction of upflow velocity, it can improve solid retention in the reactor. At the same time, for having funnel it enhanced solids separation from the outward flowing wastewater. Biomass was formed as granules matrix and it flooding as suspension and could control upflow velocity. Granules appear naturally after several weeks and contain many bacteria and generate overall methane fermentation of substrates. UASB reactors are chosen for many reasons: low retention time, elimination of the packing material cost, high biomass concentrations

(30,000–80,000 mg/L), excellent solid/liquid separation, and operation at very high loading rates [37]. If feedstock concentration is too high (e.g., distillery wastewater), it is diluted with water in the ratio of 1:2. The organic loading rate of the diluted distillery spent wash is found to be 1.68 kg COD/m^3 per day with hydraulic retention time (HRT) of 30 days and flow rate of 0.23 ml/min. OLR can be increased to 3.36 kg COD/m^3 per day at a relatively uniform rate in the next 30 days. After 60 days, the reactor can run with the real raw spent wash, thus increasing its organic loading rate to 5.04 kg COD/m^3 per day and COD removal efficiency of 92% [9].

17.5 Application of Biopolymer and Biocomposite in Wastewater Treatment

Biopolymers such as polysaccharides have various applications in medicine, food, and petroleum industries [38]. Biocomposites are a combination of materials covering one or more phases derived from a biological origin [39]. Polymer composites have at least one component that is bio-based or biodegradable [40]. Derivatives of cellulose, alginates, carrageenan, lignins, proteins, chitosan, and chitin are included in biopolymeric materials as they have a number of different functional groups of hydroxyls and amines to which the metal ions can bind either by chemisorption or by physisorption [10]. To improve the strength of composites, fibers are included from cotton, flax, hemp, recycled wood, waste paper, or byproducts of food crops [39]. In the last few decades, the fundamental role of replacing conventional polymer composites in various applications has been played by composites produced with renewable resource materials [40].

17.5.1 Application of Chitosan in Wastewater Treatment

Chitosan, a natural cellulose-like copolymer of glucosamine and N-acetyl-glucosamine, has the ability of biodegradation and it is a more ecofriendly coagulant for water and wastewater treatment [41]. Chitosan produced from shrimp shells can be used to remove heavy metals from wastewater. But the adsorption rate of metal ions on chitosan depends on the degree of de-acetylation of chitosan and initial pH value of chitosan solution. A chitosan membrane can be prepared by making a 3 wt% chitosan solution and then adding 6 wt% silica particles (40–63 μm) and using a flat polycarbonate surface and dried at 60°C for 12 h [42]. The objectives of using chitosan in wastewater treatment are flocculation, coagulation, and removal of heavy metals. In treatment of Beni-Amrane dam water, two methods are used. In the first method only chitosan is used and in the second method chitosan is used as the primary flocculant and aluminum sulfate is used to aid coagulation. On evaluating the performance of the two processes, the first and the second methods reduced the turbidity of water by 85% and 97%, respectively. The dosing rate of chitosan was 0.15 and 0.2 mg/L and that of aluminum sulfate as coagulant was 0.02 mg/L. Low doses of aluminum sulfate is not only good for effective flocculation and coagulation but also poses less danger to aquatic environment due to the reduced quantities of dissolved aluminum. Use of aluminum sulfate also enhances coagulation and flocculation and reduces chitosan consumption [43].

Chitosan is also used in the case of bagasse-based paper and pulp industry wastewater. The process takes place in a batch reactor with different operating conditions such as agitation time (15–25 min), initial pH (4–8), chitosan dose (1.2–2.0 g/L), and settling time (40–80 min). Sulfuric acid (0.1 M) or sodium hydroxide solution (0.1 M) is used for adjusting pH. The optimal conditions for wastewater treatment are agitation time of 20 min, initial pH of 6, a chitosan dose of 1.8 g/L, and settling time of 60 min. Then the removal efficiencies of turbidity, BOD, and COD are 84, 93, and 90%, respectively [44].

In the textile industry, chitosan has been used to study the effect of coagulation with various dosage, pH, and mixing time. The optimum performance is 72.5% of COD reduction and 94.9% of turbidity reduction under condition of 30 mg/L of chitosan dosage, pH 4, and mixing with 250 rpm for 20 min, 30 rpm for 1 min, 30 rpm and 30 min of settling time. Since chitosan is insoluble in pH 6, a pH less than 6 should be used. Chitosan is an effective coagulant having the capability to reduce the level of COD and turbidity in textile industry wastewater [37]. The optimum pH for using alum, chitosan, and ferric in settling water turbidity was 5.5–6.0. Lead (II) adsorption by chitosan has been studied by treatment of lead (II) solution (84.53 mg/L) with variable dosages of chitosan powder

(40–60 g/L) at pH 6. The result showed that the adsorption ratio decreases from chitosan dosage with 10.76 to 2.07 mg of lead/g of chitosan [45].

Moreover, chitosan membrane and power are used to study the adsorption of Cu(II) (various concentration from 20–50 ppm) at various reaction times (30–240 min). The results showed that this type of membrane is more effective than powder because the membrane swelled on contact with liquids. Increasing the membrane volume increases the mobility of the polymer chain, so it is more powerful for the penetration of solvent. Moreover, chitosan is used as a surface coating of ceramic membrane to remove nickel. It is prepared by dissolving 250, 500, and 1000 mg chitosan flakes in each 250 ml of 1% (v/v) acetic acid solution, which is then stirred using a magnetic stirrer at 1200 rpm for 1 h. After the preparation of chitosan solution, the ceramic membrane is dipped into the chitosan solution for 2 min. The membrane is dried in an oven at 60°C for 15 min. This process is repeated 10 times, and the membrane is kept in a desiccator before use. When the experiment is run, the film becomes thicker and smoother as the chitosan loading increases. Removal of nickel can be varied by flow rates. The flow rate is set at 2.5 ml/min, and at 10, 15, and 20 mg chitosan loadings, the amounts of Ni removed are 89.0, 85.1, and 74.2 mg/g chitosan, respectively. When the flow rate is doubled, the amount of Ni removed also increases (123.0, 113.8, and 100.6 mg/g chitosan). The removal amount of Ni increases with an increase in flow rate due to larger flow, but decreases with an increase in the amount of chitosan loading, indicating that adsorption takes place mainly on the surface of the chitosan film, which, in turn, is controlled by the surface area of the membrane [46].

17.5.2 Application of Alginate in Wastewater Treatment

Alginate, a natural biopolymer, is gaining momentum due to its extraordinary affinity toward adsorption of heavy metal ions. Especially in the hydrogel form, the uptake is comparable or even better than that of commercial ion exchange resins [47]. Alginate is used as flocculants and adsorbents. Composite flocculants are prepared using sodium alginate, poly-aluminum ferric chloride, and cationic polyacrylamide and used in wastewater treatment in paper industry. Flocculant which composite with sodium alginate, poly-aluminum ferric chloride and cationic polyacrylamide had the removal efficiencies of 89.6% for COD and 99.2% for turbidity. Optimal condition dosage range of flocculant was 20 mg/L, pH 7–8, with slow mixing 200 rpm for 2.5 min and rapid mixing 40 rpm for 9 min and settled down 30 min [48].

Moreover, sand coated with chitosan and calcium alginate beads are also used as adsorbents. First, 1 g of chitosan powder is added to 100 ml of 5% acetic acid solution, which is then stirred and left overnight for dissolving completely. Second, 10 g of dried sand is added to the solution of chitosan and continuously stirred for 6 h. The sand is then transferred to a vacuum oven at 60°C for curing. After curing, the sand particles are dropped in 100 ml of 1 M sodium hydroxide solution and stirred overnight for chitosan coating. Chitosan-coated sand particles are dried and washed. The dried chitosan-coated sand particles are sieved, and a homogenous particle size of 0.50 mm is obtained, which are ready to use for removing heavy metals. Although chitosan-coated sand has many steps, calcium alginate has only two steps. A 1% solution of calcium alginate is prepared and added dropwise to a 0.1 M $CaCl_2$ solution to obtain beads. Homogeneous beads are obtained using a syringe and constant stirring. The beads are washed with and stored in distilled water. Now both of them are ready to be tested to find which one is better. It is observed that chitosan-coated sand and Ca–Alg both remove heavy metal ions such as chromium (40% and 61%) and iron (21% and 62%). According to the results, Ca–Alg removes higher amount of chromium and iron than chitosan [47].

17.6 Agriculture Byproducts as Low-Cost Biosorbent for Wastewater Treatment

Some biopolymers can be used as low-cost adsorbents. They can be divided into five categories: (1) household waste, (2) agricultural products, (3) industrial waste, (4) sea materials, and (5) soil and ore materials. Household wastes consist of fruit waste, coconut shells, and scrap tires. Agricultural products contain bark and other tannin-rich materials, saw dust, and other wood-type materials, rice husk, and other agricultural waste. Industrial wastes are petroleum wastes, fertilizer wastes, fly ash, sugar industry wastes, and blast furnace slag. Sea materials are chitosan and seafood processing wastes, sea weed and algae, peat moss, and miscellaneous waste. Soil and ore materials consist of clays, red mud, zeolites, sediment and soil, ore minerals, and metal oxides and hydroxides (Pollard et al., 1992, cited in Ref. [1]).

Among these wastes, tamarind fruit shells can be used as a low-cost adsorbent. The method of preparing adsorbents from tamarind fruit shells has eight steps: (1) washing tamarind fruit shells; (2) setting up dryer at 90°C for 8 h; (3) selection size by hammer mill; (4) screening; (5) carbonate in furnace at 300°C for 5 min; (6) washing by hot water; (7) drying at oven 100°C for 2 h; (8) initial concentration of Cr(VI) as 0.0025, 0.005, and 0.01 g/10 ml and removal efficiencies are 50–55%, 70–75%, 80–85%, respectively. Dosages for initial concentration of Ni(II) are 0.01, 0.04, and 0.08 g/10 ml and effectiveness percentages are 20–25%, 70–80%, and 75–90%, respectively. It can be said that tamarind fruit shells used as adsorbents are more useful for removing Cr(VI) than Ni(II) [49].

For biosorption, forest wastes such as eucalyptus, neem, and mango leaves are selected as adsorbents for the removal of Cu ion. All matured leaves are collected and washed with fresh running water to remove dust and any adhering particles. The leaves are then sun dried for a few days and also dried in an oven to make them crisp. To get a powdered form, the dried leaves are blended. The powder is sieved with different mesh sizes till fine biomass powder is obtained. The fine powder is treated with 0.3 M HNO_3 solution for 24 h, and then washed with deionized water till it reaches a pH of 7.2 and dried in a 60°C oven with constant mixing. Conditions for the adsorption of Cu ion on the leave powder are as follows: pH 7; initial concentration of Cu ion: 5 mg/L; contact time: 20 min; particle size of leave powder: 75 µm; agitation rate: 150 rpm. Between pH 7 and 9, the percentage removal becomes consistent, ranging between 95 and 98.7% [50]. The pH is very sensitive due to high concentration and high mobility of H^+ ions. When pH<7, the adsorption rate is lower. Removal efficiency decreases when concentration suddenly increases (5–20 mg/L) [50].

17.7 Conclusion

This chapter reviewed different types of wastewaters, sources of industrial discharge, and effects of industrial discharge on the environment (i.e., corrosive action on human health and negative impact on the environment). Therefore, wastewater has to be treated to get a greener environment. Different ways of wastewater treatments (physical, biological, chemical), different types of reactors, and effects of biopolymers and biocomposites on wastewater treatment were reviewed. Removal of heavy metals and usage of agricultural byproducts as biosorbents were described in this chapter. Treatment methods must be chosen according to the wastewater concentration. Biopolymers such as chitosan and alginates are best for coagulation, flocculation, and adsorption of heavy metals.

Acknowledgments

The authors thank Mr. Win Myo Thu, President of Advancing Life and Regenerating Mortherland (ALARM), Yangon, for his encouragement in this work.

References

1. Tripathi, K. N., Ahmad, I., and Jamal, Y. (2015). Comparative study of 'BOD', 'DO' and pH of distillery treated and untreated waste water, *International Journal of Scientific and Research Publications*, **5**, pp. 1–7.
2. Lou, X. F., Nair, J., and Ho, G. (2012). Influence of food waste composition and volumetric water dilution on methane generation kinetics, *International Journal of Environmental Protection*, **2**, pp. 22–29.
3. Henze, M. and Comeau, C. (2008). Wastewater characterization, in *Biological Wastewater Treatment: Principles, Modelling and Design*, Henze, M., van Loosdrecht, M. C. M., Ekama, G. A., and Brdjanovic, D. (Eds.) (IWA Publishing, London), pp. 33–52.
4. Tesoro-Martinez, D., GanironJr, T. U., and Taylor, H. S. (2014). Use of fluidized bed technology in solid waste management, *International Journal of u- and e- Service, Science and Technology*, **7**, pp. 223–232.
5. Manyuchi, M. M. and Ketiwa, E. (2013). Distillery effluent treatment using membrane bioreactor technology utilising *Pseudomonas*

fluorescens, International Journal of Scientific Engineering and Technology, **2**, pp. 1252–1254.

6. Shon, H. K., Phuntsho, S., Chaudhary, D. S., Vigneswaran, S., and Cho, J. (2013). Nanofiltration for water and wastewater treatment: A mini review, *Drinking Water Engineering and Science*, **6**, pp. 47–53.

7. Pontius, F. W. (2016). Chitosan as a drinking water treatment coagulant, *American Journal of Civil Engineering*, **4**, pp. 205–215.

8. Dara, S. S. (1993). *A Text Book of Environmental Chemistry and Pollution Control* (S. Chand and Company Ltd., Ramnagar, New Delhi).

9. Lekshmi, S. R. (2013). Treatment and reuse of distillery wastewater, *International Journal of Environmental Engineering and Management*, **4**, pp. 339–344.

10. Crini, G. (2005). Recent developments in polysaccharide-based materials used as adsorbents in wastewater treatment, *Progress in Polymer Science*, **30**, pp. 38–70.

11. Sunder, G. C. and Satyanarayan, S. (2013). Efficient treatment of slaughter house wastewater by anaerobic hybrid reactor packed with special floating media, *International Journal of Chemical and Physical Sciences*, **2**, pp. 73–81.

12. Chhaya, V. and Kumar, R. (2014). Utilization of distillery waste water in fertigation: A beneficial use, *International Journal of Research in Chemistry and Environment*, **4**, pp. 1–9.

13. Tekle, D. Y., Hailu, A. B., Wassie, T. A., and Tesema, A. G. (2015). Effect of coffee processing plant effluent on the physicochemical properties of receiving water bodies, Jimma Zone, Ethiopia, *American Journal of Environmental Protection*, **4**, pp. 83–90.

14. Yans, G. P., Suyén, R. P., Hernández, J. J., and Sánchez-Girón Renedo, V. (2013). Performance of a UASB reactor treating coffee wet wastewater, *Biology and Technology*, **22**, pp. 35–41.

15. Tikariha, A. and Sahu, O. (2014). Study of characteristics and treatments of dairy industry waste water, *Journal of Applied and Environmental Microbiology*, **2**, pp. 16–22.

16. Posavac, S., Dragičević, T. L., and Hren, M. Z. (2010). The improvement of dairy wastewater treatment efficiency by the addition of bioactivator, *Mljekarstvo*, **60**, pp. 198–206.

17. Singh, N. B., Singh, R., and Imam, M. M. (2014). Waste water management in dairy industry: Pollution abatement and preventive attitudes, *International Journal of Science, Environment and Technology*, **3**, pp. 672–683.

18. Nithya, R. and Sudha, P. N. (2016). Removal of heavy metals from tannery effluent using chitosan-g-poly(butyl acrylate)/bentonite nanocomposite as an adsorbent, *Textiles and Clothing Sustainability*, **2**, pp. 1–8.
19. Ngaha, W. S. W., Teonga, L. C., and Hanafiah, M. A. K. M. (2011). Adsorption of dyes and heavy metal ions by chitosan composites: A review, *Carbohydrate Polymers*, **83**, pp. 1446–1456.
20. Harte, J., Holdren, C., Schneider, R., and Shirley, C. (1991). *A Guide to Commonly Encountered Toxics. Toxics A to Z: A Guide to Everyday Pollution Hazards* (University of California Press, Berkeley), pp. 244–247.
21. United States Environmental Protection Agency (USEPA). (2003). *Wastewater Technology Fact Sheet: Screening and Grit Removal*, EPA 832-F-03-011.
22. United States Environmental Protection Agency (USEPA). (2004). *Primer for Municipal Wastewater Treatment Systems*, EPA 832-R-04-001.
23. Samer, M. (2015). Biological and chemical wastewater treatment processes, in *Wastewater Treatment Engineering*, Samer, M. (Ed.) (InTech Open Access), pp. 1–50
24. Ganczarczyk, J., Hamoda, M. F., and Hong-Lit, W. (1980). Performance of anaerobic digestion at different sludge solid levels and operation patterns, *Water Research*, **14**, pp. 627–633.
25. Saleh, M. M. A. and Mahmood, U. F. (2004). Anaerobic digestion technology for industrial wastewater treatment, *Eighth International Water Technology Conference, IWTC8*, Alexandria, Egypt, pp. 817–833.
26. Chan, Y. J., Chong, M. F., Law, C. L., and Hassell, D. G. (2009). A review on anaerobic–aerobic treatment of industrial and municipal wastewater, *Chemical Engineering Journal*, **155**, pp. 1–18.
27. Guihong, P. E. I. and Feng, Y. U. (2016). Review on ink wastewater treatment technology, *Journal of Scientific and Engineering Research*, **3**, pp. 67–70.
28. Kupusović, T., Milanolo, S., and Selmanagić, D. (2009). Two-stage aerobic treatment of wastewater: A case study from potato chips industry, *Polish Journal of Environmental Studying*, **18**, pp. 1045–1050.
29. Yamamoto, K., (2011). Guidelines for introducing membrane technology in sewage works: The 2nd edition, *Sewage Technical Meeting on Membrane Technology*.

30. Muro, C., Riera, F., and Carmen, D. M., (2012). Membrane separation process in wastewater treatment of food industry, In *Food Industrial Processes: Methods and Equipment*, Chapter 14, pp. 253–280.
31. Xianghua, W., Chuanhong, X., and Yi, Q. (2000). Ceramic ultrafiltration membrane bioreactor for domestic wastewater treatment, *Science and Technology*, **5**, pp. 283–287.
32. Thenmozhi, N., Gomathi, T., and Sudha, P. N. (2013). Preparation and characterization of biocomposites: Chitosan and silk fibroin, *Scholars Research Library*, **5**, pp. 88–97.
33. Hassan, S. R., Zwain, H. M., and Dahlan, I. (2013). Development of anaerobic reactor for industrial wastewater treatment: An overview, present stage and future prospects, *Journal of Advanced Scientific Research*, **4**, pp. 7–12.
34. Rajeshwari, K. V., Balakrishnan, M., Kansal, A., Lata, K., and Kishore, V. V. N. (2000). State-of-the-art of anaerobic digestion technology for industrial wastewater treatment, *Renewable and Sustainable Energy Reviews*, **4**, pp. 135–156.
35. Zarrabi, M., Safari, G. H., Yetilmezsoy, K., and Mahvi, A. H. (2013). Post-treatment of secondary wastewater treatment plant effluent using a two-stage fluidized bed bioreactor system, *Journal of Environmental Health Science and Engineering*, **11**, pp. 1–9.
36. Weng, C. K., Ismail, N., and Ahmad, A. (2014). Application of partial-mixed semi-continuous anaerobic reactor for treating palm oil mill effluent (POME) under mesophilic condition, *Iranica Journal of Energy and Environment*, **5**, pp. 209–217.
37. Hassan, M. A. A., Li, T. P., and Noor, Z. Z. (2009). Coagulation and flocculation treatment of wastewater in textile industry using chitosan, *Journal of Chemical and Natural Resources Engineering*, **4**, pp. 43–53.
38. Rao, M. G., Bharathi, P., and Akila, R. (2014). A comprehensive review on biopolymers, *Science and Reverse Chemistry Communication*, **4**, pp. 61–68.
39. Fowler, P. A., Hughes, J. M., and Elias, R. M. (2006). Biocomposites: Technology, environmental credentials and market forces. *Journal of the Science of Food and Agriculture*, **86**, pp. 1781–1789.
40. Barton, J., Niemczyk, A., Czaja, K., Korach, Ł., and Sachermajewskam, B. (2014). Polymer composites, biocomposites and nanocomposites. Production, composition, properties and application fields, *CHEMIK*, **68**, pp. 280–287.

41. Frederick, W. P. (2016). Chitosan as a drinking water treatment coagulant, *American Journal of Civil Engineering*, **4**, pp. 205–215.
42. Nwe, N. (2015). *Biopolymer Based Micro- and Nano-materials* (Momentum Press), pp. 29–33.
43. Zemmouria, H., Drouicheb, M., Sayeh, A., Lounici, H., and Mameri, N. (2013). Chitosan application for treatment of Beni-Amrane's water dam, *Energy Procedia*, **36**, pp. 558–564.
44. Thirugnanasambandham, K., Sivakumar, V., and Maran, J. P. (2014). Bagasse wastewater treatment using biopolymer: A novel approach, *Journal of Serbian Chemical Society*, **79**, pp. 897–909.
45. Asandei, D., Bulgariu, L., and Bobu, E. (2009). Lead (II) removal from aqueous solutions by adsorption onto chitosan, *Cellulose Chemistry and Technology*, **43**, pp. 211–216.
46. Chooaksorn, W. and Nitisoravut, R. (2015). Heavy metal removal from aqueous solutions by chitosan coated ceramic membrane, *4th International Conference on Informatics, Environment, Energy and Applications*, **82**, pp. 36–41.
47. Pal, P. and Banat, F. (2014). Contaminants in industrial lean amine solvent and their removal using biopolymers: A new aspect, *Physical Chemistry and Biophysics*, **4**, pp. 1–5.
48. Zeng, D., Hu, D., and Cheng, J. (2011). Preparation and study of a composite flocculant for papermaking wastewater treatment, *Journal of Environmental Protection*, **2**, pp. 1370–1374.
49. Pandharipande, S. L. and Kalnake, R. P. (2013), Tamarind fruit shell adsorbent synthesis, characterization and adsorption studies for removal of Cr(VI) & Ni(II) ions from aqueous solution, *International Journal of Engineering Sciences & Emerging Technologies*, **4**, pp. 83–89.
50. Kumar, S. V., Pai, K. V., Narayanaswamy, R., and Sripathy, M. (2013), Experimental optimization for Cu removal from aqueous solution using neem leaves based on Taguchi method, *International Journal of Science, Environment and Technology*, **2**, pp. 103–114.

Index

acid 41, 78, 84, 110, 174, 184, 187, 188, 231, 232, 290, 308, 379, 409, 412, 417, 419
  α-amino 407
  acetic 303
  acrylic 41, 246, 342
  adipic 312, 315
  amino 67, 68, 78, 276, 285, 307, 353, 406, 407, 409, 410, 412–414, 417, 418, 424, 425, 427
  ascorbic 151
  aspartic 407, 415, 427
  benzoic 207
  butyric 108, 109
  camphor sulfonic 46
  D-galacturonic 345
  D-glucuronic 341, 345
  dicarboxylic 12
  dodecyl benzene sulfonic 46
  fatty 78, 83, 84, 101, 108, 111, 308
  gallic 444
  glutamic 407, 417, 429
  glutamine 418
  lactic 11, 12, 69, 141, 144, 171, 201, 206, 310, 336
  palmitic 69, 78, 83, 108, 109
  polyacrilic 150
  polylactic 12, 14, 15, 141, 257, 281, 286
  polymethacrylic 51
  proponoic 207
  sialic 411
  steric 308
  sulfuric 188, 231, 473
  terephthalic 10
  tragacanthic 345
  uric 48
activated carbon 351, 375, 386, 387, 396, 470, 471
adhesion 84, 146, 184, 233, 309, 354
  fiber matrix 8, 234
  fibroblast 428
  interfacial 334
adsorbent 201, 331, 338, 346, 351, 352, 378, 379, 381, 386, 387, 396, 474–476
adsorption 52, 335, 338, 340–344, 346, 351, 352, 354, 375, 381–383, 386–388, 394–397, 420, 421, 467, 473, 474, 476, 477
  activated carbon 381
  chemical 381, 386
  physical 381
advanced thyroid cancer cells 107
AFB see anaerobic fluidized bed
AFP see automated fiber placement
age-related illness 109
albumin 150, 286, 308, 408, 409, 422
alcohol 187, 308, 409
  polyfurfuryl 16
  polyvinyl 10, 31, 52, 80, 304, 313, 380
algae 17, 52, 163–175, 280, 284, 287, 317, 385, 424, 466, 476
  brown 167, 174, 306
  green 3, 424
  marine 167
  red 168, 169
algal fiber 164, 167, 169–171

alginate 83, 167, 168, 174, 175,
    286, 289, 306, 377, 379, 459,
    472, 474, 477
aliphatic homopolymers 315
aliphatic polyanhydrides 315
aliphatic polyesters 11, 289,
    310–312
alternating magnetic field (AMF)
    75, 98, 106, 114
AMF see alternating magnetic field
amylopectin 187, 189–191, 202,
    280, 304
amylose 187, 190, 191, 280, 304
anaerobic fluidized bed (AFB)
    457, 470
anhydrides 185, 315
    acetic 246
    maleic 13, 69, 246
    polycarbonate/polystyrene-co-
        maleic 322
    sebacic 315
    succinic 12
animal fiber 3, 137, 139, 142, 165
antibodies 51, 101, 334, 406, 410
anticancer drugs 75, 76, 149, 150
anticancer effect 81, 82, 105, 119
antimicrobial activity 38, 82, 84,
    144, 283, 284, 306, 339, 343,
    350
antimicrobial agents 82, 207, 282,
    283
    nanosized 207
    natural 207, 340
    synthetic 207
antitumor activity 107, 108, 110
aqueous solution 41, 42, 80, 102,
    104, 113, 115, 323, 324, 333,
    339–341, 344, 346, 347, 378,
    379, 382, 383, 385, 387
arginine 407, 415, 417, 427
automated fiber placement (AFP)
    319–321

backbone 12, 286, 299, 315, 414
    ester 310
    peptide 414
bacteria 3, 17, 84, 185, 206,
    279–281, 283, 284, 286–288,
    300–302, 312, 313, 317, 335,
    385, 466, 471
    drug-resistant 340
    gram-negative 38, 52, 112, 288,
        435
    gram-positive 112, 340
    green 424
    infectious 147
bacterial cellulose 286, 287, 313,
    317
bacterial infections 151, 444, 446
bamboo 9, 136, 166, 221–223,
    228, 229, 246, 259
banana 4, 5, 9, 136, 166, 167,
    221–223, 229, 253
banana fibers 1, 2, 5–7, 9, 15–17,
    224, 230, 231, 254
banana sap (BS) 1, 9, 12, 13
barriers 81, 182, 185, 205, 280
    dermal 150
    diffusion 149
    hydrophobic 6
    lipophilic 79
    mass transport 207
    steric 111
BC see block copolymers
behavior 115, 117, 219, 229, 233,
    236, 417
    hysteresis 112
    non-Newtonian flow 341
    pseudo-capacitive 49
    rheological 308, 320, 323
    supercapacitance 49
    superparamagnetic 100, 114
    viscoelastic 258
bentonite 203, 318, 338, 381, 394,
    395

biocers 172
biocompatibility 51, 52, 111, 112, 115, 116, 139, 140, 146, 148, 151, 174, 199, 208, 209, 334, 337–339, 437, 439, 440, 442, 443
biocomposites 1, 2, 14–18, 69–71, 115–117, 119, 135, 136, 163–167, 170–174, 176, 375–378, 380, 381, 394, 395, 439–441, 457–460, 472–474
  algae-based 172, 176
  biodegradable 14
  chitosan-based 71
  green 439
  lipid-based 71, 78, 79, 81, 83
  manganite-based 117
  starch-based 71
biodegradability 17, 18, 65, 69, 111, 163, 164, 207, 208, 244, 297, 298, 300, 310, 312, 314, 337, 437, 439–443
biodegradable polymers 10, 38, 69, 140, 182, 200, 298–301, 303–305, 307, 309–311, 313, 315–317, 336, 347
biodegradation 3, 99, 119, 164, 201, 206, 299, 300, 303, 305, 314–316, 395, 441, 442, 472
biofibers 3, 14, 140, 170, 249
biofilms 17, 167, 185, 190, 191, 193
biofuels 136, 164, 171
biogas 467, 470
bioink 145
biological oxygen demand (BOD) 460–463, 473
biomass 17, 163, 185–187, 298, 459, 471
  algal 164, 170
  global 303
biomaterials 65, 67, 68, 71, 73, 76, 82, 116, 118, 142, 145, 147, 148, 283, 427, 441, 446
  advanced 289
  biocomposite 441
  hybrid 74, 447
  protein-based 426
biomedicine 55, 208, 276, 289, 292, 405, 406, 430
bionanocomposites 199–201, 204–211, 298, 300, 302, 304, 306, 308, 310, 312, 316–326, 330, 332–340, 342, 343, 353, 354
biopolyesters 433–438, 440, 442, 444, 446
biopolymers 115, 116, 200, 201, 203, 204, 210, 211, 275, 276, 279, 280, 285–287, 291, 292, 297, 298, 305–307, 375–378, 393, 443, 458, 459, 472, 473
  agro-based 202
  cationic 201, 338
  hybrid 279
  hydrocolloid 304
  non-toxic 306
  plant-based 308
  starch-based 208
  synthetic 285, 286
  water-insoluble 309
  water-soluble 323
biosensors 282, 292, 347, 405, 426, 430
biosorption 376, 382, 383, 385, 387, 388, 459, 476
bleached red algae fibers (BRAF) 164
blends 69, 70, 84, 139, 148, 151, 252, 304, 305, 322, 325, 470
block copolymers (BC) 37, 39, 42, 165, 287, 288, 317
blood 68, 81, 100, 108, 111, 406, 407, 409, 411, 412, 443, 462
blood vessels 100, 429, 441
  artificial 429, 444
BOD see biological oxygen demand
bonds 171, 173, 230, 318, 366, 368, 413, 414, 421

chemical 118, 386
covalent 411, 419
disulfide 416, 428
fiber-matrix interfacial 171
glycosidic 187, 231, 411
bone 68, 73, 74, 116, 143, 144, 280, 281, 429, 462
bone marrow 144, 149, 410
bone regeneration 74, 119, 144, 291
bone repair 74, 428, 438
bone replacement 200, 209, 211
bone tissue 71, 73, 74, 144, 173
bovine serum albumin (BSA) 149, 310
BRAF *see* bleached red algae fibers
BS *see* banana sap
BSA *see* bovine serum albumin

cancer 75, 81, 97, 98, 106, 111, 116, 119, 150, 389, 391, 464
   bladder 75
   bone 75
   breast 98, 149
   metastatic 282
   visceral 465
cancer cells 75, 82, 98, 100, 106, 109, 110, 150, 282
carbon nanotube (CNT) 204, 208, 317, 318, 331, 430
carrageenan 78, 169, 472
cartilage 143, 145, 410, 429
cartilage tissue 71, 145
casein 68, 286, 309, 408, 410–412, 421, 422, 427
cashew nut shell liquid (CNSL) 11, 14, 15
cassava 187, 189, 190, 194
catalysis 202, 289, 333, 349, 418
   hydrogen peroxide 376
   photochemical 284
catalyst 36, 115, 210, 255, 283, 299, 311, 339, 350

cells 36, 51, 72, 73, 75, 77–79, 106, 107, 143, 144, 169, 281–283, 289, 306, 334, 411, 418, 428
   bacterial 283, 335, 435
   cotyledon 423
   diseased 108
   embryonic 74
   epithelial 438
   fibroblast 77
   liver 109
   osteoblast 74
   osteosarcoma 75
   senescent 109
   smooth muscle 74
   stromal 149
   tumor 106, 107, 110, 111
cellulose 3–5, 7, 168, 200–202, 204, 218, 228, 230, 241, 244, 245, 285–287, 302–305, 317, 318, 347–351, 377, 378
cellulose chain 171, 231, 303, 324, 347
cellulose fibers 67, 170, 171, 173, 184, 232, 241, 261, 303, 349
cellulose fibrils 3, 303, 317, 318
cellulose nanocomposites 347, 351, 352
cellulose nanocrystals 70, 317, 348
cellulose nanofibers 201, 290, 348, 350
chemical oxygen demand (COD) 459–463, 473, 475
chemicals 139, 265, 303, 304, 363, 364, 387
   toxic 301, 351
chemisorption 352, 381, 386, 472
chitosan 38, 77, 113, 147–149, 201–203, 285, 286, 305, 306, 333, 337–340, 342, 343, 377–384, 393–395, 428, 458, 459, 472–477

chitosan bionanocomposites 201, 337, 339–342
cholesterol 83, 84, 110, 411
chromium 334, 335, 340, 342, 350, 376, 378, 379, 390, 463, 464, 475
clay
 cloisite-Na⁺ 336
 hydrophilic 33
 moist 318
 organic 206
CMR *see* complete mixed reactor
CNSL *see* cashew nut shell liquid
CNT *see* carbon nanotube
coagulation 98, 376, 381, 383, 385–387, 395, 412, 419, 468, 473, 477
coating 37, 52, 81, 99, 101, 108, 109, 111, 113, 115, 119, 168, 184, 185, 207, 308, 316
 anti-corrosion barrier 354
 latex 6
 layer-by-layer 114
 non-polar 101
 optical 349
 polymeric 112
 solar anti-reflective 55
COD *see* chemical oxygen demand
coir 9, 137, 138, 166, 220–223, 229, 232, 245, 246, 264
collagen 65, 67, 68, 74, 75, 77, 147, 280, 281, 285, 307, 353, 409, 410, 415, 427, 428
complete mixed reactor (CMR) 468
composite materials 3, 9, 14, 66, 100, 101, 116, 118, 136, 140, 164, 173, 241, 244, 246, 247, 257, 258
 bio-based 439
 fiber-filled 241
 nanoclay-reinforced 321
 protein-based 427, 429
 wild silk-based 427

compression molding 171
contaminants 330, 331, 338, 339, 346, 351
 chemical 331
 inorganic 349
copolymers 4, 169, 201, 288, 291, 305, 311, 312, 315, 344, 364, 472
crop 138, 203, 228, 229
 food 4, 189
 rain-fed 138
 root 181, 187
 tuber 194
cytotoxicity 75, 112, 150, 444

DBSA *see* dodecyl benzene sulfonic acid
defects 74, 144, 222, 250, 254, 320, 323, 425
digestion 104, 406, 418, 467
 aerobic 375, 466, 467
 anaerobic 375, 385, 466, 467
diseases 75, 80, 105, 145, 406, 426, 462, 465
 coronary heart 109
 hazards-induced 391
 iron deficiency 84
 oncological 118
 skin-related 83
 vascular 465
 waterborne 466
dodecyl benzene sulfonic acid (DBSA) 46, 47
doxorubicin 75, 107, 110
drug carriers 51, 107, 111, 167, 173, 174
drug-delivery system 75, 79, 85, 149, 291, 306, 319, 325, 330, 354
drugs 51, 79–83, 85, 97, 101, 107, 112–115, 119, 148, 150, 151, 282, 291, 308, 311, 314
 antibiotic 82
 anti-inflammatory 151

antitumor 115
chiral 352
cisplatin 75
hydrophobic 80
labile 111
lipophilic 80
liquid 174
non-emulsion 80
ophthalmic 81
dyes 44, 45, 54, 175, 184, 203, 324, 338, 340, 341, 375–377, 379, 391–397, 463, 468
 cationic 324, 341, 393
 natural 463
 organic 354
 synthetic 391, 463

ecosystem 44, 186, 194, 229, 262, 301, 376, 378
effluents 381, 397, 461, 463, 467, 471
 colored 463
 industrial 346, 376
 inorganic 381, 386, 398
EGF *see* epidermal growth factor
elastin-like polypeptides 427
elastins 148, 427, 429
electrophoresis 47, 417
environment 2, 33, 34, 65–67, 76, 135, 136, 141, 142, 182–184, 186, 194, 208, 256, 278, 301, 397, 398, 441
 acidic 38, 201, 283, 303
 aquatic 473
 chemical 394
 culture 440
 greener 477
 marine 353
 oral 146
 osteogenic 144
 oxygen-free 102
 simulated body 115

enzymes 101, 251, 285, 300, 305–307, 315, 333, 406, 409, 410, 412, 417, 418, 422, 441
 antioxidant 110
 endogenous 175
 proteolytic 308, 418, 420
epidermal growth factor (EGF) 77, 148
Escherichia coli 148, 340, 343
expanded granular sludge bed 470

fabric 136, 203, 222, 224, 225, 229, 252, 254, 255, 261, 266, 320, 391
feather fiber 147
fiberglass 248, 254–256, 266
fiber loading 15, 16, 226, 227, 250
fibers 2–9, 34, 136–140, 165, 166, 171–173, 218–222, 224–226, 228–236, 241, 242, 244–246, 250, 251, 257, 262–264, 266, 350
 abaca 138
 algae-derived 165
 alkali-treated 233
 bamboo 10, 426
 biocomposite 176
 biodegradable 72
 carbon 9–11, 219
 cellulose-based 218, 235
 chicken feather 136
 collagen protein 116
 electrospun 34
 ferromagnetic 116
 flax 15, 138, 141, 142, 222, 247–249, 257, 261
 glass 3, 9, 142, 146, 219, 234, 236, 248, 249, 252, 354
 grass 9
 hemp 11, 14, 69, 70, 138, 140, 261
 human-made 218
 hydrophilic 9

kenaf 7, 225, 226, 234, 261
kenaf and sisal 254
leaf 229
lignocellulosic 2, 3, 5–7, 9, 17, 347
marine 165
multicellular 141
nanoparticle-spun 34
natural 1–3, 9, 14, 69, 70, 135–151, 164–167, 173, 217–222, 229, 230, 234–236, 238–246, 250, 252, 257–259, 262–266
natural cellulosic 379
natural protein 429
oil palm 9, 261
piezoelectric 175
pineapple 147
plant 3, 4, 137, 139, 217–220, 222, 224, 226, 228, 230, 232, 234–258, 260, 262, 264, 266
protein-based 147, 165
ramie 70, 166, 261
rayon 392
resin-impregnated 320
rice husk 261
silane-treated 233
sisal 8, 137, 140, 222, 254, 261
synthetic 3, 140, 166, 218, 241, 243, 254, 266
textile 137, 309
vegetable 3, 137, 228, 231
vine 229
wool 150
fibrin 65, 74, 76, 77
fibrinogen 74, 76
fibroblasts 76, 146
fibroin 139, 408, 410, 428
fillers 30, 33, 35, 42, 43, 66, 70, 71, 146, 164, 199, 206, 210, 334, 337, 365, 366, 368
carbon nanotube 28
inorganic 337
magnetic 116, 117
metallic nanoparticle 30

mineral 116
nanosized 337
nanostructured 208
thermally conductive 237
versatile 142
films 12, 46, 65, 70, 168, 193, 209–211, 237, 303, 305, 306, 308, 309, 316, 363, 364, 405, 426
adhesive 237
agricultural mulch 305
biodegradable 192, 309
casein-based edible 309
electric conductive gold 193
high-temperature resistant 236
nanoclay-based wheat gluten 426
nanocomposite 46, 48, 168
porous 305
sensor 46
standalone 236
starch-based 181
water-soluble 304
zein 308
flocculant 314, 344, 346, 458, 473–475
flocculation 346, 383, 385, 395–397, 468, 473, 477
food industry 164, 168, 202, 458, 459
food product 182, 183, 189, 309, 446
Fourier transform infrared spectroscopy (FTIR) 339, 340, 342, 343, 346, 347, 382
FTIR *see* Fourier transform infrared spectroscopy
fungi 17, 185, 284, 285, 300, 302, 303, 305, 424, 466

GAC *see* granular activated carbon
gelatin 65, 67, 73, 74, 76, 77, 147, 285, 286, 290, 307, 421, 428
genes 68, 79, 109

geotextiles 138, 261, 262
glass substrate 46, 47, 51
glassy carbon electrode 47
gliadins 68, 308, 423, 426
globular proteins 408, 410
globulins 308, 309, 408, 409, 422
glucose 5, 7, 12, 13, 44
glutenins 68, 308, 409, 426
glycerol 38, 69, 70, 308
glycine 307, 315, 407, 415, 427
gold nanoparticles 81, 279, 282
granular activated carbon (GAC) 470, 471
granules 172, 189, 190, 202, 304, 435, 471
  energy-storage 312
  intracellular 435
  semi-crystalline 187
  subcellular 423
green composites 14, 16, 201, 236, 439, 445
growth factors 149, 446
  epidermal 77, 148
  human beta-nerve 73
  nerve 149
  vascular endothelial 77
gum 139, 175, 341, 344, 345
  ghatti 341, 345, 346
  guar 344–347
  karaya 341, 344–346

heat deflection temperature 70
heavy metal 338, 350, 351, 375–390, 392, 394, 396–398, 412, 419, 457, 458, 464, 465, 469, 472, 473, 477
heavy metal ions 306, 324, 346, 351, 352, 354, 463, 474, 475
hemicellulose 3–5, 7, 8, 218, 223, 230, 231, 233, 241, 244, 245, 250, 303, 347
hemoglobin 290, 406, 408, 412, 413

hemp 11, 15, 67, 69, 136, 137, 140–142, 165, 166, 218, 220–223, 228, 229, 242, 245–247, 259, 262–264, 266
histones 409, 412
holes 17, 53
hollow fiber 469
HRT *see* hydraulic retention time
hybrid composites 9, 166, 246, 340
hybrid nanocomposites 46, 48, 55, 56, 340
hydraulic retention time (HRT) 470, 472
hydrocarbons 104, 174, 185
hydrogels
  agarose 145
  biocompatible crosslinked 429
  biodegradable 308
  nanocomposite 38
hydrogen bond 7, 68, 317, 414, 415, 419, 421
hydrogen bonding 6, 7, 38, 40, 69, 309, 337, 352, 414, 415
hydrolysis 31, 41–43, 192, 231, 233, 303, 306, 308, 310, 313, 406, 408–410, 412, 418, 420
hydroxyapatite 73–75, 97, 116, 289
hyperthermia 97, 98, 100, 105, 106, 114, 118, 119

industrial wastewater 376–385, 387, 389, 392–397, 457, 458, 460, 462, 464, 466, 468, 470, 472, 474, 476
infection 77, 82, 84, 147, 444, 465
injection molding 225, 236, 239, 240, 248, 265, 304, 322
insulin 149, 406, 408, 410
interactions 15, 29, 31, 43, 69, 70, 99, 108, 136, 232, 250, 319, 352

cell   440
chemical   31, 42, 351, 460
covalent   352
electrostatic   38, 40, 42, 69, 333, 341, 352, 386, 415
filler-polymer   366
hydrophobic   309, 335, 415, 419
intermolecular   337
interparticle   101
ionic   113
molecular   352
nanofiller   346
non-covalent   307, 352
phase   69
size-dependent   283
interpenetrating polymer network   429

kenaf   15, 136, 137, 166, 218, 220–223, 229, 235, 242, 245, 253, 254, 259, 264
keratin   68, 69, 150, 408–410, 428

Langmuir constant   352
Langmuir isotherm   346, 352
layered silicates   201, 207, 321, 322, 336
lecithin   78, 82, 84, 286, 411
life cycle assessment   15
lignin   3–5, 7, 8, 11, 138, 201, 218, 221, 230–233, 244, 245, 250, 303, 304, 347, 348, 472
lipoproteins   411, 422
liposomes   101, 106–108
  magnetic cationic   105
  water-based   151
liver   143, 390, 391, 412
lysine   307, 407, 415, 417, 418, 422, 423, 425

macroalgae   169, 172
maghemite   103, 114, 117, 394
magnetic cationic liposomes (MCLs)   105, 106, 288, 465

magnetic nanoparticles (MNPs)   37, 97–102, 108–112, 114, 334, 341, 346, 379
magnetite   37, 75, 100, 102, 104–106, 117, 379, 380, 429
maize   68, 187, 189, 190, 194, 202
MCLs *see* magnetic cationic liposomes
microbes   83, 283, 341, 423, 435, 466
microemulsions   80, 82, 103, 104
microorganisms   276, 279, 283, 288, 299–301, 303, 305, 306, 312, 313, 345, 418, 439, 441, 462, 466, 470
micropollutants   44, 338, 354
minimum inhibitory concentration   112
mixed plug flow reactors   468
MNPs *see* magnetic nanoparticles
moisture   68–70, 77, 171, 245, 266, 300, 304
moisture absorption   3, 6, 16, 69, 203, 218, 257, 260
mold   171, 236, 238–240, 251, 255, 256, 319, 320
monomers   14, 40, 42, 107, 277, 280, 306, 314, 315, 436
  algae-derived   165
  furanic   16
  hydroxyalkanoate   288
  organic   278
  synthetic   176, 310
  vinyl   43
  vinyl acetate   314
montmorillonite   28, 70, 201, 203, 206, 210, 211, 318, 321, 322, 338, 380, 394
muscles   281, 406, 422, 429
  biomimetic   430
  paravertebral   74
  reddish-brown   422
  skeletal   422

nanoclay 28, 54, 70, 203–205,
  208, 210, 318, 322
nanocomposites 27–36, 38–56,
  73, 82, 83, 199–204, 206, 276,
  277, 297, 298, 329–331, 333,
  335, 336, 342–344, 346–354,
  364–368, 372, 373
  bio-based 348
  cellulose-based 349
  clay 33, 319, 322, 330, 333, 354
  drug-loaded 81
  halloysites-based 204
  hybrid polyamide 29
  mesoporous 51
  metal matrix 331
  nylon 28
  organoclay 322
  polymeric 333
  protein-based 70
  silica-based 36, 40
nanofillers 201, 204, 208, 210,
  316–320, 322, 323, 332, 366
nanofiltration 34, 383, 387, 458,
  459, 468
nanosilica 364–373
nanostructured lipid carriers 81
natural biopolymers 278, 285,
  286, 307, 474
natural fiber composites 142, 218,
  235, 236, 243, 247, 248, 266
natural polymers 3, 52, 70, 186,
  199, 200, 218, 277, 301, 354,
  377
natural resources 17, 163, 164,
  229, 262, 304, 317, 319
nerve growth factor 73, 149
nervous system 82, 146, 390, 391,
  465
nutrients 77, 169, 285, 289, 308,
  324, 388, 406, 446, 460

oil 6, 78, 141, 261, 308, 311, 313,
  353, 363, 364, 425, 457, 461,
  462, 469, 470

castor 11
citronella 80
coconut 78
corn 78
cottonseed 76
crude 17
olive 76
palm 12
pine 11
soybean 11, 309
vegetable 67, 315
organ 78, 97, 98, 100, 101, 143,
  428, 429
organic loading rate 467, 471, 472
organisms 143, 299, 424
  biological 376
  living 67, 99, 285, 306, 334,
    376, 377, 388
  non-target 52
  spoilage 418
organoclay 28, 202, 322, 353
ozonation 375, 377, 395, 397

paper industry 172, 175, 230,
  390, 423, 475
Parkinson's disease 47
pectin 3, 4, 7, 201, 245, 303, 304,
  348
peptide bond 68, 413–415, 418,
  420
permeability 185, 209, 219, 222,
  253, 254
pesticide 44, 201, 280, 339, 342,
  351, 376, 383, 389, 390, 464
phosphoproteins 309, 412, 422
photocatalysis 52, 342, 388, 397
plastics 2, 141, 166, 183–185,
  200, 209, 239, 249, 280, 284,
  299, 309, 376, 391, 396
  biocompatible 281
  biodegradable 69, 299–301
  compostable 17
  fiber-reinforced 254
  green 240

Index | 493

laminated 184
non-biodegradable 186, 446
synthetic 166
plug flow reactors 458, 468
pollutant 330, 331, 335, 352, 354, 376, 386, 457
 air 46
 cationic 324
 inorganic 351
 toxic 45
poly(3-hydroxybutyrate) 288, 433, 436, 437
polyacrylamide 101, 458, 474, 475
polyacrylonitriles 53, 392, 469
poly-alkyl-cyanoacrylates 286
polyamide-amine-epichlorohydrin 348
polyamides 185, 243, 286, 315, 392, 469
polyamidoamine 79
polyanhydrides 286, 315
polyester 2, 36, 73, 218, 247, 250, 281, 286, 288, 364, 392, 435
 jute fiber 142
 natural 437
 synthetic 336
polyethylene 10, 14, 35, 185, 249, 313, 315, 468
polyhydroxyalkanoates 14, 174, 279, 288, 291, 433, 435
polymer 27–31, 33–42, 44, 48–53, 66, 67, 69, 112, 113, 200, 201, 203, 204, 238, 301, 302, 304–308, 310–316, 319–323, 368
 alcohol-soluble 308
 aliphatic 12
 amorphous 3
 anionic 305
 bio-based 16, 441
 bio-derived 209
 bionanocomposite 204
 bioorganic 116

branched 441
carbohydrate 302
cationic 305
cellulose esters 202
chitosan-based 329
fiber-reinforced 147
fossil-derived 330
hydrocarbon 3
hydrophilic chitosan 113
hydrophobic 322
non-biodegradable 14, 147, 201
petroleum-based 325
synthetic 147, 218, 301, 308, 325, 330, 437, 438, 441
ultrathin 32
vinyl 286, 313
polymerization 15, 40, 42, 43, 54, 107, 202, 204, 278, 291, 312, 321, 335
polypeptide 68, 405, 406, 412
polypropylene 14, 141, 164, 174, 185, 238, 243, 247, 249, 313, 437, 469
polysaccharide 3, 4, 11, 101, 167–169, 186, 202, 204, 205, 285, 286, 289, 302, 308, 336, 341, 344, 351, 352
polyurethane 40, 142, 173, 237, 248, 314, 365, 394, 395
polyvinylchloride (PVC) 185, 249, 379, 380
precursor 16, 30, 110, 113
 inorganic 32, 41
 silica gel 41
 solution phase 31
proline 307, 407, 415, 427
proteins 65, 67–73, 75, 78, 84, 85, 101, 108, 109, 285, 286, 307, 309, 337, 338, 353, 405–428, 430, 435
blood 113
bone morphogenetic 74, 144, 149

catalytic 408
cereal 423, 425
conjugated 408, 410, 411
contractile 408
corn 68
dietary 425
endosperm 423
fibrous 408, 410, 414, 415
fish 422
gel-forming 421
germ 422
heme 290
keratinous 444
leaf 424
muscle 422
nut 425
pulse 411, 425
seed 409, 423
serum 36
single-cell 423
soy 68–71, 167, 308, 309, 426
soybean 427
tissue 426
tropoelastin 427
viral 109
zein 308
pulp 15, 169, 261, 376, 391, 464, 466
PVC *see* polyvinylchloride

quartz 318, 471

ramie 137, 165, 166, 220–223, 228, 229, 245, 246, 264
reactive oxygen species (ROS) 54, 109, 144, 334
reactors 457–459, 468, 470–472, 477
anaerobic baffled 467
anaerobic expanded bed 467
mixed flow 458
reagent 35, 104, 170, 246, 250, 397, 412

relative humidity (RH) 34, 193, 246, 324
resin 7, 10–13, 16, 17, 84, 116, 142, 146, 147, 171, 247, 254, 255, 320, 325, 474
resin film infusion (RFI) 319, 320
resin transfer molding (RTM) 245, 252, 254, 256, 266, 319, 320
resistance 34, 46, 50, 70, 138, 139, 141, 184, 225, 260, 283, 314, 366
ablation 298
chemical 16
fatigue 66
radiation 368–371, 373
sensor 47
weather 281
reverse osmosis (RO) 11, 208, 376, 382, 387, 459, 469
RFI *see* resin film infusion
RH *see* relative humidity
RO *see* reverse osmosis
ROS *see* reactive oxygen species
RTM *see* resin transfer molding

saturated fatty acid (SFA) 108, 109
scaffold 72–74, 76, 79, 119, 139, 143–145, 147–149, 281, 289, 311, 325, 434
artificial bone 174
conductive 291
silk collagen 429
silk fibroin 149
seeds 137, 138, 144, 187, 228, 229, 345, 423
sensor 28, 45–47, 200, 208, 209, 276, 289
chemical 46
chemiresistive 35
sepsis 77, 145, 147
sericin 139, 148, 149
serum albumin 149, 310, 409
SF *see* silk fibroin

SFA *see* saturated fatty acid
shell   116, 305, 337, 378
  biocompatible   112
  capsule   114
  cashew nut   14
  hazelnut   16
  polymeric   38
  shrimp   472
  tamarind fruit   476
silane   171, 218, 233, 334
silk   135–137, 139, 142, 143,
    145–149, 166, 218, 307, 391,
    392, 406, 408, 410, 427, 428,
    430
  dragline   139
  electrospun   150
  mulberry   139
  non-cytotoxic   149
silk fibroin (SF)   76, 142–150, 427,
    429
sisal   9, 136, 137, 140, 147, 166,
    172, 218, 220–223, 228, 229,
    235, 244–246, 251, 264, 266
skin   15, 65, 83, 143, 150, 229,
    236, 280, 281, 390, 406, 408,
    410, 415
SLN *see* solid lipid nanoparticle
sludge   324, 387, 388, 468, 470
soil   301, 323, 375, 438, 441, 475,
    476
solid lipid nanoparticle (SLN)
    80–84
species   2, 138, 285, 421, 423, 435
  microscopic   169
  nanoscopic   298
  reactive oxygen   54, 109, 144,
    334
  straw   302
  timber   11
sponge   76, 165, 166, 307, 428
starch   11, 65, 67, 78, 82, 181, 186,
    187, 189–194, 200–202, 204,
    285, 286, 302, 304, 305, 333,
    336

biodegradable   182
cassava   78
dry   202
synthetic   470
tapioca   189
thermoplastic   325, 336
surfactant   33, 81, 83, 84, 103,
    104, 111
suspension   192–194, 283, 288,
    346, 348, 379, 471

TDS *see* total dissolved solids
tensile strength   9, 10, 15, 16, 70,
    71, 140, 142, 169, 172, 206,
    220, 221, 225–227, 250, 312,
    336, 337, 363, 364, 368–371
textiles   14, 55, 136, 142, 168, 175,
    261, 262, 265, 303, 313, 337,
    344, 391, 394–396, 405
  commercial   141
  flax-based   142
  linen   165
therapy   98, 111, 112, 114, 145
thermoplastics   14, 33, 140, 142,
    217, 235, 236, 238, 247, 249,
    250, 312, 321, 330, 365, 427,
    436, 437
thermosets   14, 140, 142, 217,
    224, 235, 237, 238, 251, 365
tissue   69, 71–74, 98, 100, 101,
    143, 145, 147, 209, 211, 281,
    282, 289, 311, 405, 406,
    428–430, 443, 444
  animal   108, 280
  connective   307, 422, 428
  corneal   146
  diseased   100
  microscale   429
  morphological   422
  tumor   98, 106
total dissolved solids (TDS)   460,
    461, 463
toxicity   41, 80, 82, 111, 115, 164,
    310, 349, 388, 389, 458, 471

toxins 186, 418
tumor 76, 98, 100, 101, 105–107, 111, 151, 282
turbidity 461, 463, 473, 475

UA *see* uric acid
UASB *see* upflow anaerobic sludge blanket
upflow anaerobic sludge blanket (UASB) 468, 471
uric acid (UA) 48, 108, 110, 188, 231, 473

vacuum-assisted resin transfer molding (VARTM) 245, 252, 266, 319, 320
variable range hopping 44
VARTM *see* vacuum-assisted resin transfer molding
volatile fatty acids 467

waste 164, 171, 186, 266, 289, 300, 388, 464, 470, 476
  agricultural 1, 18, 351, 459, 476
  arsenic-containing 464
  citrus peel 348
  fertilizer 476
  food-packaging 182
  forest 476
  industrial 164, 475, 476
  miscellaneous 476
  oily liquid 394
  pine oil 11
  seafood processing 476
  sugar industry 476
  wastewaters 329–331, 334, 338–341, 346, 349–351, 353, 354, 375–382, 386, 387, 389, 391, 392, 395–397, 458–466, 468, 470, 477
  colored 391, 395
  distillery 459, 472
  dyeing 468
  pulp industry 473
  septic tank 458
  slaughterhouse 462
  synthetic 324
  textile industry 376, 473
wastewater treatment 329–332, 334, 336, 338, 340, 342, 344, 346, 348, 350–354, 391, 458, 459, 468–475, 477
wound 76, 77, 147, 148, 350
  chronic 76
  spiral 469

Young's modulus 71, 141, 206, 219, 227, 263, 287, 288

PGMO 04/27/2018